"Packed with cutting-edge evidence and insights from experts across the field, this remarkable book will inform thinking and practice in child protection for years to come."

—***Professor Robbie Gilligan****, School of Social Work and Social Policy, Trinity College Dublin*

"This is an excellent collection of significant international relevance. The book's 20 chapters bring together leading scholars from across the globe to address critical issues in child welfare and protection. Chapters cover key elements of the child protection process, whilst at the same time underscoring the central role that family networks play in providing care and protection for children. Given the book's comprehensive scope, it will be of considerable value to social work educators, students and practitioners alike."

—***Professor Karen Broadhurst****, Director: Centre for Child and Family Justice Research, Department of Sociology, Lancaster University, UK*

"This carefully curated volume includes an impressive array of internationally renowned scholars who grapple thoughtfully and constructively with the theoretical and practice dilemmas inherent within the child protection and child care continuum. The accomplished editors pull the diverse threads of knowledge, theory and practice together to achieve better understanding, assessment and decision making for children and their families, not just in Australia but globally."

—***Marian Brandon****, Professor of Social Work and Director of the Centre for Research on Children and Families, University of East Anglia, UK*

"This book is essential reading for practitioners and students working with children, young people and families involved with child protection systems. The editors present contributions from leading international researchers to offer an evidence-informed and practice-based approach to better practice from early intervention to protective care. The approach is child-centred, family-inclusive and culturally sensitive. I strongly recommend this book."

—***Professor Karen Healy****, AM, Head of Discipline for Social Work and Counselling, The University of Queensland, Australia*

Child Protection and the Care Continuum

This important new book critically examines the complex policy and practice issues surrounding child protection, including the impact of theoretical orientations, contemporary debates, policy initiatives and research findings, and maintains an emphasis on the ethics and values underpinning child welfare interventions.

The book introduces policies that are central to understanding the position and needs of children and young people, and how policy and practice have been influenced by developments including the children's rights agenda. It also explores the most significant issues in child welfare. These include: the experience of maltreatment by children, the systems of child protection to safeguard them, the methods and challenges of risk assessment, and the wide range of policy and therapeutic interventions to respond to children's needs. The book also examines family support to promote children's wellbeing before considering provision for children and young people who are looked after in out-of-home care. There is also a final section that focuses on best practice in communicating and working with children and young people, drawing on participatory, rights-oriented and resilience-based approaches, and supporting foster and adoptive carers and biological parents.

Contributing in a substantive and clear manner to a growing international conversation about the present function and future directions for child welfare in contemporary societies, this textbook will be of interest to undergraduate and postgraduate social work students and those from allied disciplines, and professionals who are engaged in child welfare services.

Elizabeth Fernandez is Professor of Social Work, School of Social Sciences, University of New South Wales, Australia. She teaches courses in Life Span Development, Child and Family Welfare Practice and Research. Her research focuses on child and family poverty, early intervention and family support, pathways and outcomes for children in care, including reunification of separated children and outcomes of care leavers. She has led several Australian Research Council funded research studies focusing on these themes and has published widely. She is Associate Editor for *Children and Youth Services Review* and *The Journal of Child and Family Studies*. She is recipient of the 2019 International Society for Child Indicators (ISCI) Award in honour of Alfred J. Khan and Sheila Kamerman in recognition of outstanding contribution to the field of child indicators research from an international perspective.

Paul Delfabbro completed his PhD in Psychology in 1998 and has been employed by the School of Psychology at the University of Adelaide, Australia, since 2001 in a combined teaching and research position. He was appointed to Professor in 2014. His principal research areas are behavioural addictions, applied cognition and child protection. He has published over 250 refereed journal articles and another 100 government reports, book chapters and conference papers.

Child Protection and the Care Continuum

Theoretical, Empirical and Practice Insights

Edited by
Elizabeth Fernandez and Paul Delfabbro

Routledge
Taylor & Francis Group
LONDON AND NEW YORK

First published 2021
by Routledge
2 Park Square, Milton Park, Abingdon, Oxon OX14 4RN

and by Routledge
52 Vanderbilt Avenue, New York, NY 10017

Routledge is an imprint of the Taylor & Francis Group, an informa business

British Library Cataloguing in Publication Data
A catalogue record for this book is available from the British Library

Library of Congress Cataloging-in-Publication Data
Names: Fernandez, Elizabeth, 1942- editor. | Delfabbro, Paul H. (Paul Howard), editor.
Title: Child protection and the care continuum : theoretical, empirical and practice insights / edited by Elizabeth Fernandez and Paul Delfabbro.
Description: Milton Park, Abingdon, Oxon ; New York, NY : Routledge, 2021. | Includes bibliographical references and index.
Identifiers: LCCN 2020028420 (print) | LCCN 2020028421 (ebook) | ISBN 9781760529680 (paperback) | ISBN 9780367639174 (hardback) | ISBN 9781003121305 (ebook)
Subjects: LCSH: Child welfare. | Children–Social conditions. | Children–Services for.
Classification: LCC HV713 .C362628 2021 (print) | LCC HV713 (ebook) | DDC 362.7–dc23
LC record available at https://lccn.loc.gov/2020028420
LC ebook record available at https://lccn.loc.gov/2020028421

ISBN: 978-0-367-63917-4 (hbk)
ISBN: 978-1-760-52968-0 (pbk)
ISBN: 978-1-003-12130-5 (ebk)

Typeset in Sabon
by Taylor & Francis Books

Contents

List of illustrations ix
List of contributors x
Foreword xv
Acknowledgements xvii

PART 1
The context of child and family welfare **1**

1 Policy and trends in child welfare in Australia and the global context 3
ELIZABETH FERNANDEZ AND PAUL DELFABBRO

2 Theoretical and value frameworks underpinning work with children and families 27
ELIZABETH FERNANDEZ AND PAUL DELFABBRO

3 Children's rights and the protective care continuum 52
JENNIFER DRISCOLL

PART 2
Child abuse and neglect **65**

4 Working with cases of neglect and emotional abuse 67
ALICE LOVING AND DAVID SHEMMINGS

5 Child sexual abuse 79
DALE TOLLIDAY

6 Assessment in child protection 96
ELIZABETH FERNANDEZ

7 Child protection and the role of the Children's Court 123
ROSEMARY SHEEHAN

8 Therapeutic approaches to children and families in child protection contexts 134
PAUL DELFABBRO AND ALEXANDRA OSBORN

PART 3
The protective care continuum 149

9 Prevention and early intervention with children, young people, and families 151
CARMEL DEVANEY

10 Foster family care as a response to child maltreatment 163
JUNE THOBURN

11 Kinship care in Australia and the United Kingdom 175
MEREDITH KIRALY AND ELAINE FARMER

12 Therapeutic residential care 192
KENNY KOR AND PATRICIA MCNAMARA

13 Educational interventions that improve the attainment and progress of children in out-of-home care 209
JUDY SEBBA

14 Reunification in out-of-home care 223
ELIZABETH FERNANDEZ AND PAUL DELFABBRO

15 Creating a family life for a child through adoption 241
JOHN SIMMONDS

16 Beyond care: Identities, transitions and outcomes 252
PHILIP MENDES AND JADE PURTELL

PART 4
Children, parents and carers as stakeholders 269

17 Child protection and child participation 271
JAN MASON AND TOBIA FATTORE

18 The right of Aboriginal and Torres Strait Islander children and families to effective child protection services 289
CLARE TILBURY AND NATALIE LEWIS

19 Engaging first mothers, fathers and grandparents in the care continuum 300
ELIZABETH FERNANDEZ AND ROS THORPE

20 Responding to carers' needs 318
JILL DUERR BERRICK

Index 332

Illustrations

Figures

10.1 The special needs of children who are looked after by the local authority 169
14.1 North Carolina Family Assessment Scale 232

Tables

10.1 0–1 Percentages of those entering care by age group. Data for Australia, England and USA from 2016 to 2017 and for other countries from 2010 to 2013 164
10.2 0–2 Percentages of children in care in different placement types. Data for Australia, England and USA from 2016 to 2017 and for other countries from 2010 to 2013 165
12.1 Key results of the pilot program group vs. the general residential care group in the Victorian Therapeutic Residential Care (TRC) evaluation 196
12.2 Summary of the milieu-based models evaluated in the Northern Ireland study 198

Boxs

3.1 Supporting parents 58
3.2 Respecting children's participation rights in court proceedings 60

Contributors

Elizabeth Fernandez is Professor of Social Work, School of Social Sciences, University of New South Wales, Australia. She teaches courses in Life Span Development, Child and Family Welfare Practice and Research. Her research focuses on child and family poverty, early intervention and family support, pathways and outcomes for children in care, including reunification of separated children and outcomes of care leavers. She has led several Australian Research Council funded research studies focusing on these themes and published books, book chapters and journal articles from her research. She serves on the Boards of the International Society for Child Indicators (ISCI) and of the International Association for Outcome Based Evaluation and Research on Family and Children's Services (IAOBERfcs). She is recipient of the 2019 International Society for Child Indicators (ISCI) Award in honour of Alfred J. Khan and Sheila Kamerman in recognition of outstanding contribution to the field of child indicators research from an international perspective.

Paul Delfabbro completed his PhD in Psychology in 1998 and has been employed by the School of Psychology at the University of Adelaide, Australia, since 2001 in a combined teaching and research position. He was appointed to Professor in 2014. His principal research areas are behavioural addictions, applied cognition and child protection. He has published over 250 refereed journal articles and another 100 government reports, book chapters and conference papers.

Jill Duerr Berrick serves as the Zellerbach Family Foundation Professor in the School of Social Welfare at U.C. Berkeley, USA. Berrick's research focuses on the relationship of the state to vulnerable families, particularly those touched by the child welfare system. She has written on topics relating to family poverty, child maltreatment and child welfare services. Berrick's research approach typically relies upon the voices of service system consumers to identify the impacts of social problems and social service solutions in family life.

Carmel Devaney is Lecturer and Course Director of the Master's Degree in Family Support Studies at NUI Galway, Ireland. Carmel has a longstanding interest in and commitment to supporting and protecting children and young people within their family context. Carmel was Principal Investigator on several research projects under the Partnership, Prevention and Family Support programme for Tusla, the Child and Family Agency and has recently completed an Irish Research Council funded feasibility study on conducting a longitudinal study on children in care or leaving care in the Irish context.

Jennifer Driscoll runs the MAs in Child Studies and International Child Studies at King's College London, UK, and was previously a Family Law barrister specialising in child protection. Her academic interests are at the intersection of children's rights and child protection, including child protection systems, outcomes for care leavers and ethics of research with young people. Current research includes an ESRC-funded project with the Social Care Workforce Research Unit at King's on the role of schools in safeguarding and a Leverhulme-funded study of the interaction between formal and informal child protection arrangements in Uganda.

Elaine Farmer is Emeritus Professor of Child and Family Studies in the School for Policy Studies at the University of Bristol, UK, prior to which she spent several years as a social worker in England and Australia. She has directed 11 major studies, most in programmes funded by the Department of Health or the Department for Education. She has researched and published widely on child protection, fostering, residential and kinship care, adoption and reunification. She is author or co-author of ten published books, six online books or reports and many articles and book chapters. Elaine is a Trustee for Grandparents Plus.

Tobia Fattore is a Senior Lecturer in the Department of Sociology, Macquarie University, Australia. His empirical research is in the broad areas of the sociology of childhood and sociology of work. This includes a sociological examination of children's wellbeing, that analyses children's understandings of wellbeing and how this reflects processes of modernisation; and understanding how the everyday politics of worker practices in out-of-home care institutions are informed by historically constructed understandings of childhood.

Meredith Kiraly is a psychologist with over 30 years' experience specialising in child and family welfare, and particularly in kinship care. She is an Honorary Research Fellow in the Social Work Department at the University of Melbourne, Australia, and has a small consultancy in human services. Her numerous research projects and consultancies have covered a range of human service areas with a focus on vulnerable children and families, and out of home care.

Kenny Kor is a social work educator, practitioner and researcher with over 17 years' frontline and management experience in child protection, out-of-home care, family violence and mental health. Specialised in prevention, response and treatment of child maltreatment in out-of-home care settings, Kenny's research examines young people's lived experience in residential care and therapeutic residential care development and implementation.

Natalie Lewis is a descendant of the Gamilaraay (Kamilaroi) Nation and is the Commissioner, Queensland Child and Family Commission. She was previously CEO of the Queensland Aboriginal and Torres Strait Islander Child Protection Peak and served on the National Executive of SNAICC – National Voice for our Children, and co-chairs Family Matters: Strong Communities, Strong Culture, Stronger Children, the national campaign to eliminate the over-representation of Aboriginal and Torres Strait Islander children in statutory child protection systems. For over 20 years, her experience has been called upon in Australia and the USA in youth justice and child protection for Indigenous peoples, providing direct services, programme and policy development, and organisational leadership.

Alice Loving is Curriculum Lead for the Parenting curriculum delivered by Frontline and honorary lecturer for the Centre for Child Protection at Kent University, UK. She also works independently, completing assessment and intervention work for local authority child protection teams and has ten years of experience working in this field. Alice has recently completed her PhD within the Social Care department at Royal Holloway University, UK, focused on exploring influencing factors on the outcomes of intervention, with a particular interest in the impact of childhood trauma on parenting capacity.

Jan Mason is Emeritus Professor at Western Sydney University, Australia, where she was Foundation Professor of Social Work. She was also Foundation Director of the Childhood and Youth Policy Research Unit and then the Social Justice and Social Change Research Centre. Jan's early career, in the state child welfare department, informs her academic work which focuses on linking theory, policy and practice on children's issues. She has published on child welfare and protection, child and family policy, child–adult relations, children's needs in care, kinship care, child wellbeing and researching with children.

Patricia McNamara is an experienced teaching and research academic, currently based at the University of Melbourne as a Senior Fellow in Social Work (Hon). She worked for many years as a teacher, social worker and family therapist. Patricia is widely published and has frequently been invited to present internationally. Her current research interests are therapeutic approaches to residential and foster care and education in out-of-home care.

Philip Mendes is Director of the Social Inclusion and Social Policy Research Unit in the Social Work Department at Monash University, Australia. For the last 20 years, he has been engaged in ongoing research on young people transitioning from out-of-home care. He is a member of the Transitions to Adulthood for Young People Leaving Public Care International Research Group, and has completed a number of major leaving care studies pertaining to youth justice, disability, Indigenous care leavers, and mentoring and employment programs.

Alexander Osborn holds a PhD in psychology from the University of Adelaide and completed a Master of Clinical Psychology. She has worked in clinical practice for almost a decade and specialises in the treatment of mood disorders, trauma and a range of other conditions. Her PhD and published research focused specifically on the needs of children in out-of-home care, therapeutic approaches, services and supports.

Jade Purtell is currently undertaking a PhD study in the Department of Social Work at Monash University on care leavers, family and early parenting. She is an Out-of-Home Care and Transitions from Care researcher as well as a Youth Participation consultant. Jade has worked collaboratively with the Children, Youth and Families sector to promote young people's participation in research and increased involvement of young people in policy and key decision making by government and the community sector. Jade has assisted the Victorian Commission for Children and Young People in the development of their youth engagement framework and recent inquiries.

Judy Sebba is at the Rees Centre for Research on Fostering and Education at the University of Oxford, UK. The Centre involves education professionals, carers and care experienced young people in setting priorities, undertaking research and dissemination. Her current role at the Rees Centre includes supporting others designing research and evaluations in children's services, mainly on education–social care linkage, mental health, fostering/adoption and UASC. She was awarded an OBE in 2018 in the New Year's Honours list.

Rosemary Sheehan teaches mental health in the postgraduate social work programme and is Co-ordinator of the Higher Degrees by Research programme at the Department of Social Work at Monash University. She was previously a Dispute Resolution Convener in the Children's Court of Victoria, dealing with disputes between families and the child protection service. She was awarded the Order of Australia in 2014 for services to children and the law. Her published research covers child welfare and the law, family violence, mental health, judicial and corrections responses to offenders, with reference to women offenders and ageing offenders.

David Shemmings is Emeritus Professor of Child Protection Research at the University of Kent, UK and Visiting Professor of Child Protection Research at Royal Holloway, University of London. David is the author of over 70 articles, books and chapters on relationally based theory, research and practice. Finally, he was co-Director, with Prof Jane Reeves, of the online International Centre for Child Protection at the University of Kent where they established a multidisciplinary and international distance-learning MA in Advanced Child Protection.

John Simmonds is Director of Policy, Research and Development at CoramBAAF, formerly the British Association for Adoption and Fostering. Previously, John was head of the social work programmes at Goldsmiths College, University of London. He is a qualified social worker and has substantial experience in child protection, family placement and residential care settings. He is currently responsible for CoramBAAF's contribution to the development of policy and practice in social work, health, the law and research. He was awarded an OBE in the New Year's Honours list 2015 and an honorary doctorate in Education from the Tavistock NHS Foundation Trust/University of East London.

June Thoburn is Emeritus Professor of Social Work at the University of East Anglia, UK. She practiced as a child and family social worker in England and Canada before becoming a social work educator and researcher. She has practiced, lectured and researched and published across the whole area of child and family welfare services, including neighbourhood-based family support, intensive family casework, family court work, and services for children in care or placed for adoption. She was awarded a CBE for services to social work in 2002.

Ros Thorpe is Emeritus Professor of Social Work at James Cook University, and, since her retirement at the end of 2010, she is President of and a volunteer community social worker with The Family Inclusion Network, a service user support and advocacy organisation in which families and supportive professionals work together to achieve greater social justice for children and families caught up in the child protection system. Ros has had significant practice experience in family casework and group-work in child welfare and has an international reputation for her research with children in out-of-home care, their parents, and their foster carers.

Clare Tilbury is the Leneen Forde Chair of Child and Family Research and Professor in the School of Human Services and Social Work at Griffith University. Her research expertise relates to child protection systems, performance measurement, accountability and racial disparities. She has led significant national child protection research projects and publishes extensively about child protection and family support in Australian and international scholarly journals. Prior to entering academia in 2004, Clare worked for 20 years in child and family direct practice, policy, management and research roles.

Dale Tolliday is NSW Health Senior Clinical Advisor on Sexual and Violent Behaviour and Clinical Advisor to NSW Health's New Street Services. New Street Services are an integrated network of health services for children who have engaged in harmful sexual behaviour delivered across NSW. Dale is based at the Sydney Children's Hospitals Network and NSW Ministry of Health. Dale's work with people who have sexually harmed others spans over 30 years. Prior to this, Dale worked in a variety of child, adolescent and family mental health settings.

Foreword

This book offers proof positive that the universe of international child welfare is at once expanding and contracting. Author/editors Elizabeth Fernandez and Paul Delfabbro are seasoned and senior child welfare scholars and researchers well qualified to paint in broad strokes the complex and multidimensional landscape within which child protective services resides in contemporary Australian society. With their impressive and varied cohort of contributing authors, they have produced a work that holds great promise as a sourcebook in child welfare and child protection. I have little doubt that its varied and detailed twenty chapters will yield insights and valuable knowledge for beginning students in social work and related disciplines, as well as for seasoned practitioners, senior administrators and child welfare researchers. The contents of this richly detailed compendium – *Child Protection and the Care Continuum: Theoretical, Empirical and Practice Insights* – draws equally from value, empirical and theoretical sources. The scaffolding erected by the editors – policy, practice and research – allows for fluid transmissions within and between these domains and illustrates both in broad themes and specific exemplars the interpenetration within and between all three.

International child welfare scholars will quickly discover familiar pathways and signposts here, in lucid discussions of such familiar topics as "privacy", "setting a threshold for state intervention in family life", "permanency", "evidence-based practice" and the "role of parents, children and carers as stakeholders". In fact, this last topic constitutes an entire section of the book and illustrates the central and continuing role of parents, children and caregivers in choosing, shaping and implementing both particular interventions and broad policy initiatives. That the examples offered here reflect sensitivity to both the challenges of multi-generational parenting and parenting needs and strengths within communities of color suggests both the value of richly textured indigenous initiatives and the folly of "one-size-fits all".

One final note: Fernandez and colleagues contribute in a substantive and clear manner to a growing international conversation about the present function and future directions for child welfare in contemporary societies. If there is indeed an Australian template here, perhaps its ultimate benefit to those of us outside may be in identifying how a society examines values, data and circumstances similar in many ways to our own and comes up with different policy, practice and research priorities. Rigorous, cross-national analyses must constitute a key element in our future child welfare reform initiatives. This book serves as a stimulus and catalyst to just such an exercise.

James K. Whittaker, PhD
Charles O. Cressey Endowed Professor Emeritus
School of Social Work
The University of Washington, Seattle, USA

Acknowledgements

This work is the outcome of the generosity and commitment of many individuals who must be acknowledged. Special thanks are due to Professor James Whittaker for writing the foreword to this book, bringing to it insights based on his international understandings of research, policy and practice developments and challenges in this field.

Special thanks are due to Professor Paul Delfabbro for his collaboration as co-editor and his commentary on chapters. This collection has been made possible by the expertise of the contributing authors and their commitment to scholarship and the book's vision. Thanks go out to all authors who have provided unique cross-national perspectives on advancing the care and protection of children and the wellbeing of their caregivers. Their patience and cooperation with the editorial process are acknowledged.

The themes presented in this book have benefited from collaboration and exchange. Conversations with colleagues in Australia and overseas have afforded a wellspring of ideas. Students, practitioners, academics and researchers have enriched this work immeasurably over the years. It has been invaluable to exchange ideas with researchers at seminars hosted by the International Association of Outcome Based Evaluation and Research in child and family services (IAOBERfcs), and national conferences of the Association of Children's Welfare Agencies (ACWA).

Thanks are due to Routledge UK for the opportunity to publish this volume, in particular, to Catherine Jones, Editorial Assistant, who has kept the book on track and steered it through the production process to completion, and Jane Fieldsend for her thorough copy-editing to ensure consistency in presentation. I would like to acknowledge Elizabeth Weiss who provided valuable editorial guidance in the early development of this volume.

I would like to acknowledge P. Suyat and Dr Nicole Saintilan, Education Developer, UNSW for facilitating the development of the cover design. I thank Szilvia Kovacs for her research assistance and for formatting the manuscript with exceptional skill and care.

A great deal of commitment and forbearance have been necessary in our respective families who have been a source of strength and support. I thank my husband, Carl, for his patience, understanding and nurture throughout the writing of this book. I express appreciation to my parents who rose above many adversities to support my education. Through their energy and curiosity, Sienna, Antonia and Quinn challenge my thinking about children and keep me critical. It is hoped this collection contributes in some measure to supporting the rights and wellbeing of children and families served by the child welfare system and makes a difference to outcomes.

Elizabeth Fernandez

Part I

The context of child and family welfare

Chapter 1

Policy and trends in child welfare in Australia and the global context

Elizabeth Fernandez and Paul Delfabbro

Introduction

Family and child welfare policy and practice reflect society's organised concern about the intrinsic worth of the child and the family, and the rights of the child as a developing person and citizen. The field of family and child welfare is confronted with challenges to respond to complex problems, including the increased official reporting of child abuse and neglect and the care and protection of children and young people. Evidence of community outrage at media accounts of children who have been abused physically, emotionally and sexually, or neglected, and the inability of the child welfare system to prevent maltreatment or protect children either in their own families or in public care have influenced directions of child welfare policy and practice. However, the child protection system operates in a complex environment where decision making often requires interdisciplinary knowledge; legal understanding; psychological and sociological insights; analytical skills; and, reflective ethical practice. As will be shown in this book, the policies and services designed to protect children and support families are constantly evolving in response to these challenges and debates. Policymakers and practitioners are confronted with difficult decisions that have far reaching consequences for children and families.

Safeguarding children who are maltreated and who need protective care is a central element of child welfare. For example, the definition and scope of maltreatment, its cause, and how it should be responded to are the subject of continuing international and national debate. At what point or threshold should care be considered inadequate or abusive? Some commentators have argued that the definitions of maltreatment applied to families are too broad, exposing families to unwarranted intrusion through investigative processes (Besharov 1985; Gibbons, Conroy & Bell 1995; Munro 2011), whereas others have argued that many families do receive adequate interventions. These dilemmas confront child protection systems internationally and are equally relevant to child protection policy and practice in Australia.

The child welfare continuum

Child welfare systems are often described as providing a 'continuum' of services and supports for children affected by child abuse and other related problems. The term continuum refers to the scope and intensity of the intervention or the degree to which the state is required to intervene to protect children from harm. The priority in this continuum is the provision of family-based services to enable families and children to remain together. Interventions can range from the notification or recording of abuse incidents; to investigations and substantiations; to the provision of services that involve the state in the lives of children and families, including removal of children from their families and placement into other arrangements. Interventions often involve a range of parties including the court system, child welfare services, non-government organisations and those who provide the care itself (e.g. foster carers and kinship carers and adoptive parents). Even within these different levels of the system there can be variations in what might be considered a 'continuum' of service options. For example, in out-of-home care, children can be placed with their relatives or with strangers (foster care), but there are also more institutional forms of care (group homes, residential care) where the environment is less similar to the child's home or family environment. Services can also vary in terms of the level of resources applied to each case or intensity of intervention provided (Whittaker, del Valle & Holmes 2015). Some children may go into out-of-home care with few additional supports, whereas others may receive therapeutic interventions and a constellation of different services.

Child maltreatment

In the last five decades of child welfare history and policy, child maltreatment has been a major focus of concern. The 'discovery' and growth in concern about child abuse since the 1960s has been the subject of an expanding international literature which has documented the emergence of it as a social concern and how it might be addressed. In the 1960s Henry Kempe and his colleagues, focusing on extremely brutalised young children, drew attention to what was labelled the 'battered child syndrome' (Krugman & Korbin 2013). Initial conceptualisations of the problem of maltreatment as 'the battered child' syndrome in the 1960s reflected a narrow definition of child maltreatment. This definition has since expanded to include physical neglect, emotional abuse, sexual abuse and organised abuse. Constantly widening definitions of child abuse have seen the phenomenon of physical battery expand to include neglect, emotional abuse and sexual abuse (Cooper 1993) and a consequent expansion of the grounds on which the state may intervene.

A further influential factor in the mobilisation of the child protection agenda was the rise of the 'women's movement' in the late 1970s. This movement added political momentum to the recognition of the problem of sexual abuse (Finkelhor 1996) and resulted in greater recognition of the importance of family safety and domestic violence (Parton 1990). As women's representation in the government and higher status professions such as medicine, law and health increased, they brought with them their interest in children and sensitivity to child welfare concerns increased. The children's rights movement of the 1980s gave further impetus to the child protection agenda. Other important developments have been the effect of children's exposure to domestic violence and parental drug and alcohol misuse (Cleaver et al. 2007) as well as recognition of the simultaneous exposure of children to multiple forms of maltreatment or polyvictimisation (Clemmons et al. 2007).

A large body of international research has shown that childhood exposure to physical, sexual and emotional abuse impacts developmental outcomes and contributes to impaired mental health in adulthood (Buckingham & Daniolos 2013; Fernandez & Lee 2017; Finkelhor et al. 2007; Gilbert et al. 2009; Nurius et al. 2007). Trauma from childhood maltreatment causes debilitating emotional and behavioural difficulties in children and can affect their ability to cope while in care, and can lead to adverse outcomes for older youth transitioning out of the care system (McMillen et al. 2005). In support of this view, Australian research quantifying the burden of psychological disturbance attributable to multiple forms of maltreatment concludes that a significant proportion of depressive and anxiety disorders and intentional self-harm is attributable to maltreatment in childhood (Moore, McArthur & Noble-Carr 2015).

All of these developments have occurred in the context of ongoing debate about the definitions and causes of abuse. The international child welfare literature is replete with definitions and typologies of specific types of maltreatment (Corby et al. 2012). These definitions, often presented in statutes and in the literature, are usually descriptive of incidents constituting abuse. In a legal context, the definitions adopted can influence reporting requirements; decisions about state intervention involving removal of children to care; and, even the termination of parental rights. More broadly, the definitions and understanding of child abuse have expanded beyond the family to encompass internationally recognised problems such as child sexual exploitation, child pornography, child trafficking and institutional abuse.

Meanwhile, at a basic practice level, child neglect continues to be the most frequently occurring form of abuse faced by child protection systems. The psychological and physical consequences of neglect are widely documented (Erickson & Egeland 2002). Neglect has had a low profile in professional and public awareness relative to physical and sexual abuse, with neglect cases often being filtered out of the system at various thresholds. Further, neglect has been portrayed as almost indistinguishable from the effects of poverty (Stevenson 1989). Research repeatedly highlights the association between maltreatment and low-income families and neighbourhoods and the potential for social inequalities to have an impact on the incidence of maltreatment, and for service responses to reinforce and exacerbate such inequities for children and families (Bunting et al. 2018; Bywaters et al. 2015; Coulton et al. 2007; Donelan-McCall, Eckenrode & Olds 2009).

The broad association of poverty with increased rates of neglect as well as other forms of abuse draw attention to the fundamental importance of understanding the extent to which abuse arises from structural or broader socio-economic factors as opposed to those which are attributable to individual characteristics of families: their decisions, choices, behaviours and disposition. For example, if abuse is seen to arise largely from structural factors, it implies that significant improvements might be achieved through preventive and supportive approaches. Accordingly, there have been calls for child protection systems to respond differentially to cases involving substantial risk and those situations where families are in need of services and family-based interventions. Such tensions are evident in the literature relating to the definition and causes of abuse. For example, early discussion of abuse favoured definitions that illuminate abuse at the institutional and structural levels as opposed to the exclusive legal focus on individual culpability. Abuse was defined as 'inflicted gaps or deficits between circumstances of living which would facilitate the optimal development of children to which they should be entitled and their actual circumstances, irrespective of the sources or agents of the deficit (Gil 1975: 346). Such a broader approach to definition highlights the structural bases of maltreatment and has the potential for intervention that enhances the quality of life for all children. The link between structural disadvantage and child maltreatment has been underscored. That child maltreatment occurs across the spectrum of family income and education, or that some forms of child maltreatment are more explicitly linked to socio-economic stress is acknowledged (Pelton 2015; Welbourne 2012). However, through the 1990s commentators have affirmed the need for a more comprehensive strategy which is child-centred, family-focused and neighbourhood-based (Berger & Slack 2014; Garbarino & Barry 1997; Melton & Barry 1994) and which involves a range of systems: physical and mental health, education, justice, housing and income support, in achieving a broader safety net for all children.

Historical context and trends in child protection

In the mid-1970s there was a re-emergence of state and media interest in the incidence and severity of child maltreatment, and children at risk of abuse became a major focus of all Statutory Departments. In response to the increased identification of child abuse and well publicised cases of maltreatment, such as Colwell in Britain (Parton & Martin 1989) and Montcalm in Australia (Lawrence 1983), a strong interventionist stance re-emerged and there was a proliferation of directives and safeguards to ensure early detection and prompt action in dealing with child abuse and neglect. Despite the broader long-term trends, there can be significant variations between jurisdictions based upon the drawing of thresholds. Nevertheless, it is thought that there has been a lowering of thresholds for defining abuse and sanctioning intervention over time; an outcome resulting from increasing emphasis on children's rights, the influence of the feminist theories about victimisation and societal expectation and endorsement of state intervention in family life (Fernandez 2005). One of the particularly influential factors has been the adoption of the policy of mandatory reporting which has been an integral part of the child welfare agenda to further ensure children's safety and wellbeing.

In support of this view, the pattern of reporting abuse and neglect reflects a striking increase over time. In Australia over 2017–2018 396,000 notifications or reports of child abuse were recorded. An estimated 245,000 children were the subject of these notifications (AIHW 2019). Children may be involved in multiple statutory notifications in a year. During the period 2012–2013, 272,980 notifications were received involving 184, 216 children, and representing a 98% increase in reports over a decade (AIHW 2014). Of the notifications in 2017–2018, 37% (146,000) were judged to require further investigation, while 63% were referred to support services. The rate of children who were subject of notifications rose from 37.8 per 1000 children in 2013–2014 to 44.4 per 1000 children in 2017–2018. Other statistics show that the rate of children who were subject of a substantiated notification rose from 7.2 per 1000 children in 2013–2014 to 8.5 per 1000 children in 2017–2018 (AIHW 2019). Children who were subjects of substantiation were most likely to be from the lowest socio-economic areas (36% in contrast to 5% in the highest). Aboriginal and Torres Strait Islander (ATSI) children are vastly overrepresented in substantiations at 42 per 1000 children compared with 6.5 per 1000 for non-Indigenous children, reflecting seven times the rate of non-Indigenous children.

In 2017–2018 emotional abuse was the most common primary type of abuse substantiated (59%), followed by neglect (17%), physical abuse (15%) and sexual abuse (9%). Variations are evident in the substantiations of different types of abuse in different states with differential policies across state jurisdictions accounting for variations. While these data point to a perceived escalation in the incidence of maltreatment, they are indicative of increasing professional and community awareness of the vulnerabilities of children and increased commitment to protect the rights of children.

Regardless of jurisdictional differences between the states, in general in situations where the harm, or the risk of harm, is serious or when parents need relief for a period of time, the authorities may apply to the Children's Court for Care and Protection Orders. An overview of the structure and decision-making processes of Children's Courts in different states is available in Sheehan (Chapter 7). Care and Protection Orders may vary from highly interventionist orders involving transfer of legal guardianship to the State Department; to Third Party, Parental Responsibility Orders involving transfer of guardianship to a relative or carer; to less interventionist orders such as supervisory orders where children continue to be under the custody and responsibility of parents with the State Department supervising and monitoring the quality of care (AIHW 2014). Placement in out of home care is considered as an intervention of last resort. When children are placed in care the policy emphasis is on reunification. The number of Australian children on Care and Protection orders following substantiated abuse has been steadily rising. At June 2018, 56,400 children were on Care and Protection Orders. A rate of 10.1 per 1000 children (AIHW 2019), rising from 8.2 per 1000 in 2012–2013 (AIHW 2014). Indigenous children are vastly overrepresented on Care and Protection Orders at 68.5 per 1000 children (AIHW 2019).

In Australia, as is the case overseas, child protection systems are reviewed periodically. A major driver of policy change has been a series of child abuse tragedies and alleged negligent practice. Media archives document scandals, and errors in judgement and management that have exposed vulnerable children to extreme maltreatment and even death. While the development and refinement of child protection systems have brought greater numbers of children and families to the attention of child protection authorities, there is a trend of ignoring vulnerable families of children in need, until there is demonstrated risk. Further, the unintended consequences have been an avalanche of child abuse reports transforming the nature of child welfare in that statutory child welfare systems have been consigned to receiving, investigating and substantiating child abuse reports as a restricted paradigm of responding to children and families (Fernandez 2014; Worley & Melton 2013).

Particular discourses have emerged around the operation of child protection systems and their impact on children and families and the need to strike a balance between protection and prevention. There have been portrayals of the child protection system as being either under protective or overly intrusive (Ainsworth & Hansen 2005; Gibbons, Conroy & Bell 1995; Hutchinson 1990). Other commentators have drawn attention to the forensically dominated responses to child protection in recent years, where monitoring and surveillance have dominated and social work with children and families is increasingly portrayed in legal and procedural terms (Parton 1997). The preoccupation with a child protection focus has had wide-ranging impacts on service delivery to families. The systems and practices developed to respond to the escalating notifications of abuse had implications for responses to children and families generally and not only those who were abused or at risk of abuse. Many who met the threshold did not receive the appropriate service or received no service at all.

Ensuring effective protective and supportive responses to the needs of children, young people and their parents is an ongoing challenge in the design and delivery of child protection and welfare systems worldwide. The distinction between, and merits of a Child Protection or Family Support orientation (Gilbert, Parton & Skivenes 2011) are widely debated. An appraisal of the child protection orientation and protective care systems have identified several deficits and inadequacies including:

- Responses being incident focused, forensically driven, defensive and reactive and dominated by surveillance and monitoring (Buckley 2011; Parton 2006).
- Inadequate responses to families experiencing different vulnerabilities including entrenched poverty, isolation, family violence and physical and mental health challenges which are overlooked until there is demonstrated risk (Morris et al. 2018; Parton 2014; Pelton 2015; Welbourne 2012).
- Preoccupation with investigation and validation of reports and failure to engage with families resulting in alienation of families and their reluctance to approach welfare and other services (Munro 2008; Waldfogel 2008).
- The continued over presentation of Aboriginal and Torres Strait Islanders in child protection notifications, substantiation and in care systems resulting from the slow recognition of Aboriginal self-determination and reluctance of welfare authorities to accept intrinsic differences in family structure and child rearing practices between Aboriginal and non-Aboriginal societies and appreciation of the legacy of the Stolen Generations (Atkinson 2011; Blackstock, Trocme & Bennett 2004; Lavarch 1995; Tilbury 2015).
- Paucity of 'early' intervention and supportive services to prevent entry to protective care, and to facilitate reunification with families when care is needed (Delfabbro et al. 2013; Higgins & Katz 2008; Devaney 2016; Parton 1997).
- Marginalisation of the views of young people and parents in decision making (Buckley, Carr & Whelan 2011; Thorpe 2008).
- An overburdened system posing challenges in workforce retention and relational continuity for clientele (Healy & Oltedal 2010).
- Lack of evaluative research to establish the efficacy of child protection interventions relative to other modes of intervention (Price-Robertson, Bromfield & Lamont 2014).
- System and service failures reflected in the revolving door of re reporting and re substantiation (AIHW 2019; Bentley et al. 2017; Fluke et al. 2008) highlighting inadequacies in assessment and/or inadequacies in response to ameliorating the circumstances of vulnerable children and families (Higgins et al. 2019).

The current system mostly responds to allegations of risk and harm, rather than needs. The impact on children and families of being drawn into, and subsequently filtered out of the child protection net when claims of abuse are dismissed has been noted. Large numbers of children and families notified do not receive even the pretence of any service other than investigation (Cooper 1993; McCurdy & Daro 1993; Melton & Barry 1994; Thompson 1994). This investigative focus detracts from the more fundamental development of policy and practice to prevent initial or further harm.

Preventative and supportive services for all children and families receive lower priority. Vulnerable families in need of services are likely to be caught in the net of child protection in order to access services. The preoccupation with investigation and validation and failure to engage with families to address their needs had the effect of alienating and deterring families from approaching welfare services (Fernandez 2005; Munro 2008; Waldfogel 2008). The effectiveness and impact of child protection interventions have also been called into question by researchers including (Campbell et al. 2010) who found no improvement in risk factors experienced by investigated families. Issues of family functioning, lack of social supports, poverty and children's emotional and behavioural problems persisted and were comparable to families who were not investigated.

For the most part, child maltreatment has been attributed to parental inadequacies compounded by pitfalls in child protection systems, but the causes are often more complex and arise from a combination of personal, social and broader structural factors. Despite developments in public health and preventative approaches, much of the focus of child protection policy has been on the residual, protective and coercive dimensions of statutory social work at the expense of family support services. Such approaches position practitioners in child protection as agents of social control, with intervention being focused at the tertiary level after abuse has occurred. Pelton (1989), critical of the residual focus of child protection interventions, advocates rethinking our collective responsibility for children by addressing wider social and economic problems which families face. In a similar vein, Frost and Stein (1989) advocate policies of 'structural prevention' and a child welfare practice that acknowledges and responds to divisions of class, ethnicity and gender (Lee & Fernandez 2019).

Over the past 15 years several state or territory public inquiries into the operation of child protection systems have been undertaken in a number of jurisdictions reflecting strong public interest in child protection outcomes for children (AIHW 2012; Commission for Public Administration 2004; Commission of Inquiry into Abuse of Children in Queensland 1999; Crime and Misconduct Commission 2004; Ford 2007; Mulligan 2008; Northern Territory Government 2010; Nyland Royal Commission (SA) 2016; Wood 2008).

In calling for a paradigm shift in the operation of child protection systems to generate better responses to, and outcomes for vulnerable children and families, these inquiries have triggered major changes in policy and practice in the respective jurisdictions. Different states have responded to the acknowledged need for major system-wide reform in different ways. Some states have embarked on large-scale reform of legislation and policy following major Inquiries, in order to strengthen child protection and/or strengthen family-based services (Wise 2019). One example has been the recommendation to introduce more early intervention strategies as based on a more public health approach to child welfare. Early intervention and family support programs are designed to enable parents to provide a nurturing environment for children and reduce the likelihood of children entering public care. Family-based, early intervention is particularly important in promoting a safe and stable environment for children exposed to issues of parental drug and alcohol misuse, domestic violence, mental health concerns, and who are in general at imminent risk of abuse and neglect and removal to care (Fernandez & Atwool 2013).

At a Federal level, in Australia, an overarching child protection national policy is represented in a National Framework for Protecting Australia's Children 2009–2020 (Council of Australian Governments, (COAG) 2009) developed through a consultative process with states and territories and significant stakeholders including children and young people. This framework, grounded in the principles of the UN Convention on Rights of the Child and endorsed by the Council of Australian Governments (AIHW 2013) reflects national leadership in the sphere of safeguarding children and provides impetus for changes across systems. Discussion is also directed towards the value of public health approaches to child protection, with an emphasis on primary prevention.

Central to this model is a focus on intervening early in children's lives to identify needs and problems to ensure they do not escalate and responding to families in supportive ways. The emphasis is on reducing risk factors and optimising children's developmental outcomes through universal primary preventive services delivered to all families, with additional services targeted to those in special need (Tomison 2004; Wulczyn et al. 2005).

Instead of focusing on children at risk, a public health approach would entail reorienting universal and secondary services towards working at the community level to proactively nurture and support children and families in their everyday lives (Melton 2014. This shift in thinking has prompted discourses about 'balancing' and 'refocusing' services and redefining concerns from 'child protection' to 'safe guarding' (Daro & Benedetti 2014; James & James 2008; Parton 2006).

Public health approaches underscore the importance of extending the focus of child protection responses from detection of cases and removal to out-of-home care to prevention. This paradigm argues that resources can be more effectively allocated to the primary strategies that examine the underlying causes of child protection involvement (e.g., social disadvantage, the number of children, sources, and the availability of services and supports). Such approaches encourage practices that look to support families at times of vulnerability to reduce the likelihood of abuse occurring and to provide more supportive, rather than punitive service responses. Approaches favoured under this paradigm include intensive family preservation services; home-visiting services; community support programmes; mentoring and other interventions that are directed towards the communities and families at greatest risk of child protection involvement. Such approaches are not, however, without challenges. Daro and Karter (2019) draw attention to the challenges and requisites for transitioning from targeting prevention services to a universal platform for all parents and children, while Parton (2019: 76) introduces a note of caution suggesting that 'at a time when many of the long term universal welfare services are being cut back and withdrawn altogether we need to be careful about what we do in the name of public health and prevention'.

Out-of-home care

Increasing use of Care and Protection Orders coincides with increases in out-of-home care. Integral to Australian child protection is out-of-home care provision for children, where reports of abuse and neglect are substantiated and where children cannot live safely with their families. At June 2018, nationally approximately 45,800 children were in out-of-home care, a rate 82.2 per 1000 children; 93% of children were in home-based care (kinship care and non-relative foster care) and about 6% in residential care. The pattern of disproportionality is further evident in the rate of Indigenous children in out-of-home care, 59.4 per 1000 children, 11 times the rate for non-Indigenous children (AIHW 2019) and showing steady increases since 2009 from 44.8 per 1000 children.

The reasons for this increase are likely to reflect changes in the broader child protection system, but also reflect broader issues in society including increasing drug and alcohol use by parents, increasing exposure of children to domestic violence and abuse, implementation of policies of mandatory notification, and increasing levels of poverty and deprivation in families.

In response, there are a range of options available for children who are unable to be cared for by their parents temporarily or permanently. These include formal and informal care arrangements. Formal care options include foster care with non-relatives, kinship care, adoption and residential care, the latter comprising institutions, boarding schools, small group homes, and youth hostels and shelters. Family-based foster care remains the dominant form of out-of-home care for maltreated and dependent children in most developed countries. Other increasingly important forms of care are kinship foster care placements (which now comprise around 50% of all placements) and more intensive approaches to care, including treatment foster care placements. Such new 'professionalised' or intensive forms of care have emerged to replace more institutional or congregate forms of care that have declined over the last few decades due to concerns about quality, child abuse allegations and links to the 'Stolen Generation' policies. Placement of this nature are often more expensive and are frequently provided by external organisations in the form of 'care packages' that often involved significantly increased levels of resourcing (Delfabbro, Osborn & Barber 2005). The organisation and outcomes of these initiatives will be of substantial interest to readers in Australia and across the world as will the outcomes that are being achieved.

Principal issues in out-of-home care

Outcomes

The system of out-of-home care has been subject to research scrutiny to identify outcomes experienced by children, and the practices and policies that underpin its operation (Fernandez & Atwool 2013). Internationally, studies allude to the serious difficulties children in care experience (Doyle 2007), exacerbated by the instability they experience through breakdown of placements (McDowall 2013; Oosterman et al. 2007; Sinclair et al. 2004; Wulczyn 2003). A number of studies have demonstrated the low priority out-of-home care systems give to education and schooling and the barriers to educational attainment that children in care experience as a result of changes of placement and schools, and low expectations by teachers and carers (Sebba et al. 2015; Townsend 2012) and children's vulnerability to mental health concerns (Fernandez 2008; Tarren-Sweeney & Hazell 2006).

The goals of out-of-home care interventions

There have also been debates about the broader ideological goals of child protection, particularly in relation to the debate concerning the goals of family preservation, child protection and permanency and stability. In recent years child welfare policy has extended its focus from child safety to child permanency (Maluccio, Fein & Olmstead 1986). Such approaches involve early intervention and family support to prevent entry to care as a priority, and when care is essential to the child's safety to facilitate reunification with families from care. When reunification is not considered a viable pathway, a care plan must propose a suitable long-term placement or adoption. The goals of safety, stability and permanence have dominated out-of-home care systems. While these are acknowledged as important and laudable goals they are limited in their reach. Though there has been some emphasis on broadening child welfare policy to incorporate child wellbeing as a central goal policy, specifying child wellbeing as an explicit outcome has not been stressed. A broader focus is needed that targets overall wellbeing of children (Wulczyn et al. 2005) encompassing education, health, emotional, social and relational outcomes as part of the metrics by which out-of-home care is evaluated. An integrated and holistic approach to children's wellbeing in care enhances the prospects of safety and permanence, and their later wellbeing (Courtney 2009).

Leaving care

The challenges experienced by young people leaving the care system have received wide attention in research and policy. Evidence from research suggests they confront major difficulties in securing educational, vocational, housing, employment and other opportunities integral to their transition out of care. Australian studies have documented their severely reduced life chances, noting they are more prone to experiencing substance abuse and mental health problems, marginal educational and employment outcomes, homelessness and becoming parents at an early age (Cashmore & Paxman 2007; McDowall 2013; Okpych & Courtney 2014; Pecora et al. 2006).

Inter-generational abuse

Another significant issue is the historic abuse experienced by adults who as children lived in institutional and other forms of care during the twentieth century and experienced harsh punishment and sexual abuse that were reported to be common experiences impacting on their current mental health (CLAN 2008; Fernandez et al. 2016; McKenzie 2003; Penglase 2005). Currently national concern about how children were treated whilst in 'care' instigated the Australian Government's Royal Commission into Institutional Responses to Child Sexual Abuse particularly in relation to organisations with responsibility for children in their care. In addition to the public acknowledgement of 'wrongs' perpetrated against children, the evidence emerging from proceedings should inform policy and practice to enhance the safety of contemporary systems, a theme addressed in this book in Chapter 5 by Tolliday.

Policy and practice issues

Recognition of child rights and listening to children

There is increasing recognition of the need to enhance participation of children in the services they receive. The discourse of child welfare has shifted internationally in the last century from one of child rescue, in which the child is viewed as vulnerable and dependent and in need of adult protection, to that of children's rights, focusing on the child's capabilities, strengths and agency, and recognising the child as an active participant in decisions affecting them (Mayall 2002). This raises implications for privileging children's rights in the operation of the protective care continuum. Participation by children in matters which affect them is a reflection that children as individuals have views and opinions which cannot be represented by parents or professionals. The past decade has seen changes to legislation which place specific statutory duty on Community Service Departments to ascertain the wishes and feelings of the child and to take these into account when making decisions. Children's participatory rights have been enhanced by the establishment in Australia of the CREATE Foundation (www.create.org.au) and a national Commissioner for Children to engage and empower young people in participating actively in decisions which affect their lives.

Indigenous children

The overrepresentation of Aboriginal and Torres Strait Islander children in the child welfare system is a major policy challenge for many countries with colonised indigenous populations. In Australia the legacy of colonisation is evident in large gaps between indigenous and non-indigenous wellbeing on several social and economic indices. These inequities are also evident in the child welfare system with indigenous families much more likely to be subject to child protection interventions and removals to care. Earlier in Australia's history, processes of colonisation involved regulation of family life and childhood through forcible separation of children from their families, institutional care, assimilation and denial of cultural identity, stolen childhoods and intergenerational trauma. Entrenched problems of poverty, social exclusion, lack of resources and reluctance of main-stream welfare authorities to accept differences in family structure and child rearing practices between Aboriginal and non-Aboriginal societies contributed to an over-representation of Aboriginal children in care. This pattern of over-representation and disadvantage continues today even after formal recognition of the tragic mistakes of previous policies and practices. The trauma associated with the severance of parental and family relationships, the added alienation from culture and the attempted erasure of Aboriginality has had a severe and long-lasting impact on the 'stolen generations' and their descendants. The legacies that created the policies of the stolen generations continue to be felt by Aboriginal communities across Australia. This history compels critical analysis of the dimensions of indigenous disproportionality in the child welfare system and the need for alternative models of service delivery which respond to the wellbeing of indigenous children and families and support their cultural identity. The need for special attention to policy and practice in relation to Indigenous children is reflected in the Aboriginal Child Placement Principle, now entrenched in legislation. It emphasises a preference for the placement of Aboriginal and Torres Strait Islander people with their indigenous people who may include the child's extended family, its Indigenous community or other Indigenous people in that order of preference.

Structure of the book

The book will examine research, policy and practice in the area of family and child welfare. It is designed to acquaint practitioners and students with key policy and practice issues in relation to working with children and families in special need and their underlying assumptions. The impact of theoretical orientations, contemporary debates, policy initiatives and research findings on policy and practice will be examined, in addition to the ethics and values that underpin child welfare interventions. Emphasis will be on critical analysis of the context, issues and constraints that shape policy and practice. For the purpose of this book, child welfare denotes services provided to children and families whose needs arise from confirmed abuse and neglect or the vulnerability to its occurrence. A focus is given to the spectrum of services that are conceptualised as being on a continuum of prevention, early intervention and family support at the front end, and protective care through fostering, group care and adoption as indicated by the child's need for safety and permanency.

The core knowledge, skills and values of family-centred and child-focused practice will be explored in this book, engaging with core areas of knowledge, policy and practice related to families and children, including:

- Theories and research on the causes and consequences of child maltreatment;
- Legal and political structure of child welfare and the extent to which child welfare systems provide a continuum of care and prevent, or perpetuate, the oppression of children, women and disadvantaged groups;

- Preventative and supportive interventions to strengthen and support families, promote the healthy development of children and reduce risks, and maintain connections with community institutions and neighbourhood;
- Protective interventions focused on families whose children have experienced physical, emotional, and sexual abuse and neglect. Interventions including investigation, risk assessment, and thresholds for socio-legal interventions;
- Protective care for children whose families are unable to maintain an adequate and safe environment in the home. Out-of-home care with non-related foster parents, relatives or kinship care and residential care as integral aspects of protective care, and adoption for children in need of permanency.

Many of these topics will be explored from an international perspective, with some chapters providing comparative analyses of how specific policies and practices vary across countries, while others involve case studies based on individual countries. What should become clear to readers is that, despite variations in policy and legislative environments, there are many commonalities that can be observed. These include: the prevailing concern about the prevalence of child maltreatment and the complex factors that are contributing to its occurrence; the growing interest in how child protections are positioned in relation to other government service areas; and the emergence of a public health perspective that balances reactive interventions against the need to prevent the occurrence of abuse or to minimise harm through early interventions. Readers will observe that these themes are emerging, despite differences in the administrative structures prevailing in different countries (e.g., whether child protection is centrally administered as is the case in some European countries) and more state and province based as would be observed in Australia, the United States and Canada.

This volume is organised in four sections addressing core areas of policy and practice.

Part 1: The context of child and family welfare

This section provides a contextual introduction exploring the history of child welfare, theories underpinning childhood and development. It introduces key policy developments that are central to understanding the position and needs of children and young people, and how policy and practice have been influenced by significant developments, including the children's rights agenda.

Having outlined policy and trends in child welfare in Australia and the global context in this chapter, Chapter 2 discusses key theoretical and value orientations underpinning work with children and families. It is essential for anyone undertaking work with children to understand developmental processes and factors in the family and social environment which promote or inhibit children's development. Such a perspective provides a way to focus interventions and to target services to enhance children's developmental outcomes. In this chapter Fernandez and Delfabbro address the theoretical and ideological foundations of child welfare policy and practice as a context for understanding the diverse areas addressed in this volume. A number of important areas of conceptual understanding are discussed, drawing upon multi-disciplinary knowledge arising from psychology, psychiatry, sociology, social work and other allied areas. The chapter underscores the importance of taking a 'developmental perspective' when working with children. Important developmental theories and perspectives are discussed to show how understanding of key milestones and developmental capacity are often important considerations in determining how service responses can meet the changing needs of children. Other important themes discussed in this chapter include the importance of a social ecological perspective that provides a multi-level analysis of how children's outcomes are influenced by individual, family, neighbourhood, community and broader social factors, the importance of cultural sensitivity; the study of trauma and risk and protective factors; the nature and importance of resilience; and strengths vs deficits approaches. Finally, the concept of the 'best interest of the child', a crucial standard to be operationalised in child welfare decision making, is critically examined.

In Chapter 3 Driscoll outlines the development of the United Nations Convention on the Rights of the Child (UNCRC) and the range of rights it assures to children in relation to the operation of the protective care continuum, and illustrates the significance of a rights-based approach through consideration of three areas of Australian policy and practice. First, the state's duty under the UNCRC to support the care of children within their family is considered in the context of recent political influences on Australian family support and early intervention services. Second, the way in which the UNCRC's guiding principles support decision making in the protective care continuum is discussed with particular reference to the importance of children's views in ascertaining their best interests. Third, a rights-based approach to alternative care provision highlights the poor life outcomes of care leavers and tensions arising in relation to preservation of culture in care placements. Recent theoretical work drawing on the capabilities approach and notions of relational autonomy are used to address concerns that a rights-based approach accords insufficient attention to the importance of personal relationships in the care and welfare of children.

Part 2: Child abuse and neglect: causes and consequences

This section explores the most significant issue in child welfare, the experience of maltreatment by children, the methods and challenges of risk assessment, the systems of child protection to safeguard them and the wide range of policy and therapeutic interventions to respond to their needs. The challenges arising from the dominance of child protection interventions and the need for prevention and early intervention strategies to support parenting capacity and child and family wellbeing are canvassed.

Working with cases of emotional abuse and neglect is the focus of the first of the chapters in this section. Loving and Shemmings begin by defining neglect and emotional abuse within the context of child protection, acknowledging the existence of this type of abuse within non-familial settings such as online and within-gang grooming and cases of sexual exploitation. A 'trauma-informed' perspective is proposed in order to provide a deeper understanding of the key pathways and mechanisms that can contribute to neglect and/or emotional abuse, supported by the relevant research in these areas. Two key concepts are discussed in relation to factors that may impact directly on caregiving behaviour. The first is 'unresolved' attachment-based trauma, alluding to the parent's inability to process and make sense of their own childhood traumatic relational experiences that leaves them vulnerable to being triggered when caring for their own child. The second factor is the parental 'capacity to mentalize' – a parent's ability accurately to consider what the child is thinking and feeling and how this may be influencing their child's behaviour. The chapter concludes with a look at current evidence-based interventions for families aimed at helping to resolve previous trauma as well as increasing mentalising capacity. The authors discuss issues such as the definition of abuse; chronic vs. acute episodes of abuse; cultural issues to do with definition of neglect and links with social disadvantage; co-morbid risk factors such as domestic violence, substance use and mental health issues; demographic correlates, cumulative effects of abuse and the longer-term consequences of specific types of abuse on children.

In the next chapter Tolliday introduces the reader to the sexual abuse of children. In recognition of the high prevalence rate of this form of abuse, attention is therefore directed towards questions such as: Where is the risk? Are there some children more vulnerable to others? Who sexually abuses children? How do they do it? Answers to these questions include identifying child sexual abuse as being most commonly perpetrated by people closely related or well known to the child and surprising to some, in a substantial proportion of cases, possibly 50% or more, by children and young people who are under 18 years old. In focusing on children and young people who have engaged in harmful sexual behaviour, their own developmental histories, including whether they have experienced trauma is considered, as well as challenges young people face in sexual development through new technologies, social media and access to pornography. The work of the Australian Royal Commission into Institutional Responses to Child Sexual Abuse is referenced as well as noting some of its limitations. The chapter concludes with a focus on promising developments in the Australian context.

In Chapter 6 Fernandez examines how child protection systems assess and respond to needs and risk and how decisions are made concerning case management and intervention. Discussion focuses on the issue of reporting systems, the prioritisation of cases, the range of child protection decisions and service responses and how these decisions are made. It explores the role of practice-based decision making, developments in assessment frameworks and actuarial models that allow identification of vulnerable areas of families. The chapter also considers the complexity of family need and how this can be assessed in an ecological context and directed towards timely decisions about family-based interventions, placement in care and permanency, including family reunification and adoption.

Chapter 7 then focuses on the socio-legal context of child protection decision making. This chapter highlights the extent to which the legal systems influence the child protection system in Australia and examines how legislation and legal process specifically direct system and service responses. Sheehan highlights the differences between legal and child welfare systems across Australia, combined with the complexity and uncertainty of child protection work and the absence of shared frameworks, frustrate the development of agreed approaches about risks and consequences of maltreatment. She advocates a more holistic and collaborative approach that offers a more effective response to families where children are referred to the Children's Court. It is argued that approaches that rely solely on legal and rights-based approaches to child protection fail to accommodate the broader understanding needed to deal with the social concerns and specific issues confronting children and families in the child protection system. The chapter concludes that child protection legislation and the legal process must be better grounded in understanding factors that influence children's outcomes and work collaboratively to improve the living circumstances of vulnerable children.

The principal focus in Chapter 8 is on evidence informed 'therapeutic' methods which encourage healthier psychological and social functioning in children, while also helping to foster the development of skills in parents that enhance parental ability to have productive and healthy interactions with their children. Delfabbro and Osborn elaborate on commonly used psychological approaches (e.g., cognitive-behavioural therapy); Multi-Dimensional Treatment Foster Care or social skills training which focus on addressing the immediate behavioural, psychological, and social needs of children are discussed, followed by elaboration of approaches that attempt to address the experience of trauma and harm often arising from exposure to abuse. Important areas discussed include trauma-based therapies, play and activity therapies and those informed by an attachment perspective. Focusing more specifically on the needs and skills of parents and carers, approaches such as Parent Child Interaction Therapy, Positive Parenting Programs, *The Incredible Years*, Multi-systemic therapy are examined for their potential value in enhancing the ability of parents and caregivers to maintain stable and nurturing home environments.

Part 3: The protective care continuum

Family-based services as core policy and practice in the continuum of supports in promoting children's wellbeing will be addressed in this section as a prelude to considering provision for children and young people who are unable to live with their families and who are looked after in out-of-home care. Pathways into care, the various care types children might experience, and the processes that are integral to good practice in care are explored, including the engagement with health and educational needs and attainment of children and the challenges and opportunities in facilitating optimal outcomes for children. Leaving care trajectories and the policies and services available to young people transitioning out of care are examined. The chapter also examines concepts of open and closed adoption and the socio-legal context of good practice.

In Chapter 9, Devaney highlights the need to ensure supportive services are available to children and young people as early as possible in the genesis of a difficulty they may be experiencing, as risk factors for child maltreatment can be cumulative in nature. Drawing on the Irish context where formal Family Support is an accepted policy and practice choice in the continuum of available services and supports, Devaney details a national programme for Prevention, Partnership and Family Support (PPFS) within the statutory child protection and welfare context. This chapter considers the potential of a Family Support approach to support children and young people who are at risk of involvement in the child protection and welfare system. In doing so it draws on the evidence underpinning the Meitheal model of prevention and early intervention located within the PPFS programme. The impact of this model on the outcomes of children, young people and parents and their associated experiences is exemplified to highlight the possibilities in supporting parenting capacity and child and family wellbeing. Central to the Meitheal model are core features of Family Support; a focus on individual strengths, participatory practices with family members, the provision of accessible supports through the collaboration of a range of services and a pool of multi-disciplinary practitioners. This chapter also considers the position of Family Support and the PPFS programme within a public health approach and advocates greater population-wide awareness and responsibility with regard to responding to families who are in need of support and assistance.

Turning to foster care as a response to maltreatment, Chapter 10 provides an overview of the cross-national knowledge base on family foster care. Thoburn describes the different ways in which foster family care may contribute to the service to maltreated children and their families. It examines broad trends in the provision of foster care services, including the prevalence of foster care in different countries relative to other forms of care describing the different types of roles of foster care. It outlines what is known about the foster care recruitment, monitoring, matching and support processes in different jurisdictions, but with a particular focus on England. It provides information on the numbers and ages of children entering care and placed in foster family care in a sample of countries with developed welfare policies. The chapter shows that the rates of those entering care (whether voluntary or court-mandated), and rates in care at any one time, vary considerably as does the age range of those entering care and the types of care. Australia, like the USA and UK nations, is a low user of residential care, with the result that foster carers provide short- or long-term homes for children with a wide range of needs. Thoburn cautions that while we can learn much from the international trends, an understanding of context is essential when considering whether approaches and methods from one country can be transferred across national boundaries.

In Chapter 11 Kiraly and Farmer document the increasingly important role of kinship care in the continuum of protective care in Australia and elsewhere, providing definitions of statutory and informal kinship care. They discuss the prevalence of this form of care, demographic characteristics of carers, and the different types of kinship placement (e.g. family care or community kinship). Important topics addressed include differences in child outcomes associated with kinship care, including stability and quality of care, prospects for reunification with parents, family contact, and risk of re-exposure to traumatic experiences within children's families. They draw attention to challenging issues relating to kinship care, including the vulnerability and resourcing of kinship carers, the level of recognition and support given to kinship carers and children; assessment and care planning; and the complexities for carers associated with having both a familial as well as a statutory carer role in relation to children and the children's parents.

Therapeutic residential care is a recent development on the Out-of-Home Care (OOHC) service landscape both in Australia and internationally. In Chapter 12, Kor and McNamara review the research evidence on therapeutic residential care for children and young people in OOHC. In response to persistent concerns regarding inconsistent service quality and outcomes in general residential care, therapeutic residential care aims to move away from basic support and accommodation to specialised models of care underpinned by trauma-informed principles. The authors identify three main approaches to therapeutic residential care: a home-grown therapeutic residential care program in Australia, milieu-based models in Europe and mental health treatment approaches in the USA. Key findings related to the effectiveness of these three approaches are reviewed in this chapter, showcasing the promise they hold and outlining their limitations. Implications for practice and policy are discussed.

Given the dearth of robust evaluations of educational interventions for children and young people in out-of-home care, Sebba's chapter provides a review of the research evidence on the effectiveness of educational interventions aimed at improving the outcomes of children in care. The emphasis is limited to educational interventions during the school years, focused specifically on children in OOHC. It draws on previous analyses which has shown that children in OOHC do better in those schools that are higher performing for children in general, while some research suggests they are over-represented in under-achieving schools. Reflecting this potential role of schools in outcomes, the chapter looks first at systemic interventions involving whole-school approaches before considering the individual interventions targeting children in OOHC specifically, and then those interventions targeting their foster carers. Finally, the implications from the evidence reviewed for policy and practice are drawn out.

In Chapter 14 Fernandez and Delfabbro examine the importance of reunification in out-of-home care: how this is defined, measured and researched. Positioned within the context of policy concern relating to the increasing number of children coming into care and the slower reunification rates being observed, the chapter examines the nature of reunification and the methodological and conceptual factors that underpin reunification trajectories, including the active or passive nature of reunification and the legal status and duration. Predictors of reunification such as the severity of the factors associated with the entry into care; the length of time children have been in care; and, the quality and frequency of family contact, as well as the child's ethnicity or cultural background are discussed. The chapter emphasises the importance of clear base-line assessments; the importance of building relationships between different parties in the care system (e. g., families, case-workers and carers); the role of trust and collaboration; and, the importance of specific services and supports during the reunification process. The chapter concludes with the observation that there are relatively few internationally recognised services available to facilitate reunification for children who have been in long-term out-of-home care.

In Chapter 15 Simmonds traces the development of adoption policy and practice as it has evolved significantly over decades and the wide range of needs and issues it seeks to address. While these issues have evolved over time, the focus of adoption has changed as well, with international adoption highly significant but falling in numbers, children placed for adoption where their birth mother decides that they cannot care for them and children who have been abused and/or neglected. Simmonds notes that adoption is a contested area that reflects a wide range of views about its appropriateness, effectiveness and outcomes. In his chapter he explores the various factors that have come to influence these issues with a specific focus on the child – their rights, needs, circumstances and developmental outcomes. The argument made is that for legislators, policymakers and practitioners, the child must be the key concern – both in the immediate present and for the rest of their lives.

In Chapter 16, Mendes and Purtell examine the policy and practice challenges associated with leaving out-of-home care. It is recognised that many young people are not well prepared to leave care and that effective preparation, transition and ongoing support services are essential to facilitate better life outcomes. Studies have shown that many young people experience difficulties in accessing stable housing, participating in ongoing education or employment, and developing supportive social connections. This chapter draws on a recent evaluation of the Berry Street *Stand by Me* leaving care program in the State of Victoria to highlight principles for effective leaving care policy and practice.

Part 4: Children, parents and carers as stakeholders

The final section turns to best practice in relation to communicating and working with children and young people drawing on participatory, rights-oriented and resilience-based approaches to enable children to participate in current and future plans. It explores the key issues in working with children and families from diverse backgrounds and models for culturally competent practice. It also addresses the complex needs of foster carers and birth parents and strategies to support them.

The focus of Chapter 17 is on the conjunction between the *protection* and *participation* rights enshrined in the UNCRC and the tensions inherent in this conjunction when translated into child protection policy. Mason and Fattore analyse the meanings of *protection* and *participation* of children as codified in the Convention and how participation and protection principles intersect in child protection legislation and practice. This analysis provides a starting point for identifying different constructions of the child and associated discourses that characterise advocacy for the protection and participation of children, with particular attention directed to issues of risk, vulnerability and agency. Some of the practice strategies and issues that are at the centre of discourses relating to children's participation in child protection are identified. Framing participation around the concepts of relational participation, advocacy coalitions and deliberative democracy, the extended analysis takes account of the role of power in the relationship between participation and protection in child protection processes, while also alerting readers to the significance of the third principle in the United Nations Convention on the Rights of the Child, that of *provision*, as inherent in service and policy-level practices.

The entrenched and increasing over-representation of Australian Aboriginal and Torres Strait Islander children in the child protection system shows that government strategies aiming to address this structural social inequality have failed. In Chapter 18 Tilbury and Lewis firstly provide an overview of the scale and nature of over-representation in Australia, using administrative data. They go on to propose a rights-oriented theoretical framework for Aboriginal and Torres Strait Islander child wellbeing to replace the current child protection orientation, whereby families are more likely to be investigated than helped or supported. Advocating a commitment to self-determination that is the foundation for change, they reiterate the importance of applying the five elements of the Child Placement Principle – prevention, partnership, placement, participation, connection – in legislation, policy, programs, processes and practice across the child protection continuum. Investment in both universal (e.g., early childhood education, child and maternal health) and targeted (e.g., housing, mental health) measures are stressed to enhance access to needed services. The authors make the case for expansion of community-led Aboriginal and Torres Strait Islander services and a reconceptualised child protection framework to ensure the right of Aboriginal and Torres Strait Islander families and communities to have children brought up safe and cared for within their own family, community and culture.

In the context of the current risk aversive child protection approach in which biological or first parents experience marginalisation in decision-making processes, Chapter 19 presents the case for building bridges with parents of children on the edge of care or in care. Fernandez and Thorpe describe the profiles of parents of children in public care, highlighting that a disproportionate number of them come from disadvantaged socio-economic backgrounds, with single-parent female-headed households and materially unfavourable environments. They often have significant health problems, confront threatened or actual violence and lack social and emotional supports. Consigned to the position of having their children removed to care, they confront challenges to their parental identity and experience a sense of loss, powerlessness and exclusion. The authors emphasise the need for case planning that balances the child's need for permanency with preservation of links with parents through meaningful contact. The importance for case workers to develop trusting and supportive relationships with parents, explore strategies and services that enable children to be looked after in their families where possible and safe to do so, and stay connected to their families, culture and community when in out-of-home care is stressed.

For children in out-of-home care who cannot be raised by parents or extended family, non-relative foster carers are central to their experience. Foster carers serve as the backbone of most nations' child welfare systems. These individuals provide daily support to children during the days, months or sometimes years that they live away from their parents. Children in foster care have especially high needs and many of them have experienced trauma in their home of origin. Identifying and supporting caregivers who can be responsive to these children on an everyday basis is one of the highest priorities for any child welfare system. In Chapter 20 Berrick lays out a 'roadmap' to get there, ensuring that foster carers are selected carefully, comprehensively trained, and thoughtfully supported. This chapter draws upon international literature to showcase research evidence about the characteristics of carers and their needs. The chapter describes the types of support caregivers need in order to thrive, outlining some of the unique challenges associated with this responsibility. Finally, research evidence is used to show how the field could improve foster carer capacity and strengths by focusing efforts on recruitment, screening, support and retention.

References

AIHW, 2012, Child protection Australia, 2010–11. Canberra: Australian Institute of Health and Welfare.

AIHW, 2013, Child protection Australia: 2011–2012. Canberra: Australian Institute of Health and Welfare.

AIHW, 2014, Child protection Australia: 2012–2013. Canberra: Australian Institute of Health and Welfare.

AIHW, 2019, Child protection Australia: 2017–18. Canberra: Australian Institute of Health and Welfare.

Ainsworth, F. & Hansen, P., 2005, 'A dream come true – no more residential care. A corrective note', *International Journal of Social Welfare*, vol. 14, pp. 195–199.

Atkinson, J., 2011, *Trauma trails recreating song lines: The transgenerational effects of trauma in Indigenous Australia*, North Melbourne: Spinifex.

Bentley, H., O'Hagan, O., Brown, A., Vasco, N., Lynch, C., Peppiate, J., Webber, M., Ball, R., Miller, P., Byrne, A., Hafizi, M. & Letendrie, F., 2017, *How safe are our children? The most comprehensive overview of child protection in the UK 2017*, London: National Society for the Prevention of Cruelty to Children.

Berger, L.M. & Slack, K.S., 2014, 'Child protection and child well-being', in A. Ben-Arieh, F. Casas, I. Frønes & J. Korbin (eds), *Handbook of child well-being*, Dordrecht: Springer.

Besharov, D.J., 1985, 'Abuse: The need to narrow the grounds for state intervention', *Harvard Journal of Law and Public Policy*, vol. 8, no. 3, pp. 539–588.

Blackstock, C., Trocmé, N. & Bennett, M., 2004, 'Child welfare response to Aboriginal and non Aboriginal children in Canada: A comparative analysis', *Violence Against Women*, vol. 10, no. 8, pp. 901–917.

Buckingham, E.T. & Daniolos, P., 2013, 'Longitudinal outcomes for victims of child abuse', *Current Psychiatry Reports.*, vol. 15, no. 2, pp. 342.

Buckley, H., 2011, 'Child protection and the proposed legislation: oil and water or an opportunity for positive change?', *Irish Journal of Family Law*, vol. 30, no. 3, p. 57.

Buckley, H., Carr, N. & Whelan, S., 2011, '"Like walking on eggshells": Service user views and expectations of the child protection system', *Child & Family Social Work*, vol. 16, no. 1, pp. 101–110.

Bunting, L., Davidson, G., Mccartan, C., Hanratty, J., Bywaters, P., Mason, W. & Steils, N., 2018, 'The association between child maltreatment and adult poverty: A systematic review of longitudinal research', *Child Abuse & Neglect*, vol. 77, pp. 121–133.

Bywaters, P., Brady, G., Sparks, T., Bos, E., Bunting, L., Daniel, B., Featherstone, B., Morris, K. & Scourfield, J., 2015, 'Exploring inequities in child welfare and child protection services: explaining the 'inverse intervention law', *Children and Youth Services Review*, vol. 57, pp. 98–105.

Campbell, K.A., Cook, L.J., LaFleur, B.J. & Keenan, H.T., 2010, 'Household, family, and child risk factors after an investigation for suspected child maltreatment: A missed opportunity for prevention', *Archives of Pediatrics & Adolescent Medicine*, vol. 164, no. 10, pp. 934–949.

Cashmore, J. & Paxman, M., 2007, *Wards leaving care: Four or five years on. A longitudinal study*, Sydney: Social Policy Research Centre, University of New South Wales.

CLAN, 2008, *A terrible way to grow up: The experience of institutional care and its outcomes for care leavers in Australia*, Sydney: CLAN.

Cleaver, H., Nicholson D., Tarr, S. & Cleaver, D., 2007, *Child protection, domestic violence and substance misuse*, London: Jessica Kingsley.

Clemmons, J.C., Walsh, K., DiLillo, D.K. & Messman-Moore, T.L., 2007, *Unique and combined contributions of multiple child abuse types and abuse severity to adult trauma symptomatology*, London: Faculty Publications, Department of Psychology.

Commission of Inquiry into Abuse of Children in Queensland (Forde Inquiry), 1999, 'Report of the commission of inquiry into abuse of children in Queensland institutions', Brisbane: Queensland Government.

Commission for Public Administration, 2004, 'The territory as a parent: a review of the safety of children in care in the ACT and of ACT child protection management', Canberra: Commissioner for Public Administration.

Cooper, D., 1993, *Child abuse revisited: Children, society and social work*, Buckingham, UK: Open University Press.

Corby, B., Shemmings, D. & Wilkins, D., 2012, 'Defining child abuse', in D. Wilkins, D. Shemmings & C. Pascoe (eds), *Child abuse: An evidence base for confident practice* (4th edn), Maidenhead, UK: Open University Press, pp. 83–101.

Coulton, C.J., Crampton, D.S., Irwin, M., Spilsbury, J.C. & Korbin, J.E., 2007, 'How neighbourhoods influence child maltreatment: A review of the literature and alternative pathways', *Child Abuse & Neglect*, 28, 771–784.

COAG (Council of Australian Governments), 2009, Protecting children is everyone's business: National framework for protecting Australia's children 2009–2020, Canberra: Commonwealth of Australia.

Courtney, M.E., 2009, 'Beyond safety and permanency: Making well-being a focus of child welfare policy and practice for children in state care', *Children Australia*, vol. 24, no. 1, pp. 15–20.

Crime and Misconduct Commission, 2004, 'Protecting children: An inquiry into the abuse of children in foster care', Brisbane: CMC.

Daro, D. & Benedetti, G., 2014, 'Sustaining progress in preventing child maltreatment: A transformative challenge', in A. Ben-Arieh, F. Casas, I. Frønes & J. Korbin (eds), *Handbook of child well-being*, Dordrecht: Springer, pp. 281–300.

Daro, D. & Karter, C., 2019, 'Universal services: The foundation for effective prevention', in B. Lonne, D. Scott, D. Higgins & T.I. Herrenkohl (eds), *Re-visioning public health approaches for protecting children*, 113–126, Cham, Switzerland: Springer Nature.

Delfabbro, P., Fernandez, E., McCormick, J. & Kettler, L., 2013, 'Reunification in a complete entry cohort: A longitudinal study of children entering out of home care in Tasmania, Australia', *Children and Youth Services Review*, vol. 35, pp. 1592–1600.

Delfabbro, P., Osborn, A. & Barber, J., 2005, 'Beyond the continuum: new perspectives on the future of out-of-home care in Australia', *Children Australia*, vol. 30, no. 2, pp. 11–18.

Devaney, C. 2016, 'Promoting children's welfare through family support', in P. Dolsan & N. Frost (eds), *A global reader in child welfare*, London: Routledge, pp. 99–109.

Donelan-McCall, N., Eckenrode, J. & Olds, D.L., 2009, 'Home visiting for the prevention of child maltreatment: Lessons learned during the past 20 years', *Pediatr Clin N Am*, vol. 56, pp. 389–403.

Doyle, J.J., 2007, 'Child protection and child outcomes: Measuring the effects of foster care', *American Economic Review*, vol. 97, no. 5, pp. 1583–1610.

Erickson, M.F. & Egeland, B. 2002, 'Child neglect', in J.E.B. Myers, L. Berliner, J. Briere, C.T. Hendrix, C. Jenny & T.A. Reid (eds), *The APSAC handbook on child maltreatment*, Thousand Oaks, CA: Sage, pp. 3–20.

Fernandez, E., 2005, 'The challenge of child protection', in M. Alston & J. McKinnon, *Social work fields of practice*, Melbourne, Oxford: Oxford University Press, pp. 176–193.

Fernandez, E., 2008, 'Unravelling emotional, behavioural and educational outcomes in a longitudinal study of children in foster care', *British Journal of Social Work*, vol. 38, pp. 1283–1301.

Fernandez, E., 2014, 'Child protection and vulnerable families: Trends and issues in the Australian context', *Social Sciences*, vol. 3, no. 4, pp. 785–808.

Fernandez, E. & Atwool, N., 2013, 'Child protection and out of home care: Policy, practice, and research connections Australia and New Zealand', *Intervención Psicosocial (Psychosocial Intervention)*, vol. 22, no. 3, pp. 175–184.

Fernandez, E. & Lee, J.S., 2017, 'Experiences and outcomes of adults who endured maltreatment as children in care in Australia in the twentieth century', in A.V. Rus, S.R. Parris & E. Stativa (eds), *Child maltreatment in residential care history, research, and current practice*, Dordrecht: Springer, pp. 419–460.

Fernandez, E., Delfabbro, P., Ramia, I.O. & Kovacs, S., 2019, 'Children returning from care: The challenging circumstances of parents in poverty', *Special Issue, Children and Youth Services Review*, vol. 97(C), pp. 100–111.

Finkelhor, D., 1996, 'Introduction', in J. Briere, L. Berliner, J.A. Bulkey, C. Jenny & T. Reid (eds), *The APSAC handbook on child maltreatment*, Thousand Oaks, CA: Sage.

Finkelhor, D., Ormrod, R.K. & Turner, H.A., 2007, 'Re-victimization patterns in a national longitudinal sample of children and youth', *Child Abuse & Neglect*, vol. 31, pp. 479–502.

Fluke, J.D., Shusterman, G.R., Hollinshead, D.M. & Yuan, Y.T., 2008, 'Longitudinal analysis of repeated child abuse reporting and victimization: Multistate analysis of associated factors', *Child Maltreatment*, vol. 13, no. 1, pp. 76–88.

Ford, P., 2007, *Review of the Department for Community Development Review report*, Perth: Department of the Premier and Cabinet.

Frost, N. & Stein, M., 1989, *The politics of child welfare: Inequality, power and change*, London: Harvester/Wheatsheaf.

Garbarino, J. & Barry, F., 1997, 'The community context of child abuse and neglect', in J. Garbarino, & J. Eckenrode (eds), *Understanding abusive families: An ecological approach to theory and practice*, San Francisco, CA: Jossey-Bass.

Gibbons, J., Conroy, S. & Bell, C. 1995, *Operating the child protection system*, London: HMSO.

Gil, D.G., 1975, 'Unravelling child abuse', *American Journal of Orthopsychiatry*, 45, pp. 346–356.

Gilbert, R., Spatz, C., Browne, K., Fergusson, D., Webb, E. & Janson S., 2009, 'Burden and consequences of child maltreatment in high-income countries', *The Lancet*, vol. 373, no. 9657, pp. 68–81.

Gilbert, N., Parton, N. & Skivenes, M. (eds), 2011, *Child protection systems: International trends and orientations*. New York: Oxford University Press.

Gil, D.G., 1975, 'Unravelling child abuse', American Journal of Orthopsychiatry, vol. 45, pp. 346–356.

Healy, K. & Oltedal, S., 2010, 'An institutional comparison of child protection systems in Australia and Norway focused on workforce retention', *Journal of Social Policy*, vol. 39, no. 2, pp. 255–274.

Higgins, D. & Katz, I., 2008, 'Enhancing service systems for protecting children: Promoting child wellbeing and child protection reform in Australia', *Family Matters*, vol. 80, pp. 43–50.

Higgins, D., Lonne, B., Herrenkohl, T.I. & Scott, D., 2019, 'The successes and limitations of contemporary approaches to child protection', in B. Lonne, D. Scott, D. Higgins & T.I. Herrenkohl (eds), *Re-visioning public health approaches for protecting children*, Cham, Switzerland: Springer Nature, pp. 3–18.

Hutchinson, E.D., 1990, 'Child maltreatment: can it be defined', *Social Service Review*, March, pp. 60–78.

James, A. & James, A., 2008, *Key concepts in childhood studies*, London: Sage.

Krugman, R.D. & Korbin, J.E., 2013, *C. Henry Kempe: A 50 year legacy to the field of child abuse and neglect*, New York: Springer.

Lavarch, M., 1995, *Bringing them home: National inquiry into the separation of Aboriginal and Torres Strait Islander children from their families*, Sydney: Human Rights and Equal Opportunity Commission.

Lawrence, R.J., 1983, *Responsibility for service in child abuse and child protection*, Sydney: Government Printer.

Lee, J-S. & Fernandez, E., 2019, 'Critical multicultural practice with ethnic minority children and their families', in S. Nippress & C. Williams (eds), *Critical multicultural practice in social work: New perspectives and practices*, Sydney: Allen & Unwin.

Maluccio, A.N., Fein, E. & Olmstead, K.A., 1986, *Permanency planning for children concepts and methods*, London and New York: Routledge, Chapman & Hall.

Mayall, B., 2002, *Towards a sociology for childhood: Thinking from children's lives*, Buckingham, UK: Open University Press.

McCurdy, K. & Daro, D., 1993, 'Child maltreatment: A national survey of reports and facilities', *Journal of Interpersonal Violence*, vol. 9, pp. 75–94.

McDowall, J., 2013, *Experiencing out of home care in Australia: The views of children and young people* (CREATE Report card 2013), Sydney: CREATE Foundation.

McKenzie, R.B., 2003, 'The impact of orphanages on the alumni's lives and assessments of their childhoods', *Children & Youth Services Review*, vol. 25, pp. 703–753.

McMillen, J.C., Zima, B.T., Scott, L.D., Auslander, W.F., Munson, M.R., Ollie, M.T., & Spitznagel, E.L., 2005, 'Prevalence of psychiatric disorders among older youth in the foster care system', *Journal of the American Academy of Child and Adolescent Psychiatry*, vol. 44, no. 1, pp. 88–95.

Melton, G.B., 2014, 'Strong communities for children: 'A community wide approach to child maltreatment', in J. Korbin & R.D. Kruger (eds), *Handbook of child maltreatment*, New York: Springer, pp. 329–339.

Melton, G.B. & Barry, J.D. (eds), 2014, *Protecting children from abuse and neglect: Foundations for a new national strategy*, New York: Guilford Press.

Moore, T., McArthur, M. & Noble-Carr, D., 2015, *Taking us seriously: Children and young people talk about safety and institutional responses to their safety concerns*. Melbourne: Institute of Child Protection Studies, Australian Catholic University.

Morris, K., Mason, W., Bywaters, P., Featherstone, B., Daniel, B., Brady, B., Bunting, L., Hooper, J., Mirza, N., Scourfield, J. & Webb, C., 2018, 'Social work, poverty, and child welfare interventions', *Child and Family Social Work*, vol. 23, pp. 364–372.

Mulligan, E.P., 2008, *Children in state care: Commission of inquiry*, Adelaide: Office of the Commissioner.

Munro, E., 2011, Munro review of child protection: Final report – A child-centred system, London: Department of Education.

Munro, E., 2008, 'Lessons from research on decision making', in D. Lindsey & A. Shlonsky (eds), *Child welfare research: Advances for practice and policy*, Oxford: Oxford University Press, pp. 194–200.

Northern Territory Government, 2010, Growing them strong, together: Promoting the safety and wellbeing of the Northern Territory's children, Report of the Board of Inquiry into the child protection system in the Northern Territory 2010, Darwin: Northern territory Government.

Nurius, P.S., Green, S., Logan-Greene, P. & Borja, S., 2007, 'Life course pathways of adverse childhood experiences toward adult psychological well-being: A stress process analysis', *Child Abuse & Neglect*, vol. 45, pp. 143–153.

Nyland Royal Commission (SA), 2016, Child Protection Systems Royal Commission, the life they deserve: Child Protection Systems Royal Commission Report, Volume 1: summary and report, Sydney: Government of South Australia.

Okpych, N.J. & Courtney, M.E., 2014, 'Does education pay for youth formerly in foster care? Comparison of employment outcomes with a national sample', *Children and Youth Services Review*, vol. 43, pp. 18–28.

Oosterman, M., Schuengel, C., Slot, W., Bullens, R.A.R. & Doreleijers, T.A.H., 2007, 'Disruptions in foster care: A review and meta-analysis', *Children & Youth Services Review*, vol. 29, pp. 53–76.

Parton, C., 1990, 'Women, gender, oppression and child abuse', in The Violence Against Children Study Group (ed.), *Taking child abuse seriously: Contemporary issues in child protection theory and practice*, London: Unwin Hyman, pp. 41–62.

Parton, N. (ed.), 1997, *Child protection and family support: Tensions, contradictions and possibilities*, London: Routledge.

Parton, N., 2006, *Safeguarding childhood: Early intervention and surveillance in a late modern society*, Basingstoke, UK: Palgrave Macmillan.

Parton, N., 2014, *The politics of child protection: Contemporary developments and future directions*, Basingstoke, UK: Palgrave MacMillan.

Parton, N., 2019, 'Changing and competing conceptions of risk and their implications for practice', in B. Lonne, D. Scott, D. Higgins & T.I. Herrenkohl (eds), *Re-visioning public health approaches for protecting children*, Cham, Switzerland: Springer Nature, pp. 65–78.

Parton, N. & Martin., 1989, 'Public inquiries, legalism and child care in England and Wales', *International Journal of Law and the Family*, 3, pp. 21–39,

Pecora, P.J., Williams, J., Kessler, R.C., Hiripi, E., O'Brien, K. & Emmerson, J., 2006, 'Assessing the educational achievements of adults who were formerly placed in family foster care', *Child & Family Social Work*, vol. 11, no. 3, pp. 220–231.

Pelton, L.H., 2015, 'The continuing role of material factors in child maltreatment and placement', *Child Abuse & Neglect*, vol. 41, pp. 30–39.

Pelton, L.H., 1989, *For reasons of poverty: A critical analysis of the public child welfare system in the United States*, New York: Praeger.

Penglase, J., 2005, *Orphans of the living: Growing up in "care" in twentieth-century Australia*, Fremantle, WA: Fremantle Arts Centre Press.

Price-Robertson, R., Bromfield, L. & Lamont, A., 2014, International approaches to child protection: What can Australia learn? (CFCA Paper no. 23), Melbourne: Australian Institute of Family Studies.

Sebba, J., Berridge, D., Luke, N., Fletcher, J., Bell, K., Strand, S., Thomas, S., Sinclair, I. & O'Higgins, A., 2015, *The educational progress of looked after children in England: Linking care and educational data*, Oxford/Bristol: The Rees Centre/University of Bristol.

Sinclair, I., Barker, C., Wilson, K. & Gibbs, I., 2004, *Foster children: Where they go and how they get on*, London: Jessica Kingsley.

Stevenson, O., 1989, 'Multidisciplinary work in child protection', in O. Stevenson (ed.), *Child abuse: Public policy and professional practice*, Hemel Hempstead, UK: Harvester-Wheatsheaf, pp. 173–203.

Tarren-Sweeney, M. & Hazell, P., 2006, 'Mental health of children in foster and kinship care in New South Wales, Australia', *Journal of Paediatrics and Child Health*, vol. 42, pp. 89–97.

Thompson, R.A., 1994, 'Social Support and Prevention of Maltreatment', in G.B. Melton & J.D. Barry (eds), *Protecting children from abuse and neglect: Foundations for a new national strategy*, New York: Guilford Press.

Thorpe, R., 2008, 'Family inclusion in child protection practice: Building bridges in working with (not against) families', *Communities, Families and Children Australia*, vol. 3, pp. 4–18.

Tilbury, C., 2015, 'Aboriginal and Torres Strait Islander families in Australia: Poverty and child welfare involvement', in E. Fernandez, A. Zeira, T. Vecchiato & C. Canali (eds), *Theoretical and empirical insights into child and family poverty*, Dordrecht: Springer.

Tomison, A.M., 2004, *Current issues in child protection policy and practice: Informing the NT Department of Health and Community Services child protection review, National Child Protection Clearinghouse*, Melbourne: Australian Institute of Family Studies.

Townsend, M., 2012, *Are we making the grade? The education of children and young people in out of home care*, Sydney: NSW Department Family and Community.

Waldfogel, J.C., 2008, 'The future of child protection revisited', in D. Lindsey & A. Shlonsky (eds), *Child welfare research: Advances for practice and policy*, New York: Oxford University Press, pp. 235–241.

Welbourne, P., 2012, *Social work with children and families: Developing advanced practice*, London and New York: Routledge.

Whittaker, J.K., del Valle, J.F. & Holmes, L. (eds), 2015, *Therapeutic residential care for children and youth: Developing evidence-based international practice*, London: Jessica Kingsley.

Wise, S., 2017, *Developments to strengthen systems for child protection across Australia.* Melbourne: Australian Institute of Family Studies.

Wood, J., 2008, *Report of the Special Commission of Inquiry into child protection services in NSW*, Sydney: State of New South Wales.

Worley, N.K. & Melton, G.B., 2013, 'Mandated reporting laws and child maltreatment: The evolution of a flawed policy response', in C. Henry Kempe (ed.) *A 50 year legacy to the field of child abuse and neglect*, Dordrecht, Heidelberg, New York, London: Springer, pp. 103–118.

Wulczyn, F., 2003, 'Closing the gap: Are changing exit patterns affecting the time African American children spend in foster care relative to Caucasian children', *Children & Youth Services Review*, vol. 25, no. 5/6, pp. 431–462.

Wulczyn, F., Harden, B., Barth, R.P. & Landsverk, J. (eds), 2005, *Beyond common sense: Child welfare, child well-being, and the evidence for policy reform*, Piscataway, NJ: Transaction Publishers.

Chapter 2

Theoretical and value frameworks underpinning work with children and families

Elizabeth Fernandez and Paul Delfabbro

In this chapter some of the theoretical concepts and frameworks relevant to interventions with children and families will be reviewed. In undertaking work with children and families it is important to understand children's development and the factors in the child's environment that promote or inhibit their developmental potential. Such a knowledge base is essential to plan interventions based on targeting factors that are significant. Howe (1995) maintains that all practice is inescapably theoretical and that different theories lead to different explanations about individuals and society. The range of theory discussed will include theories for practice including psychological and sociological perspectives and practice theory. The chapter will provide an overview of theories that illuminate psychosocial development of children and offer insights into their socio-emotional, cognitive and social development. It will address developmental approaches, concepts of attachment and bonding, trauma, and social ecological theories which emphasise a multi-interactional view of needs and problems and the interaction of individuals and their environments.

The population of children who come into contact with the child welfare system is highly diverse. They differ in age, gender, cultural background and also in terms of their family background. As a result, the type of services and practice approaches appropriate for each child may differ significantly. The needs of a teenager, for example, are likely to differ significantly from younger children. Similarly, those children who come into out-of-home care because of abuse, who have disabilities or other complex problems, may face different challenges from those who do not have these characteristics. For these reasons, one of the most important elements of working effectively with children in a way that best assists them is to adopt a developmental approach. In essence, this means that workers should be mindful of the development status and history of the child or young person under their care. In our view, this has three important elements. The first is recognition of the critical importance of the pre-natal, neonatal and early childhood years in influencing subsequent development and psychosocial functioning. The second is to understand the normative course of human development so as to understand what is expected at each age. The third is to understand that children's development needs change over time, so that what might appear to be a less important development need at a particular age might become more important when the child grows older. We will discuss each of these in turn.

An important trend in the developmental literature concerns the concept of 'stage' and its significance in conceptualising developmental processes of personality and thinking. There are a number of proponents of stages of development including Piaget (1963),

Freud (1932 cited in Hoffnung et al. 2019) and Erikson (1965). (Detailed overviews of these theories can be found in Hoffnung et al. 2019; Nicholson 2014; O'Brien 2016; Peterson 2014).

Freud identified personality traits associated with either excessive frustration or overly indulged gratification at each of various psychosexual stages, suggesting children become 'fixated' at one or other stage with residues of this process reflected in the adult personality (Peterson 2014).

Piaget's stage theory concerns the development of intelligence from birth to maturity based on the interrelated processes of assimilation and accommodation. Assimilation entails the child's adaptation of the environment to the self, while accommodation involves the impact of the environment on the child. The Piagetian description of a complex schematic structure implies the child's cognitive development depends on a range of environmental stimuli for the child to assimilate and which correspondingly induces accommodation (Fernandez 2013; Peterson 2014).

Piaget proposed identifiable stages of cognitive development and introduced the notion of readiness – the outcome of a combination of brain development and exposure to new experiences. His four key stages of cognitive development include:

- Sensorimotor development: birth to 2 years, focusing on developing gross and fine motor skills
- Preoperational: 3 to 7 years, when the ability to reason begins to surface
- Concrete operations: 7 to 11 years, marking emergent ability for logical thinking
- Formal operations: 12 years to adulthood, reflecting developing capacity for competence in abstract thinking.

Piaget's theories, built on assumptions that children make mistakes and experiment as they form their ideas, reminds us that the emotionally abused child who is responded to negatively, humiliated and labelled by adults will be inhibited in experimenting with ideas or behaviours and be stifled in their cognitive development. A neglected child who is offered little stimulation and encouragement is unlikely to develop age appropriate thinking or motor skills.

The main points to draw from the theory is that children's capacities need to be understood relative to their age and in the context of any delays. Younger children are typically more concrete in their thinking, have less ability to consider the motives and feelings of others, and often have a more transactional sense of morality (i.e., what is punished vs what is not). As a result, they often do not understand the bounds of appropriate or socially acceptable behaviour. When these children are exposed to abuse or other developmental trauma, their development will be delayed so that workers cannot assume that children who have a given chronological age are necessarily at this developmental level.

Erikson's developmental theory sets out further developmental tasks. In Erikson's (1963) eight epigenetic stages of development, the individual is confronted with a potential crisis or conflict between opposite poles to be resolved through reciprocity between self and others. Illustratively, in the first four years Erikson suggests that the child needs to develop a sense of trust as opposed to distrust, and later, a sense of autonomy and independence as opposed to self-doubt and inadequacy; the acquisition of these developmental tasks being based upon feeling loved and accepted and experiencing continuity of care giving and responsiveness to their needs. Threats to the child's perception of security and personal adequacy can evolve from experiencing neglect, abuse, inconsistency and instability in caregiving environments. Consistent with the predictions of Erikson's developmental theory, children under 12 are generally more preoccupied with building confidence and competencies. A fuller account of Erikson's life stages is available in Fernandez (2016) Hoffnung et al. (2019) and Peterson (2014).

Erikson's core messages from the theory are that children who experience trustful relationships with their carers will explore their environments, confidently display initiative in learning and acquire the skills to build a positive identity. They will transition to adolescence and adulthood to form and sustain close relationships and nurture the next generation. Erikson's theorising on identity resonates with practitioners who work with young people in care for whom issues of identity are compounded by the experience of abuse and neglect or prejudice and stigmatising attitudes towards their care status. For example, children who might have previously been very stable in care, could start to show greater interest in re-establishing ties with their families and communities. In Australia, such needs may be particularly strong in Aboriginal young people who have been removed from their 'country' or community of origin (Fernandez, Lee & McNamara 2018; HREOC 1997).

In addition to understanding how children's developmental needs change over time, it is also important to understand points of transition and opportunities for intervention. While there is general agreement that the first few years of life can have a critical influence on subsequent development, there are other important points of intervention or transition that may also provide opportunities to provide services and supports. These important points include the transition to school (age 5–6), the transition to adolescence (age 10–12) as well as the transition to adulthood (age 15–17).

The age of 5–6 is generally the age at which children with development delays or problems first start to display difficulties with school tasks and socialisation. This age, therefore, provides the first opportunities for workers to engage with educators and psychologists to identify more common developmental disorders (e.g., Autism Spectrum Disorders, Speech delays, Sensory integration problems, Attachment difficulties and Attention-Deficit problems). Early intervention and support at this age is important for assisting workers in working out what type of placement, schooling environment or services will be needed for the child. Similar issues apply at age 10–12, but this age also is the age where children are at risk of more serious behavioural problems that may have longer-term consequences. Problems with socialisation or behaviour, including engagement in early offending behaviour or substance use can often emerge during this period, so that interventions directed at this point can be beneficial for preventing more serious problems emerging and becoming more serious and entrenched during the teenage years. Finally, the age of 15–17 is the period when young people are close to making a transition to independent living (whether they are in care or living at home). At this point in their lives, much more focus therefore needs to be given to life skills, the availability of social supports and networks, and greater consideration given to education and employment opportunities and the capacity to live independently.

Attachment and bonding

An important perspective on development emerges from research into early child parent attachment and bonding. The theories of maternal infant attachment of the 1940s and the subsequent concept of maternal bonding of the 1970s and 1980s have attracted considerable theoretical and research attention and exerted major influence on intervention with children and families (Corby 2006) and the care of separated children (Aldgate 1988). They have also been subject to reappraisal in the context of contemporary thinking (Aldgate et al. 2006; Bretherton 1992; Rutter 1999; Sroufe 1989).

Bowlby (1951) formulated his controversial maternal deprivation thesis based on WHO sponsored research into the psychological outcomes of homeless children. He proposed infants need the consistent care of their mother during early months and that the absence of such constant care would result in long-term negative effects. Bowlby's early work on maternal deprivation emphasised the primacy of the child's early experience for his/her later development, identifying different forms of maternal deprivation: failure to make bonds (inadequacy of care); disruption of bonds (discontinuity of care); distortion of bonds (distorted relationships); dispersal of bonds (multiple caretaking) (Fernandez 1996). Clarke and Clarke (1976), critical of the treatment of maternal deprivation as an all-encompassing concept subsuming discrete elements of separation, attachment and deprivation, concluded from their studies that there was no evidence to support the view that attachment of the child to one person is essential to optimum development. Anthropological evidence indicates that multiple attachments can develop, given that children in many non-Western cultures are raised in the context of multiple caregiving (Werner 1979).

Rutter (1972) concluded after studying various types and lengths of parental separation that young children can be separated from their parents with minimal long-term effects. He suggested that factors associated with the negative effects of separation relate to the age of the child at separation and the quality of caregiving relationships experienced before and after separation. Implied here, for instance in the context of care, is that insufficiency and instability of care may be more significantly associated with deleterious effects rather than the separation itself.

Attachment refers to the enduring bond that develops between an infant and caregiver during the first year of life that the child uses as a secure base to explore the environment. Attachment patterns are claimed to be long term, being reflected in successive generations of parents and children. As Bowlby used the term in the 1950s and 1960s, it referred to a process which generally became apparent when the infant was around six months of age, the height of attachment occurring around nine months as evidenced typically by high stranger anxiety at this time.

There has been much theorising about the purpose and process of development of attachment in infancy and beyond. From these efforts have emerged four schools of thought: ethological, psychodynamic, cognitive and learning theory. Ethologists such as Bowlby suggest that the ability to form an attachment bond with the mother increases the infant's prospects of survival and protection, providing a secure base to explore the physical and social environment. The psychoanalytic approach emphasises instincts and maintains that, as children's instinctual needs are met by the mother in the early stages of infancy, bonds of attachment with the mother strengthen and provide the foundation for ensuing relationships. Cognitive theories view attachment and proximity seeking behaviours as the outcome of cognitive awareness of the perceptual differences between the mother and others in the environment. It is claimed that attachment is strengthened because of the child's ability to construct a mental image of the mother's distinguishing characteristics and understand the notion of person permanence, a concept closely related to object permanence.

Learning theorists see attachment as a learned rather than innate process, the mother being associated with dispensing the primary reinforcers of tactile stimulation, warmth and responding to the infants needs. Researchers have observed that infants reach out actively to their environment for social contact. In turn the mother/caregiver influences the child by encouraging responses, and in subtle ways her behaviour is also shaped by the child. This two-way transaction has led developmentalists to portray the mother and child as an 'attachment system'.

Attachments develop in a series of phases including indiscriminate sociability to focused attachments at two years with increased memory and representational skills. Also noted are intervening phases such as: separation anxiety – the infant's discomfort at being separated from their caregiver at 9–18 months; stranger anxiety – wariness and avoidance of strangers at 6–9 months, the strength of these reactions depending on familiarities of the environment. Shaffer and Emerson (1964) identify specific stages of attachment: an 'asocial period' when infants respond to a variety of human and inanimate social stimuli followed by a stage of indiscriminate attachment characterised by tendencies to generalise their attachment to all humans in their environment. In a third stage of 'specific attachment' between 6–12 months infants' preferred attachment is directed to a specific person, usually the mother and will display signs of protest and distress when separated. Attachments to other persons in the environment are also in evidence and cross-cultural variations in age approximations and patterns of attachment are to be noted.

Indications of attachment are also described. Among other manifestations of attachment, such as 'selective social smiling', 'stranger anxiety' is evident at six months when the infant sees noticeable differences in the stranger compared with the mental image of the mother's features stored in its developing mind. 'Separation anxiety' another indicator of attachment evident at 12 months when separation from the attachment figure is accompanied by protest and distress.

A widely used method for studying attachment involves the 'Strange Situation' developed by Mary Ainsworth (Ainsworth 1979) which presents the child with a series of controlled separations; namely, being separated from a caregiver and meeting a stranger. The reactions of infants in the experiment formed the basis of Ainsworth's classification of attachment styles: secure attachment; anxious resistant attachment or ambivalence; anxious avoidant attachment; disorganised disoriented attachment. These conceptualisations of attachment have been researched internationally, 60–65% of children being assessed as securely attached, whereas patterns of insecure attachment are variable (Van Ijzendoorn & Kroonberg 1988). Research using the Strange Situation framework in different countries reflects marked differences in the distribution of attachment classifications across cultures (Van Ijzendoorn & Kroonenberg 1988).

Wilkins, Shemmings and Shemmings (2015) highlight the complexity of attachment behaviours that is captured by this simplistic dichotomy and cautions that, while secure attachment patterns are associated with positive outcomes, neither of the insecure patterns should be regarded as pathological. Further cross-cultural research draws our attention to cultural implications of applying attachment theory to cultures that have diverse ways of parenting and achieving attachment.

Ryan (2011) discusses the key tenets of this theory in relation to Aboriginal parenting. Ryan's review of the relevance of Bowlby's theory of attachment to Aboriginal parenting draws attention to caregiving practices in Aboriginal Communities that are at odds with key concepts of the theory. For example, the theory asserts that children who develop a secure attachment develop competence reflected in values of autonomy, independence, problem solving and resilience. In contrast to a Western orientation, Aboriginal people espouse values of interdependence, group cohesion and spiritual connectedness, with the notion that the primary caregiver is a base for the securely attached child in exploring its environment. In the Aboriginal culture, young children are carried and in the process restricted from exploration away from the caregiver (Ryan 2011). Particular parenting interventions predicated on attachment theory, such as 'Circle of Security' which focuses on the relationship between infant and mother are perceived to be ineffective for indigenous families as they fail to take into account the other caretaking relationships and supportive networks (Mildon & Polimeni 2012).

Bowlby's conceptualisations of attachment broadened in subsequent work as he described attachment as 'the propensity of human beings to make strong affectional bonds to particular others and of explaining the many forms of emotional distress .... which unwilling separation and loss gives rise to' (Bowlby 1984: 87). Attachment has been dominant in theorising of early relationships and continues to be influential in child welfare. As has been evaluated and revaluated, greater appreciation has been gained of the role and contribution of fathers, siblings and grandparents (AIFS 2015; Garbarino 2014; Grossman et al. 2002).

Attachment theory has been through different iterations and continues to be influential in multiple disciplines including social work practice where it underpins decisions about child protection and with children in care and vulnerable families. The early relationship formed with primary caregivers acts as a template for later relationships and it is critical that attachment is nurtured and supported. The importance of nurturing and supporting this critical relationship is reflected in early intervention programmes where parenting is a significant component, recognising that secure attachment is associated with optimal outcomes later in life. This framework also has relevance to child protection practice and children in care. In child protection decisions, assessments may focus on the nature of the bond with the caregiver. Decisions about contact and visitation may rest on the practitioner's assessment as to whether attachment and bonding is evident and is adequate justification for continuation of the relationship. The potential for reunification is also premised on the strengths or deficits in this relationship (Fernandez 2013).

The situation confronted by practitioners is one where established affectional bonds are disrupted at removal of children to protective care. Further challenges emerge when children experience changes in placement resulting in feelings of rejection and self-blame which often lead to children resisting the prospect of forming attachments with new caregivers (Aldgate 1991). Adcock, Lake and Small (1988) suggest that separating children from attachment figures engenders in them acute fear and the most frightening experience for children is simultaneously to be afraid and separated from attachment figures. Frequent moves in care exacerbate such fears. This points to the importance in practice of handling the early stages of the relationship sensitively when placing children with foster and adoptive parents, arranging contact and reunifying children with birth parents, and paying due attention to the impact of separation on children.

Closely related to attachment are notions of separation and loss (Bowlby 1969) encountered during the lifespan in different contexts. Several writers have drawn attention to the significance of loss in the experience of children entering care (Aldgate 1988, 1991; Schofield & Beek 2014). Children in care may grieve for the absence of their birth parents and siblings and for the loss of their previous family life and sense of normalcy. Consistent with theoretical perspectives on grief and loss they may display feelings of shock, denial, guilt and despair (Kubler-Ross, 1970; Marris 1986) and may require help from their caseworkers and new carers to express their feelings and come to terms with the experiences of separation and loss. There are also grief reactions associated with what Boss (2007) refers to as ambiguous loss which is illustrative of the experience of children and young people in care whose families are physically absent but very present in their minds.

There has been increasing interest in using an attachment perspective to understand adult responses to trauma and loss which has led to the development of the Adult Attachment Interview (AAI) (Main 1995). Designed to enable individuals to understand their lives in the context of vulnerabilities in their early relationships, Bifulco et al. (2008) have developed a suite of attachment-style interviews to capture current adult attachment style with respect to an individual's ability to access and utilise social support. These include an AAI designed for practice needs of fostering and adoption in Children's Services (Nicholson 2014).

Theorising bonding

Theories of bonding which emerged in the 1970s through the work of Klaus and Kennell (1972) have also been influential among professionals in child welfare including social workers, paediatricians, obstetricians, psychologists and nurses. Klaus and Kennell (1972) theorised the bonding process between mothers and new-born infants, claiming there was a critical period soon after birth for the formation of a bond between mother and infant. The concept holds some parallels with attachment though the two concepts are conceptually distinct. Bonding refers to the special relationship held to develop between mother and child, specifically from the mother to the child. In the initial formulation of Klaus and Kennell (1972), this bonding is believed to occur when there is close skin to skin contact between infant and mother immediately after birth and was dependant on the presence of a sensitive period in the mother for its development. It was proposed that during the first hours after birth the mother should engage in bonding with her baby through tactile and visual stimulation, and interruption of this bonding process could have negative long-term effects. This bleak view is no longer held, though the notion of maternal bonding still holds interest in child welfare. Attachment, as noted earlier is conceptualised as a two-way process, predominantly an interactional relationship between mother and child. It differs from bonding which is seen essentially as a one-way tie of mother to child that occurs immediately after birth. However, in practice and literature, it is not uncommon for the two terms to be used interchangeably and to assume their functional equivalence. Nevertheless, there are similarities to be noted. Both are seen as essential to the optimal development of the child. A further similarity derives from the long-term outcomes claimed by both proponents. For Bowlby, attachment is seen as the prototype on which all other affectional relationships are based. Klaus and Kennell stressed the centrality of the mother and that early extended contact enhances reciprocity in mother–infant interactions, ensuring positive maternal infant relationships and reducing the potential for abuse and neglect.

The empirical and sociological bases of the bonding theories have been questioned. The theory claimed the presence of a critical period for the development of the mother–infant bond, implying that if this did not occur in the specified time frame the child's subsequent attachment would be affected. The notion of a 'sensitive period' for the formation of a mother to infant bond has not been supported empirically, and later attachments can develop (Clarke & Clarke 1976; James & Fernandez 1986). In response to criticism of genderisation and ethnocentric bias, adjustments were made to the theory to reflect a focus on parent–infant bonding rather than maternal infant bonding.

Klaus and Kennell's original study involved an experimental study of 14 mothers of full-term babies who were followed up for five years to test the impact of early and extended contact on the bonding process. The experimental group received early and extended contact with their babies after birth (skin to skin contact within two hours after birth and extra exposure to their infants for the next three days) compared with routine exposure of the control group (glance at birth, visit 6–12 hours late and 20–30 minutes feed every four hours during the day). The findings of this study and a series of replication studies that followed were found to yield little support for the bonding concept due to the lack of statistical sophistication and ambiguity in the conceptual and empirical definition.

For instance, a study by Cater and Easton found that separation at birth was a common experience in their sample of 80 children who experienced abuse, combination of other stresses and circumstances including family instability, domestic violence, psychiatric disturbance and parental immaturity, making it not possible to attribute causality to any one event, including maternal–infant separation. Reviews of the evidence from various studies can be found in Sluckin, Herbert and Sluckin (1984).

In the light of the foregoing, the evidence for supporting a connection between extended contact and bonding or later attachment for mother and infant or for subsequent marginal mothering or child abuse has been regarded as scant and weak. These critical comments are not intended as an argument against infant parent contact as soon as practicable. The argument advanced is that humanising the natal and neonatal experience is a desirable goal and a right of parents and children to settings which are conducive to forging such relationships. At issue is the deterministic claims of the theory and the potential attribution that early relationships are unalterable. With almost one half of mothers in the workforce and practical issues of child care it would be crucial to promote the concept of parent–child bonds.

Child protection assessments underpinned by the theory influence strategies for intervention. However, a narrow focus on bonding and attachment to the exclusion of significant influential factors including environmental factors, the child's behaviour, the lack of formal supports, inadequacy of mental health and drug and alcohol services and structural inequalities that place parents under stress may well be overlooked and restrict the scope of assessments and interventions (Featherstone, White & Morris 2014; Fernandez, Lee & McNamara 2018).

Sociology of childhood

The developmental theories that portray childhood in universalistic terms have been challenged for their Eurocentric bias and failure to capture the diversities and complexities of childhood. Developments in the Sociology of Childhood and the discourses on the political and social context of positioning children (James & Prout 1997; Mayall 2000; Qvortrup 2004) have challenged explanations of childhood that focus on children in terms of stages they progress through in the journey towards becoming an adult (well becoming) under-emphasising understanding children's present lives (well being). The importance of understanding children in terms of the present as both being and becoming is highlighted in this paradigm (Huebner 2004; Stainton Rogers & Stainton Rogers 1992; Walkerdine 2009).

In this reframing, the conception of children as vulnerable and dependent on adults to have their needs met is contrasted with understandings of children as experts in their own lives, shifting the needs discourse to one of rights that treats children as social actors acknowledging their agency and entitlement to have a voice and participate in decisions about them (Mayall 2000; Wyse 2004). James and Prout (1997) maintain that children are not just a 'bundle of needs' that are to be met but their rights and aspirations as citizens must be recognised. These changing discourses on childhood are reflected in the child rights movement and the United Nations Convention of the Rights of the Child (UNCRC 1989) with its emphasis on 'provision of services', 'protection' from abuse and exploitation and 'participation' in decisions that affect them. Its core principles call for respecting the views of the child (article 12), acknowledging children's right to have their views heard.

These changing conceptualisations of children and childhood have been extended to the recognition of the significance of the child's perspective in research, of respecting children's ability to interpret their current lives to others and counter adults' monopoly in research (Fernandez 2006; Wyse 2004). There is a rich international literature on the methodological and ethical challenges in child-centred and child-inclusive research (Christensen & James 2000; Alderson 2000) The imperative to recognise children and young people as effective communicators of the reality of their lived experience and capable of informing policies that affect them resonates through individual chapters in this collection.

Contextual theories

Psychological theories have had a major influence on child welfare practice with little attention paid to systems surrounding individuals that influence their responses. The need to widen practitioners' conceptual lenses to include the influence of environmental factors on family functioning and address the interface between people and their environments has been advocated (Howe 2009; Laird 1979; Maluccio 1986). An important consideration for effective practice is to understand the complex contextual factors that often underlie families who come into contact with child welfare systems. In most cases, it is rare to find families who are affected by only single problems. Instead, as shown in many studies (e.g., Delfabbro et al. 2009, 2013; Fernandez 2006, 2013), children who receive notifications or substantiations for one type of abuse, very often have reports of other types. Abuse will frequently coincide with domestic violence, parental mental illness or substance misuse and all of these factors will be statistically more likely to occur in households where there are multiple children and entrenched poverty (financial problems or housing difficulties). Thus, when one is confronted with a child with complex needs, workers should not assume that the problems observed are entirely due to the individual characteristics of the children (e.g., their temperament or cognitive ability). In most cases, children will have experienced prolonged periods of living in difficult living circumstances in lower socio-economic areas that are often less safe, have fewer services or amenities and less well resourced schools. In recognition of this, many researchers understand child and family needs within the context of sociological frameworks that recognise the multiple levels of influence on children's outcomes.

There are a number of contextual approaches that have broadened our perspective on developmental influences. One influential framework is Bronfenbrenner's (1979) sociological approach that positions the individual within broader spheres of influence that range from the immediate family to include peers, school and the wider community, contributing to our understanding of how contextual relationships influence a child's development.

Bronfenbrenner views the child as developing within a complex system of interrelationships that are impacted by the surrounding environment. He portrays the environment as a series of nested structures, proposing a person's development is influenced by four overlapping and interactive levels:

- The microsystem level – interactions children have with parents, grandparents, siblings, carers, teachers, caseworkers.
- The mesosystem level – connections and relationships among the child's microsystems.
- The exosystem – the settings and systems that indirectly influence the child, e.g. parents' place of employment, school administration, statutory department.
- The macrosystem – prevailing ideologies, beliefs, values of society, cultural contexts including poverty/ethnicity and social policies that influence the individual directly or indirectly through their impact on micro- and mesosystems.
- Chronosystem – the experience of events, transitions and socio-historical occurrences over the lifespan.

Each system has an influential impact on development. The environment is regarded as a dynamic and ever-changing system where critical events, e.g. parental separation, addition of a sibling, removal to a care placement, modify relationships between individuals and their environments. This perspective enables a dual focus on the child and his/her environment, recognising that children are in constant interaction with various individual and institutional systems and intervention can be effected through any of these systems (Fernandez 1996).

Bronfenbrenner's ecological thinking has been influential on social work theory and practice, prompting recognition that children affect and are affected by parents, peers, school and service systems. In turn, parents and the quality of their parenting is influenced by their histories, relationships, support systems, work lives, income, housing and neighbourhoods as well as social policies (Bronfenbrenner & Morris 2007; Howe 2009) and provision of services needed to take into account larger ecosystems. The ecological approach offers us a framework which enables us to understand the many layers of influence from immediate to distal.

Maluccio (1986) has identified several ecological principles that are relevant in thinking about interventions. These include: interactionism, which emphasises that emotional and behavioural responses are not solely the function of personality or of environmental influences but are the outcome of the complex interaction of between person and environment; transactionism, which recognises individuals' agency and views them as active participants in transactions with their environments; a growth orientation that focuses on individual strengths rather than merely on deficits.

Approaches of this nature are important because they encourage workers, Courts and other decision makers to look beyond the immediate flaws of the individual and to consider the broader context. Complex behaviour is placed into a context and this serves to provide a motivation for looking for strategies that might: (a) identify risk and protective factors that either exacerbate or improve the circumstances of children and families, (b) consider services that are multi-faceted and multi-level in approach and (c) to avoid making the attribution that complex families are immutable to change. Such perspectives have been central to the development of 'wraparound' frameworks that look for opportunities to find service responses that deal with more than one problem at a time or programmes such as Multi-Systemic Therapy (MST) (Henggeler et al. 1997). Programmes therefore may include a combination of child therapy, parental support and training, community engagement as well as interventions involving schools.

Resilience and strengths-based approaches

Recently there has been developing support for resilience-led perspectives in child welfare practice to provide a balancing focus against the background of deficit-based approaches and risk assessment models that have predominated (Gilligan 1997; Luthar & Zigler 1991; Rutter 1999; Walsh 1998). A focus on strengths is central to a broader literature relating to resilience in the context of child welfare. Resilience refers to positive patterns of development or functioning in children that emerge in the face of adversity (Masten 2006). Elaborating on the concept of resilience further, Gilligan (1997) emphasises the 'qualities which cushion a vulnerable child from the worst effects of adversity … and which helps a child or young person to cope, survive, and even thrive in the face of great hurt and disadvantage'. It has been found that many people appear to be able to achieve good outcomes in life, despite having faced very difficult circumstances, which can include exposure to trauma and abuse (Werner & Smith 1982). Resilience is thought to arise from a range of different factors, including individual differences (intelligence, good self-regulation skills, positive outlook and appealing qualities, good socialisation skills); relationships (e.g., either good parenting or good relationships with certain key adults who influence the trajectory of the young person's life); and community/ structural factors including access to good schools, opportunities to develop important talents and good social/career-relevant connections (Masten 2006). None of the factors on their own are usually sufficient in that any child with the capacity to do well will struggle to do well if they do not have the appropriate supports from adults and opportunities to build upon their strengths. It is for this reason that some writers (e.g., Lalonde 2006) have emphasised the importance of avoiding what is sometimes called the 'trait trap' in which it is assumed some children possess a natural 'hardiness' or 'invulnerability'. If this logic is interpreted too narrowly, it can sometimes lead to unjustifiable inferences. The first is that some children will have the ability to deal with adversity no matter what life throws at them and so need less help. Alternatively, there might be the view that, just because young people appear superficially to be still functioning after abuse and trauma, it does not always follow that they are doing well in many other aspects of their life. A retreat to resilience logic can, therefore, lead to the belief that the main source of change should be in the individual rather than the environment or that certain children 'just cannot be helped' because they do not appear to have the qualities necessary for success.

Aligned with this perspective is Rutter's (1990) work on risk and protective factors affecting child development which demonstrates that, although the effects of risk factors may be significant, cumulative protective factors can have substantial positive effects. This highlights the valuable role that foster/adoptive carers can play in enhancing protective factors for children in order to promote an improved sense of self-esteem and self-efficacy through consistency, nurturance and predictability to diminish the traumatic impact of children's early experiences, and promote resilience (Fernandez 2006; Hughes 1997).

Strengths-based practice

Much of the research that involves vulnerable families and children adopts a child protection approach. Although broader legislative statements will refer to the 'best interests of the child' and the importance of enhancing the lives of young people, the process of child protection is often about risk management, wherein workers are often asked to use standardised decision-making tools that might require them to rate the severity of abuse; its likelihood of occurring again; or, the strengths and weaknesses of the household environment when deciding whether children can live there. In situations of this nature, where risk aversion is often elevated to the highest importance, much of the focus of the work with families and any associated research can tend to be very focused on the deficits or weaknesses of the families and the problems experienced by the children.

There is nothing inherently wrong with identifying risk factors in child welfare contexts. Such approaches can allow for the early detection of families who may need extra supports; it can help to identify the factors that reduce the chance of children of being able to go home; and, it can also be a way of identifying the children who are most likely to experience difficulties when they are placed into care. As discussed earlier in this chapter, one of the striking features of child welfare populations is that families often experience multiple problems (Delfabbro et al. 2009; 2013; Fernandez et al. 2019). At the same time, it is recognised that effective practice should not solely be about deficits. Children in care have many strengths and so do their families. The identification of these factors also plays an important role in understanding what areas might provide the basis for helping families overcome their difficulties and help children develop better lives.

Strengths-based approaches (Oliver 2017; Saleeby 2002) direct attention away from the labels applied to service users and clients and the negative identities and defects ascribed to them. The emphasis is on identifying and recognising strengths, experience, skills and supports the parent or young person draws on to cope with the challenges they face. Saleeby describes the strengths approach thus:

> the strengths perspective is about discerning those resources and respecting them and the potential they have for reversing misfortune, countering illness, easing pain and reaching goals ... clients want you to believe they can surmount adversity and begin to climb towards transformation and growth.
>
> (Saleeby 2002: 14)

Howe (2009) offers a useful summary of Saleeby's approach to eliciting client strengths and enabling them to recognise and value their competencies and resourcefulness through specific strategic questions: survival questions to explore who and what helped them in the past; exception questions inviting service users to reflect on what their experience was when things went well; possibility questions which enable them to explore the hopes and qualities that helped them move forward to realise their hopes; esteem questions which help them reflect on assets or aspects of themselves they feel proud of.

In summary, the approach encourages practitioners to see service users – parents and or young people – as more than their problems, identify their capacities and bolster their resilience. Some of the areas that might be considered include building social support networks, engaging young people in community activities, developing hobbies and interests, or providing training and education in relation to parenting or cultural activities (Fernandez, 2006).

Trauma and neurobiological perspectives

People who work with children in child welfare contexts frequently encounter complex behaviour. Children may experience difficulties forming effective social relationships; they may display aggressive, sexualised or destructive behaviours; or they may be highly anxious or depressed. Others may show clear deficits in some areas of cognitive or behavioural functioning. Although it sometimes may be tempting to merely attach a label to these children (e.g., 'complex', 'high needs' or 'difficult to place'), good practice involves trying to understand the causes of this behaviour and how it might be addressed. Extensive neurophysiological research now shows that children who were exposed to significant trauma in the early years often experience neurological harm which can affect their subsequent behaviour (Beers & DeBellis 2002; McLean 2016; Moffitt 2013; Perry 2006, 2009; Sunderland 2006). Common problems include difficulties with memory, language problems, hyperactivity, executive functioning (the inability to organise tasks and stay focused), or difficulties in emotional regulation and sensory processing.

Various neurologists have scrutinised the role of early experiences and their impact on brain development. Perry and Szalavit (2008) establish links between the brain and how attachments develop, asserting that the brain is shaped positively or negatively by our childhood relationships with caregivers. Along similar lines, Sunderland (2006) argues that if children are not met with responsive and nurturing relationships in early life they may remain poorly equipped to deal with stressful feelings in later life. Sunderland (2006), based on her work with children who have been traumatised, offers important insights into the effects of stressful early experiences on the developing brain and long-term consequences for the child. Briefly, Sunderland highlights the particular brain regions associated with stress managing functions such as the amygdala which establishes the emotional meaning of experiences and communicates with the hypothalamus, the region of the brain which triggers release of stress hormones which prepares the body for fight or flight responses. If children are not met with sensitive responses and attuned relationships in early life which prime them to deal with emotions and feelings, ineffective stress responsive systems become ingrained in the brain.

Perry and Szalavitz (2008) link the brain to processes of attachment, describing how attachment templates develop through parenting and brain development.

> Loving caregivers provide the template that you use for human relationships. Attachment, then, is a memory template for human to human bonds. This template serves as your primary world view on human relationships. It is profoundly influenced by whether you experience kind, attuned parenting or whether you received inconsistent, frequently disrupted, abusive or neglected care.

In sum, this biological explanation suggests the brain is shaped positively or negatively by our relationships in childhood with caregivers whose responses can affect brain structures or chemistry which, in turn, can affect interactions with others in later life.

In the context of trauma, stimuli such as a loud noise can trigger a stored memory and the amygdala may resultantly elicit fearful reaction in the child (Perry 2006). When maltreatment occurs, children are overwhelmed with stressful stimuli that impair or compromise the development of particular brain regions and affect their psychosocial outcomes. Further, Perry (2006) argues that children's emotional and behavioural development is nurtured by exchanges with their caregivers, strengthening their neural pathways and enabling them to regulate stress. Children who are subject to insensitive and punitive responses fail to develop effective stress responsive systems that manifest in emotional withdrawal, persistent states of anxiety, hyper arousal and lack of enthusiasm and engagement. As with attachment theorising, the emphasis is on children's relational experiences with caregivers.

Some children experience caregiving that places them at risk of poor psychological development and wellbeing. The term childhood adversity is used to describe a range of incidents that pose a threat to a child's physical and psychological wellbeing. Child abuse and neglect, parental rejection, parental separation, domestic violence, bullying, and extreme poverty are examples of childhood adversity. Such experiences are perceived to have deleterious consequences, particularly when they occur early in life, are severe and are repetitive or accumulate over time. Trauma is the potential outcome of exposure to adversity. The Adverse Childhood Experiences (ACEs) has drawn attention to the critical issue of childhood adversity and cumulative harm and its developmental impacts.

It is claimed that the effects of childhood adversity can become embedded in the early sensitive periods of brain development. Howe (2009), commenting on the impact of neglect, notes that brain cells in the young child that do not get exposed to expected sensory stimulation during those early sensitive periods of brain development are unlikely to develop the required neurological connections to achieve optimal development. On an optimistic note, recovery is seen as possible. With warm, sensitive and skilled caretakers the brain remains 'plastic', retaining the ability to 'neurologically organise and reorganise itself throughout the lifespan' (Howe 2009: 184). This introduces some caution in allowing ourselves to become deterministic in our thinking. The similar study of Felitti et al. (1998) uses the term Adverse Childhood Experiences (ACEs) to describe various adversities including emotional and physical neglect, abuse, divorce and separation and social disadvantage. Researchers found that the more ACEs adults reported from their childhoods the worse their physical and mental outcomes. Trauma is the outcome of exposure to adversity and occurs when an individual experiences an incident or set of circumstances as threatening, emotionally or physically. A child's experience of trauma is likely to be accompanied by fear and helplessness and physiological symptoms which may continue beyond the initial exposure (Bartlett & Sacks 2019).

While childhood trauma can impact different domains of development, its effects on each child varies depending on individual family and environmental risk and protective factors and each child is likely to respond in distinctive ways to the same type of adversity and correspondingly requires different responses. Caution, however, is needed to avoid exclusive focus on ACEs to the exclusion of the full range of children's needs and the variation in children's responses to adversity. Knowledge of childhood adversity and trauma has underpinned the development of interventive approaches including trauma-informed care. While the neurobiological perspective has been influential in child protection decision making, concern is levelled against the uncritical acceptance of this perspective on trauma (Bruer 1999; Munro & Musholt 2014; Teicher & Samson 2016; Wastell & White 2012), drawing attention to methodological flaws, over simplification, selective reporting and inadequate contextual interpretation. There have been some concerns about misapplication of the theory in child welfare contexts (Grandquist et al. 2017).

Bruer (1999) alludes to contradictory and inconclusive findings, indicating they are to be applied with caution and, further, expresses concern that the narrow focus on specific regions of the brain limits the potential for inferences and generalisations about the overall functioning of the brain to be drawn. Causes are multifactorial with socio-economic risks playing a key role. Teicher and Sampson (2016) draw attention to the contradictory findings reported with respect to the relationship between brain alterations and child abuse and highlight that, while some neglected children showed increased amygdala volume, contradictory findings were evident in other studies. Perry's published work portraying the juxtaposed images of a smaller brain of a neglected child and the normal-sized brain of the child who is not neglected has also attracted critical comment on the basis of the lack of methodological details and contextual formation on the nature of their care environments. The neurobiological perspective has been influential and remains a dominant theoretical approach in child welfare decision making. The empirical and scientific work underpinning the conceptualisation and the controversies around the work have been less conspicuous. In summary, the neurobiological perspective offers a useful contribution to understanding child adversity and trauma when used in conjunction with social science perspectives which point to the multifactorial circumstances including socio-economic risks that are at play.

Value frameworks underpinning child welfare decision making

Although there is usually legislation and training that governs specific areas of practice involving children and families, the way in which practitioners understand and approach their work is also likely to be strongly influenced by their broader knowledge and values (Trevithick 2008). Such understanding acts as a filter for how situations might be interpreted. For example, it can influence a worker's attitude towards families, what decisions are made, how the situation is interpreted and what service options are considered. These values can sometimes arise explicitly from education, training or life experience and are known to the worker. Other values may be implicit and only evident with reflection or from the standpoint of others. Some of these values or areas of knowledge can enhance the quality of practice by making workers more reflective, insightful and well informed, whereas others can have the opposite effect. Some workers may have well-established views that make it difficult for them to appraise each case on its merits or consider broader perspectives or approaches that might be relevant to the family.

Statutory child welfare interventions are informed by particular value orientations that point to different policy and practice directions. To examine the different values underpinning the state's relationship with families and children and interventions in child welfare it is instructive to draw on Fox Harding's (1991) fourfold classification of value positions reflected in child welfare policy: laissez faire, state paternalism and child protection, defence of the birth family and parent rights, and child liberation and children rights. A review and elaboration of these is available in Fernandez (1996).

The **laissez-faire** value position emphasises minimal intervention and intrusion into the child family relationship. Authors supporting minimalism in state intervention (Mnookin 1973; Goldstein, Freud & Solnit 1979; Wald 1982) express concerns about the limits of prediction, the quality and instability of out of home care and the issues of unlimited discretionary decision making. Goldstein, Freud and Solnit (1979: 136), emphasising continuity and constancy maintain that:

> By failing to keep families together, by failing to restrict foster care to children who have a real chance of being returned to their absent parents in a 'short time', and by failing to regard long time foster parents as autonomous, the authorities prevent feelings of security developing in either child or adult. By moving children from placement to placement in the interests of absent parents the state interferes with attachments that are essential for an individual's growth.

In contrast with the laissez-faire value position, the **state paternalism and child protection** position envisages a strong role for the state, intervening coercively in families to protect children from inadequate care or maltreatment. Fox Harding summarises this position:

> in the paternalist and child protection value perspective, those birth parents who do not bring up their children 'well' cannot expect to keep them. When they fail state power should be readily and extensively used to provide something better for the children.
>
> (Fox Harding 1991: 62)

The work of Dingwall, Eekelaar and Murray (1983), aligned with the state paternalist, concluded from their empirical work that social workers tended to resort to the 'rule of optimism' and display a preoccupation with parental rights. Emphasising children's rights and parental duties they argue:

> The parent child relationship is an unequal contract which children do not enter freely. At the same time both children and society as a whole have a vital interest in the success of that relationship in cultivating the capacity for responsible moral action.
>
> (Dingwall et al. 1983: 220)

This position has attracted criticism on the grounds of focusing on culpability of parents while overlooking wider structural factors affecting parenting environments (Featherstone et al. 2014; Pelton 2015). For example, Frost (1990) comments:

> In a divided society we cannot understand child protection work as simply being about the protection of children. Child protection practice in an environment of

> inequality and marginalisation becomes a process of judging and disciplining households defined as outside the mainstream.
>
> (Frost 1990: 39)

The **defence of the birth family and parent rights** value position summarised by Fox Harding acknowledges the notion that optimum parenting requires a materially favourable environment and inadequate care is associated with deprivation and oppression. This position favours extensive state intervention but not of the coercive kind.

> Birth families should be supported in their caring role; children should not enter substitute care except as a last resort or on a 'shared care' basis, having entered care, most of them should be kept in touch with their original family and should wherever possible return to it. The state in its child care role pays insufficient attention to upholding birth families; it also operated in a discriminatory way on the basis of social class. Most of the child care problems to which the state responds are attributable to poverty and deprivation.
>
> (Fox Harding 1991: 107)

The views represented in this position are espoused by Holman (1988), Lindsey (1994), Parton (1990) and Pelton (1989), who advocate a proactive approach to preventive and supportive work with families and children. For example, Holman's case for prevention rests on arguments for the child's right to remain with their families and their neighbourhood or wider social environment, and in relation to children placed in care advocates strongly for contact between children and their separated families, drawing a distinction between 'exclusive fostering' (excluding the child's family and kinship connections) and 'inclusive fostering' (openness to encouraging children to maintain links with parents and kinship networks).

While in the first three value positions the needs and interests of children and young persons are defined by parents/carers or state agents, the emphasis in the children's rights and child liberation position is the child's viewpoint, acknowledging the child as a separate identity. Fox Harding summarises:

> The distinguishing characteristics of this perspective .... is that the emphasis is on the child's own viewpoint, feelings, wishes, definition, freedom, choices rather than attribution by adults of what is best for the child ... Decisions should not (on the whole) be made over the child's head. Thus, the child's welfare is (at least partly) for the child herself to define.
>
> (Fox Harding 1991: 139)

Several conceptual orientations towards the rights of children exemplify this position (Eekalaar 1994; Franklin 1986; Lavery 1986; Rogers & Wrightsman 1978) and concur on the need to advance children's rights, and some acknowledge the dependence of childhood, the differences in capacities between adults and children and younger children and older children. For example, Freeman (1987: 300) asserts

> Children have not been accorded either dignity or respect. They have been reified, denied the status of participants in a social system, labelled as a problem population,

> reduced to being seen as property. Think of our attitudes towards the closure of children's homes, the criminal justice process for children, the custody decision-making process after divorce, the punishment of children and their abuse, child benefit. The list is endless.

In summary, each of these positions articulates a particular model of state/family relationship and reflects particular value stances that underpin child welfare policy and practice. While all of them can be credited with concern for children and their wellbeing, there are divergences in how the child's best interests are to be defined and operationalised.

Best interests of the child

In making decisions about child protection and protective care, professionals operationalise the values expressed in the best interests of the child standard. This standard has become significant in decision making and policy development nationally and internationally. The UN Convention on the Rights of the Child notes that 'In all actions concerning children whether undertaken by public or private social welfare institutions, courts of law, administration authorities or legislative bodies the best interest of the child shall be a primary consideration' (Article 3 (1).

Mnookin (1973) commends the principle stating 'it focuses principally on the child rather than on arbitrary legal rights of parents. It implicitly recognises that each child is unique, and that paternal conduct and home environments may have substantially different effects on different children' (Mnookin 1973: 202).

However, the complexities of this standard and the constraints in operationalising it are highlighted in the legal and social work literature (Fernandez 1996; Goldstein, Freud & Solnit 1979; Mnookin 1973; Parker 1994). Among the complexities identified are the open-endedness and indeterminacy of the concept and the lack of specific guidelines as to what set of values should be used to determine what is in a child's best interests. The issue of giving content to this standard is highlighted thus: 'it is a rationalisation by decision makers, justifying their judgements about a child's future, like an empty vessel into which adult perceptions and prejudices are poured. It does not offer guidelines about how adult powers should be exercised' (Rodham 1973: 513).

The concern is that judges and social workers predominantly from higher socio-economic groups are likely to be influenced by their own values in determining the child's best interest and, in this respect, it has the potential to provide a screen for bias and paternalism (Parker 1994), most frequently in cases involving social minorities, poor, non-white and non-conventional families (Rodham 1973).

The impact of pluralistic beliefs about child rearing and parenting on the interpretation of 'best interests' is highlighted in the experience of the Stolen Generations. Lack of understanding of the role of Aboriginal extended family networks, Aboriginal poverty and biases about Aboriginal lifestyles influenced the transfer of Aboriginal children into white care as a result of culturally based discriminatory decision making by state agents (Burns, Burns & Menzies 2004; Chisholm 1985; Fernandez et al. 2018).

The indeterminacy of the best interest principle is also related to the speculation involved in identifying probabilities and potential outcomes of decisions and attaching values to possible outcomes (Parker 1994). In this context Hubbell notes:

> each child's experience in foster care is unknown and unpredictable; it cannot be neatly plotted on a graph, it cannot be guaranteed to be loving, nurturing and to increase his (her) IQ by ten points. Lost to chance are quality of the foster home, the length of a child's tenure in that home, the number of moves a child makes from home to home, the number of different case workers a child may have while in foster care.
>
> (Hubbell 1981: 34)

Further complexities raised are whether the child should be the only object of concern and whether parents, siblings and kin are to remain peripheral, and should rights, strengths and needs of all family members be considered. Given the tensions articulated, alternative approaches to implementation of this standard are proposed. Wald (1982) proposes the focus of decision should be on 'specific harms' to the child that justify intervention rather than 'parental fault'.

Goldstein, Freud and Solnit (1979) propose in the place of the best interest standard, 'that which is the least detrimental alternative among available alternatives for the child', a reframing which introduces the notion of 'available alternatives' and has the potential to evaluate the pros and cons of each decision without getting enmeshed in the hope and magic of 'best' in a way which misleads decision makers to believe they have more power for good than for bad in what they decide (Goldstein, Freud and Solnit 1979: 25).

The conceptualisation is also linked with children's rights. Accordingly, maximising children's opportunities to develop their own perceptions of their wellbeing and increasing their capacities for choice and self determination must also be considered.

In summary, the divergent views examined introduce a note of caution and realism into the operationalisation of the best interest standard and the need for awareness of the ways in which different perceptions of the child's interest are reached and differentiated from other interests.

While this formulation appears defensible and unimpeachable it is seen as vague and malleable and subject to the personal value orientations of practitioners and decision makers (Fernandez 1996).

Balancing perspectives and the triangulation of knowledge

An important issue relates to how practitioners in the child welfare area come to understand what constitutes best practice or what sources of knowledge they should draw upon when making decisions. Although many people who work in this area receive formal university education in child welfare and child development, a question arises as to what sources of information they draw upon in their ongoing practice. To what extent do they use research evidence or principles derived from theory or frameworks (e.g., psychological theory or social work theory) as opposed to their own experience or practice 'wisdom'.

There is very likely to be no single or clear answer to these questions. Most likely the truth is that decision making is best guided by a combination of different perspectives (Trevithick 2008), and that each type of knowledge has both strengths and weaknesses when taken in isolation. For example, the adoption of broader theoretical perspectives can help to draw upon existing knowledge and frameworks and help to organise ideas. Good theories are those which help explain why certain things might occur and can be used to advance propositions or ideas that can be tested in practice. Not all people agree about the same theory and some theories can offer competing explanations.

Styles of decision making where one tries to generalise from higher level propositions to particular situations are often called 'top-down' or deductive. By contrast, there is the view that a lot of knowledge can be gained from merely working with children and families and developing a store of knowledge based on experience. Such knowledge is often called 'practice wisdom' and is more inductive or 'bottom up' in nature (one builds up a store of knowledge and may not reach any conclusions until one has observed many instances of a situation or outcome). Knowledge of this nature can be valuable in that it can be practically focused, understand the diversity of families and children and how there can be exceptions to general rules. The limitation of practice experience, however, is that individual experiences can be highly variable and it may be harder to see 'the bigger picture'. There can be a tendency for recent or highly influential cases to colour how individual workers interpret situations. Differences in perspective may also occur if people work in particular offices, or come from different countries with different policies and practice philosophies (Khoo & Nygren 2006). Another important debate in social work decision making relates to how evidence is used. Good practice is thought to arise from approaches that are 'reflective' (i.e., people think about what they did correctly or incorrectly and how they might do things differently) (Gardner 2014) or which proactively take the perspectives of different parties (e.g., children and families) into account.

Conclusion

In sum, good child welfare practice is best informed by balanced approaches that take advantage of all available evidence and which are not unduly influenced by preconceived ideas or misconceptions. The aim is to appraise needs and risk, and to be mindful of strengths and opportunities for growth and resilience without relinquishing the responsibility of practitioners to facilitate changes. Good practice should be mindful of the changes that occur in children's development and that many children in child welfare contexts may not often present in the same way as other children of their age. Although workers will often encounter children after they have already been subjected to a great deal of early harm, there are opportunities to improve children's lives by working with other professional people to provide timely assessments and interventions and to take advantage of the multiple critical phases that children pass through on their way to adulthood.

Discussion questions

- What does it mean to adopt a 'developmental approach' to child welfare?
- What are 'ecological approaches' and why are they often applied in child welfare contexts?
- In what ways can cultural biases and value judgements come into play when dealing with Indigenous or Aboriginal families?
- What is resilience? What are the strengths and limitations of adopting this approach in the child welfare context?
- What are the strengths and limitations of using practice wisdom as the basis for child welfare decision making?

References

Adcock, M., Lake, R. & Small, A., 1988, 'Assessing children's needs', in J. Aldgate and J. Simmonds (eds), *Direct work with children: A guide for social work practitioners*, London: Basford, pp. 25–35.

Ainsworth, M., 1979, 'Infant–mother attachment', *American Psychologist*, vol. 34, pp. 932–937.

Alderson, P., 2000, *Young children's rights*, London: Jessica Kingsley.

Aldgate, J., 1988, 'Work with children experiencing separation and loss: A theoretical framework', in J. Aldgate & J. Simmonds (eds), *Direct work with children: A guide for social work practitioners*, London: Basford, pp. 35–48.

Aldgate, J., 1991, 'Attachment theory and its application to child care social work: An introduction', in J. Lishman (ed.), *Handbook of theory for practice teachers in social work*, London: Jessica Kingsley, pp. 11–35.

Aldgate, J., Jones, D.P.H., Rose, W. & Jeffrey, D., 2006, *The developing world of the child*, London: Jessica Kingsley.

AIFS, 2015, The longitudinal study of Australian children annual statistical report 2014, Melbourne: Australian Institute of Family Studies.

Bartlett, J.D. & Sacks, V., 2019, 'Adverse childhood experiences are different than child trauma and it's critical to understand why', *Child Trends*, www.childtrends.org/adverse-childhood-experiences-different-than-child-trauma-critical-to-understand-why.

Beers, S.R., & De Bellis, M.D., 2002, 'Neuropsychological function in children with maltreatment-related posttraumatic stress disorder', *American Journal of Psychiatry*, vol. 159, no. 3, pp. 483–486.

Bifulco, A., Jacobs, C., Bunn, A., Thomas, G. & Irving, K., 2008, 'The attachment interview (ASI) as an assessment of support capacity: Exploring its use for adoption-fostering assessment', *Adoption & Fostering*, vol. 32, pp. 33–45.

Boss, P., 2007, 'Ambiguous loss theory: Challenges for scholars and practitioners', *Family Relations*, vol. 56, no. 2, pp. 105–110.

Bowlby, J., 1951, *Maternal care and mental health*, Geneva: World Health Organisation.

Bowlby, J., 1969, *Attachment and loss, Volume 1: Loss*, New York: Basic Books.

Bretherton, I., 1992, 'The origins of attachment theory: John Bowlby and Mary Ainsworth', *Developmental Psychology*, vol. 28, no. 5, pp. 759–775.

Bronfenbrenner, U., 1979, *The ecology of human development: Experiments by nature and design.* Cambridge, MA: Harvard University Press.

Bronfenbrenner, U. & Morris, P.A., 2007, *The Bioecological Model of Human Development, Vol. 1.*, New York: John Wiley & Sons.

Bruer, J.T., 1999, *The myth of the first three years: A new understanding of early brain development and lifelong learning*, New York: The Free Press.

Burns, A., Burns, K. & Menzies, K., 2004, 'Strong state intervention: The stolen generation', in J. Bowes (ed.), *Children, families and communities: Contexts and consequences*, London: Sage, pp. 190–209.

Chisholm, R., 1985, '*Black children: White welfare? Aboriginal child welfare law and policy*', in New South Wales, Social Welfare Research Centre Report and Proceedings No. 52, Sydney: University of New South Wales.

Christensen, P.M. & James, A., 2000, *Research with children: Perspectives and practice*, London: Falmer Press.

Clarke, A.M. & Clarke, A.D.B., 1976, *Early experience: Myth and evidence*, London: Open Books.

Corby, B., 2006, *Child abuse: Toward a knowledge base*, Maidenhead, UK: Open University Press.

Delfabbro, P.H., Borgas, M., Rogers, N., Jeffreys, H. & Wilson, R., 2009, 'The social and family backgrounds of infants in care and their capacity to predict subsequent abuse notifications: A study of south Australian out-of-home care 2000–2005', *Children & Youth Services Review*, vol. 31, pp. 219–226.

Delfabbro, P.H., Fernandez, E., McCormick, J. & Kettler, L., 2013, 'Reunification in a complete entry cohort: A longitudinal study of children entering out-of-home care in Tasmania, Australia', *Children & Youth Services Review*, vol. 35, pp. 1592–1600.

Dingwall, R., Eekelaar, J. & Murray, T., 1983, *The protection of children: State intervention and family life*, Oxford: Blackwell.

Eekelaar, J., 1994, 'The interest of the child and the child's wishes: The role of dynamic self determinism', in P. Alston, S. Parker, & J. Seymour (eds), *The best interest of the child: Reconciling culture and human rights*, Oxford: UNICEF, Clarendon Press, pp. 42–61.

Erikson, E.H., 1963, *Childhood and society* (2nd edn), New York: Norton.

Erikson, E.H., 1965, *Childhood and society*, Harmondsworth, UK: Penguin Books.

Featherstone, B., White, S. & Morris, K., 2014, *Re-imaging child protection: Towards humane social work with families*, Bristol, UK: Policy Press.

Felitti, V.J., Anda, R.F., Nordenberg, D., Williamson, D.F., Spitz, A.M., Edwards, V., ... Marks, J. S., 1998, 'Relationship of childhood abuse and household dysfunction to many of the leading causes of death in adults', *American Journal of Preventive Medicine*, vol. 14, no. 4, pp. 245–258.

Fernandez, E., 1996, *Significant harm: Unravelling child protection decisions and substitute care careers of children*, Aldershot, UK: Avebury Ashgate.

Fernandez, E., 2006, 'Growing up in care: Resilience and care outcomes', in R.J. Flynn, P.M. Dudding, & J.G. Barber (eds), *Promoting resilience in child welfare*, Ottawa: University of Ottawa Press, pp. 131–156.

Fernandez, E., 2013, 'Early childhood: dimensions and contexts of development and well-being', in A. Ben-Arieh, F. Casas, I. Frønes & J. Korbin (eds), *Handbook of child well-being*, Dordrecht: Springer, pp. 1629–1648.

Fernandez, E., 2016, 'Childhood in the context of the lifespan', in The Sage, *Encyclopaedia of early childhood education*, Dordrecht: Springer.

Fernandez, E., Lee, J.S. & McNamara, P., 2018, *Understanding the experiences and outcomes of Aboriginal and Torres Strait Islander children in out of home care in the twentieth century*, Sydney: University of New South Wales.

Fernandez, E., Delfabbro, P., Ramia, I.O. & Kovacs, S., 2019, 'Children returning from care: The challenging circumstances of parents in poverty', Special Issue, *Children and Youth Services Review*, vol. 97(C), pp. 100–111.

Fox Harding, L., 1991, *Perspectives on child care policy*, London: Longman.

Franklin, B. (ed.), 1986, *The rights of children*, London: Blackwell.

Freeman, M.D.A., 1987, 'Taking children's rights seriously', *Children and Society* 1(4), pp. 299–319.

Frost, N., 1990, 'Official intervention and child protection', in The Violence Against Children Study Group (ed.), *Taking child abuse seriously: Contemporary issues in child protection*, London: Unwin Hyman, pp. 25–40.

Garbarino, J., 2014, 'The history of fatherhood research and perspectives on father involvement', *Fatherhood: Research, Interventions, and Policies*, vol. 11.

Gardner, F., 2014, *Being critically reflective*, London: Palgrave Macmillan.

Gilligan, R., 1997, 'Beyond permanency? The importance of resilience is child placement practice and planning', *Adoption & Fostering*, vol. 21, no. 1, pp. 12–20.

Goldstein, J., Freud, A. & Solnit, A.J., 1979, *Before the best interests of the child*, London: Burnett Books.

Grandquist, P., Sroufe, L.A., Dozier, M., Hesse, E., Steele, M., van Ijzendoorn, M., 2017, 'Disorganized attachment in infancy: a review of the phenomenon and its implications for clinicians and policy-makers', *Attachment & Human Development*, vol. 19, no. 6, pp. 534–558.

Grossmann, K., Grossmann, K.E.Fremmer-Bombik, E., Kindler, H., Scheirer-English, H. & Zimmerman, P., 2002, 'The uniqueness of the child–father attachment relationship: Fathers

sensitive and challenging play as a pivotal variable a 16-year longitudinal study', *Social Development*, vol. 11, no. 3, pp. 307–331.
Henggeler, S.W., Melton, G.B., Brondino, M.J., Scherer, D.G. & Hanley, J.H., 1997, 'Multisystemic therapy with violent and chronic juvenile offenders and their families: The role of treatment fidelity in successful dissemination', *Journal of Consulting & Clinical Psychology*, vol. 65, pp. 821–833.
Hoffnung, M., Hoffnung, R., Seifert, K.L., Hine, A., Pausé, C., Ward, L., Signal, T., Swabey, K., Yates, K., Smith, R.B., 2019, *Lifespan development: A chronological approach*, 4th edn, Milton, QLD: Wiley.
Holman, B., 1988, *Putting families first: Prevention and child care*, London: Macmillan Education.
Howe, D., 1995, *Attachment theory for social work practice*, London, Macmillan.
Howe, D., 2009, *A Brief Introduction to Social Work Theory*, London: Palgrave.
Hubbell, R., 1981, *Foster care and families*, Philadelphia, PA: Temple University Press.
Huebner, E.S., 2004, 'Research on assessment of life satisfaction of children and adolescents', *Social Indicators Research*, vol. 66, pp. 3–33.
Hughes, D., 1997, *Facilitating developmental attachment: The road to emotional recovery and behavioural change in foster and adoptive children*, Lanham, MD: Rowman & Littlefield.
Human Rights and Equal Opportunity Commission, 1997, Bringing them home, Canberra, HREOC.
James, D. & Fernandez, E., 1986, 'Review and critique of bonding theory for social workers', in R. Bereen & E. Browne (eds), *Advances in social work education*, Kensington (NSW): The Heads of Schools of Social Work in Australia, pp. 79–91.
James, A. & Prout, A., 1997, *Constructing and reconstructing childhood. Contemporary issues in the sociological study of childhood* (2nd edn), London: Falmer Press.
Khoo, E.G., & Nygren, L., 2006, 'Resilient society or resilient children? A comparison of child welfare service orientations in Sweden and Ontario, Canada', in R.J. Flynn, P.M. Dudding & J.G. Barber (eds), *Promoting resilience in child welfare*, Ottawa: University of Ottawa Press, pp. 72–93.
Klaus, M.E. & Kennell, J.H., 1972, *Maternal/infant bonding*, St Louis, MO: Mosby.
Kubler-Ross, E., 1970, *On death and dying*, London: Tavistock.
Laird, J., 1979, 'An ecological approach to child welfare: Issues of family identity and continuity', in C.B. Germain (ed.), *Social work practice people and environments*, New York: Columbia University Press, pp. 174–209.
Lalonde, C.E., 2006, 'Identity formation and cultural resilience in Aboriginal communities', in R.J. Flynn, P.M. Dudding & J.G. Barber (eds), *Promoting resilience in child welfare*, Ottawa, University of Ottawa Press, pp. 52–71.
Lavery, G., 1986, 'The rights of children in care', in R. Franklin (ed.), *The rights of children*, Oxford: Basil Blackwell, pp. 73–96.
Lindsey, D., 1994, *The welfare of children*, New York: Oxford University Press.
Luthar, S.S. & Zigler, E., 1991, 'Vulnerability and competence: A review of research on resilience in childhood', *American Journal of Orthopsychiatry*, vol. 61, no. 1, pp. 6–22.
McLean, S., 2016, *The effect of trauma on the brain development of children. Evidence-based principles for supporting the recovery of children in care*, Melbourne: Australian Institute for Family Studies.
Main, M., 1995, 'Recent studies in attachment: Overview with selected implications for clinical work', in S. Goldberg, R. Muir & J. Kerr (eds), *Attachment theory: Social, developmental, and clinical perspectives*, Hillsdale, NJ: Analytic Press, pp. 407–470.
Maluccio, A.N., 1986, *Permanency planning for children: Concept and methods*, New York and London: Tavistock.
Marris, P., 1986, *Loss and change*, London: Routledge.
Masten, A.S., 2006, 'Resilience theory and child welfare policy and practice', in R.J. Flynn, P.M. Dudding & J.G. Barber (eds), *Promoting resilience in child welfare*, Ottawa, University of Ottawa Press, pp. 3–17.

Mayall, B., 2000, 'The sociology of childhood in relation to children's rights', *The International Journal of Children's Rights*, vol. 8, pp. 243–259.
Mildon, R. & Polimeni, M., 2012, Parenting in the early years: Effectiveness of parenting support programs for Indigenous families (Resource Sheet No. 16), Melbourne: Australian Institute of Family Studies.
Mnookin, R.H., 1973, 'Foster care: In whose best interests?', *Harvard Educational Review*, vol. 43, no. 4, pp. 599–638.
Moffitt, T., 2013, 'Childhood exposure to violence and lifelong health: Clinical Intervention science and stress biology research join forces', *Development and Psychopathology*, vol. 25, pp. 1619–1634.
Munro, E. & Musholt, K., 2014, 'Neuroscience and the risks of maltreatment', *Children & Youth Services Review*, vol. 47, pp. 18–26.
Nicholson, P., 2014, *A critical approach to human development*, London: Palgrave Macmillan.
O'Brien, E.Z., 2016, *Psychology for social workers*, London: Palgrave Macmillan.
Oliver, C., 2017, *Strengths-based Child Protection: Firm, Fair and Friendly*, Toronto: University of Toronto Press.
Parker, S., 1994, 'The best interests of the child: Principles and problems', in P. Alston (ed.), *The best interest of the child: Reconciling culture and human rights*, Oxford: UNICEF, Clarendon Press, pp. 26–41.
Parton, N., 1990, 'Taking child abuse seriously', in The Violence Against Children Study Group (ed.), *Taking child abuse seriously: Contemporary issues in child protection theory and practice*, London: Unwin Hyman, pp. 7–24.
Pelton, L.H., 1989, *For reasons of poverty: A critical analysis of the public child welfare system in the United States*, New York: Praeger.
Pelton, L.H., 2015, 'The continuing role of material factors in child maltreatment and placement', *Child Abuse & Neglect*, 41, pp. 30–39.
Perry, B.D., 2006, 'Applying principles of neurodevelopment to clinical work with maltreated and traumatized children: The neurosequential model of therapeutics' in N.B. Webb (ed.), *Working with traumatized youth in child welfare: Social work practice with children and families*, New York: Guilford Press, pp. 27–52.
Perry, B.D., 2009, 'Examining child maltreatment through a neurodevelopmental lens: Clinical applications of the neurosequential model of therapeutics', *Journal of Loss and Trauma*, vol. 14, pp. 240–255.
Perry, B. & Szalavitz, M., 2008, *The boy who was raised as a dog: And other stories from a child psychiatrist's notebook – What traumatized children can teach us about loss, love and healing*, New York: Basic Books.
Peterson, C., 2014, *Looking forward through the lifespan*, 6th edn, Sydney: Pearson Education.
Piaget, J., 1963, *The language and thought of the child*, London: Routledge & Kegan Paul.
Qvortrup, J., 2004, 'Childhood matters: An introduction', in J. Qvortrup, M. Bardy, G. Sgritta & H. Wintersberger (eds), *Childhood matters: Social theory, practice and politics*, Aldershot, UK: Avebury Press.
Rodham, H., 1973, 'Children under the law', *Harvard Educational Review*, vol. 43, no. 4, pp. 487–514.
Rogers, C.M. & Wrightsman, L.S., 1978, 'Attitudes towards children's rights: Nurturance or self-determination', *Journal of Social Issues*, vol. 34, no. 2, pp. 59–68.
Rutter, M., 1972, *Maternal deprivation reassessed*, Harmondsworth, UK: Penguin.
Rutter, M., 1999, 'Resilience concepts and findings', *The Association for Family Therapy and Systems Practice*, vol. 21, pp. 119–144.
Ryan, F., 2011, 'Kanyininpa (Holding): A way of nurturing children in Aboriginal Australia', *Australian Social Work*, vol. 64, no. 2, pp. 183–197.
Saleeby, D. (ed.), 1997, *The strengths perspective in social work practice*, New York: Longman.
Schaffer, H.R. & Emerson, P.E., 1964, 'The development of social attachments in infancy', *Monographs of Social Research in Child Development*, vol. 29, no. 4.

Schofield, G. & Beek, M., 2014, *The secure base model: Promoting attachment and resilience in foster care and adoption*, London: BAAF.
Sluckin, W., Herbert, M. & Sluckin, A., 1984, *Maternal bonding*, Oxford: Basil Blackwell.
Sroufe, L.A., 1989, 'Relationships, self and individual adaptation', in A.J. Sameroff & R.N. Emde (eds), *Relationship disturbances in early childhood*, New York: Basic Books, pp. 70–94.
Stainton Rogers, W. & Stainton Rogers, R., 1992, *Stories of childhood: Shifting agendas of child concerns*, Hemel Hempstead: Harvester Wheatsheaf.
Sunderland, M., 2006, *The science of parenting*, London: Dorling Kindersley.
Teicher, M. & Samson, J., 2016, 'Annual research review: Enduring neurobiological effects of childhood abuse and neglect', *Journal of Child Psychology & Psychiatry*, vol. 57, no. 3, pp. 241–266.
Trevithick, P., 2008, 'Revisiting the knowledge base of social work: A framework for practice', *British Journal of Social Work*, vol. 38, pp. 1212–1237.
UNCRC, 1989, *Convention on the Rights of the Child (UNCRC)*, New York: United Nations.
Van Ijzendoorn, M.H. & Kroonenberg, P.M., 1988, 'Cross cultural patterns of attachment: A meta-analysis of the strange situation', *Child Development*, vol. 59, pp. 147–156.
Wald, M.S., 1982, 'State intervention on behalf of endangered children: A proposed legal response', *Child Abuse & Neglect*, vol. 6, no. 1, pp. 3–45.
Walkerdine, V., 2009, 'Developmental psychology and the study of childhood', in M.J. Kehily (ed.), *An introduction to childhood studies*, 2nd edn, Maidenhead, UK: Open University Press.
Walsh, F., 1998, *Strengthening family resilience*, New York: The Guilford Press.
Wastell, D. & White, S., 2012, 'Blinded by neuroscience: Social policy, the family and the infant brain. Families', *Relationships & Societies*, vol. 1, no. 3, pp. 397–414.
Werner, E.E., 1979, *Cross cultural child development: A view from planet earth*, New York: Brooks Cole.
Werner, E.E. & Smith, R.R., 1982, *Vulnerable but invisible: A study of resilient children*, New York: McGraw Hill.
Wilkins, D., Shemmings, D. & Shemmings, Y., 2015, *A–Z of attachment*, London: Palgrave.
Wyse, D., 2004, *Childhood studies: An introduction*, Oxford, UK: Blackwell.

Chapter 3

Children's rights and the protective care continuum

Jennifer Driscoll

Introduction

A rights-based approach to work with children has been almost universally endorsed through the United Nations Convention on the Rights of the Child (UNCRC) (United Nations General Assembly 1989). This international treaty accords a wide-ranging assortment of rights to children, on a spectrum from protection to autonomy, and has cemented a shift in our perceptions of children from passive recipients of adult protection to active participants in decisions affecting them. This chapter starts by explaining the background to the children's rights movement and the development of the UNCRC. Next, it considers the implications of respect for children's rights as expressed in the UNCRC in general terms. Three areas of the protective care continuum in Australia are then reviewed through the lens of children's rights: first, the state's duties to support the care of children within their family; second, how the interaction of the guiding principles of the UNCRC can provide insight into decision making within different cultural contexts; and third, alternative care arrangements for children unable to be brought up within their birth families. Finally, the implications of commitment to the full realisation of children's rights under the UNCRC for policy and practice in the protective care continuum are discussed.

Context: Children's rights and the UNCRC

Child protection systems in advanced economies have their roots in philanthropic 'child-saving' organisations founded in the nineteenth century in response to the appalling conditions of poverty and exploitation endured by many children in the newly industrialised cities, immortalised in the case of London by the works of Charles Dickens. Early notions of child protection were therefore embedded in a patriarchal view of society which considered women and children alike as weak and vulnerable and in need of care and protection. But the civil rights movements claiming equal rights for women and racial and/or ethnic minorities led to some claims for self-determination on behalf of children, particularly in relation to the closing down of some forms of independence for older children with the newly appropriated label of adolescence (Minow 1986). In the 1970s, a group of 'children's liberationists' in the US claimed controversial rights and freedoms for children on the basis that they were an oppressed group facing similar discrimination to that of other minorities (see, for example, John Holt's *Escape from Childhood* (Holt 1974)). While the more unrealistic and potentially harmful claims of this group for children's equality of treatment compared with adults were rejected, by the time Poland proposed an internationally binding Convention on the Rights of the Child to commemorate the International Year of the Child in 1979, the twin perspectives of the protection of children as vulnerable innocents and promotion of respect for children as entitled to human rights were both well established.

The resulting Convention on the Rights of the Child is the most widely endorsed treaty in history, having been ratified by all nations except for the USA. It combines both the afore-mentioned perspectives on children, including, arguably, some claims for children's autonomy rights. As a consequence, the rights afforded to children by the Convention cannot be viewed in isolation but must be considered as interdependent. The Committee on the Rights of the Child have identified four General Principles (United Nations Committee on the Rights of the Child 1991) which are regarded as central to the operation of the Convention as a whole, namely:

Article 2: Non-discrimination
Article 3: Best interests of the child
Article 6: The right to life, survival and development
Article 12: Respect for the views of the child.

In addition, the UNCRC provides a wide range of rights covering all aspects of children's lives, including support for children's upbringing within their family (articles 9, 16, 18, 26 and 27); enjoyment of minority cultural and religious practices in community with others from their minority group (article 30); the protection of children from maltreatment within the family (articles 9 and 19); and provision of alternative care for children who cannot grow up within their birth family (articles 20, 21 (adoption) and 25).

Policy and practice focus: Do children's rights make a difference?

The significance of actively awarding rights to children is twofold. First, it recognises children as people entitled to the same respect and dignity that we would accord to adults, a status not enjoyed by children as a group historically. Adopting a 'rights-based' approach to issues affecting children means, in general terms, taking their concerns and feelings seriously and acknowledging the value of children's insights and of children themselves as members of society. Second, the elevation of an identified moral interest – such as protection from violence – to the status of a right enables the imposition of legal duties on state or other parties for its fulfilment, thereby facilitating enforcement of the duty.

Most nations have not directly incorporated the UNCRC into their domestic law and therefore the provisions are not directly enforceable by or on behalf of children. In a review of 12 developed nations, including Australia, Lundy, Kilkelly and Byrne (2013) found that article 3 was most commonly directly incorporated, followed by article 12, reflecting a primary focus on the welfare of children, but one which is tempered by recognition of the role of children's own feelings in solutions to problems that they face, a balance considered in greater detail later in the chapter. In Australia, the Human Rights (Parliamentary Scrutiny) Act 2011 requires all proposed legislation to carry a statement of compatibility with all seven human rights treaties that Australia has ratified, helping to ensure that new law does not contravene the principles of children's rights under the

UNCRC. However, there is no obligation for legislation to be amended to rectify identified concerns and the Australian Children's Commissioner has called for Australian domestic legislation to provide full conformity with its obligations under the UNCRC and impact assessments on proposed legislation affecting children's rights (Australian Human Rights Commission 2018).

But even where the provisions have not been incorporated into law, the Convention has nonetheless 'exercised an extraordinarily pervasive and significant influence on the way in which law- and policy-makers think about the status of children' (Archard 2014: 107). Davidson (2014), in an article arguing for US ratification of the UNCRC, concludes that it has not only provided the impetus for wide-ranging reforms in all areas affecting children's lives but is also 'helping countries make a collective difference in the lives of their most vulnerable children' (p. 529). One of the ways through which change is effected is the reporting mechanism established under article 44. States Parties are required to report on the progress they have made in assuring the Convention rights to children in their jurisdiction within two years of the Convention entering into force and thereafter every five years. Following further evidence gathering, the Committee on the Rights of the Child issues commentary on the reports submitted, including acknowledgement of progress made, identification of key areas of concern and recommendations for further work. The Committee published the Concluding Observations in relation to Australia's fourth periodic report in August 2012 (United Nations Committee on the Rights of the Child 2012). Australia's joint fifth and sixth report was submitted to the Committee in January 2018 (Government of Australia 2108), and the Concluding Observations followed in September 2019. The three areas considered in greater detail in the following sections are chosen as being of particular pertinence to Australian policy and practice at the current time.

The state's duties to support the care of children within their family

The preamble to the UNCRC sets out the 'conviction' of States Parties

> that the family, as the fundamental group of society and the natural environment for the growth and well-being of all its members and particularly children, should be afforded the necessary protection and assistance so that it can fully assume its responsibilities within the community.

This conviction is backed up by a number of articles in the Convention, in particular article 18, which declares that primary responsibility for the upbringing and development of the child lies with parents or legal guardians and that '[t]he best interests of the child shall be their primary concern'. Article 9 limits the circumstances in which children may be separated from their parents against their will, requiring the proper exercise of national law and procedures and a determination that separation is 'necessary in the best interests of the child'. These are generic requirements and it is for national governments to ensure that they have robust processes in place to protect children from unlawful or unnecessary removal from their parents' care.

Such processes will have been instituted in Western nations in the form of child protection laws since before the UNCRC came into force. However, these articles must be read in conjunction with others, which together make for rather more uncomfortable reading for many 'advanced' wealthy countries. In particular, article 26 requires recognition of every child's 'right to benefit from social security, including social insurance' and article 27 refers to the 'right of every child to a standard of living adequate for the child's physical, mental, spiritual, moral and social development'. While parents have the primary responsibility to ensure living conditions sufficient for the child's development, the UNCRC imposes a duty on governments to 'take appropriate measures to assist parents and others responsible for the child to implement this right and shall in case of need provide material assistance and support programmes, particularly with regard to nutrition, clothing and housing' (article 27–3). Article 18–2 is wider:

> For the purpose of guaranteeing and promoting the rights set out in the present Convention, States Parties shall render appropriate assistance to parents in the performance of their child-rearing responsibilities and shall ensure the development of institutions, facilities and services for the care of children.

This duty is to be fulfilled by nations 'in accordance with national conditions and within their means', placing greater expectations on wealthier nations to support parents in the fulfilment of their parenting duties than might be expected of less affluent countries. This approach is confirmed in article 4, which effectively requires national governments to prioritize children in their allocation of resources:

> States Parties shall undertake all appropriate legislative, administrative and other measure for the implementation of the rights recognised in the present Convention. With regard to economic, social and cultural rights, States Parties shall undertake such measures to the maximum extent of their available resources.

Political considerations are likely to determine the extent to which governments embrace the principles set out in article 4. Esping-Andersen (1990) identified three models of social policy systems. The first, the liberal model, he associated initially with Australia, Canada and the US, with Denmark, Sweden and the UK approximating to the model. In this model, market forces are allowed to operate and the role of the state is reduced, with a tendency for services to be privatised. The second, known as the corporativist or conservative model, adopts a somewhat paternalistic approach, with considerable state investment in social welfare policies and support for traditional family structures such as the nuclear family. Esping-Andersen originally identified Austria, France, Germany and Italy as conforming to this model, which is characterised by considerable investment in social welfare on the part of the state (Scruggs & Allan 2008). Potential weaknesses of the model include a tendency for services to be provided by religious or voluntary organisations (Katz & Hetherington 2006), running the risk that clear common standards are lacking (Spratt et al. 2015, referring to Germany). The third model, originally identified in Norway and Sweden and to some degree in Finland and Denmark (Esping-Andersen 1990), is the social democratic welfare model. The goal of equal opportunities drives high investment in state institutions for the direct delivery of social services under this model, although neoliberal policy has been seen to erode its operation in Nordic countries in the last decade or so (Healy & Oltedal 2010).

As a result of changes in Australian policy consequent upon neoliberal influences, Australia was later considered to represent a fourth model of social policy, not included in Esping-Anderson's original categories, but more recently still has adopted what Deeming and Smyth (2015: 307) refer to as the Australian 'social investment state'. Although in some ways the model is broadly in line with the social democratic tradition, policies badged as family-friendly are driven by economic aims such as enabling both parents to work. In addition, and in common with English-speaking Western nations more generally, Australian neoliberal influences have resulted in an increase in quasi-market policies involving public–private partnerships, competitive tendering and contracting out (Deeming 2017; Deeming & Smyth 2015). Commentators suggest that neoliberal and market-oriented policies which encourage privatisation and reduce the role of the state tend to reinforce patterns of inequality (Scruggs & Allan 2008) through reduced investment in welfare promotion and prevention work in favour of risk reduction (Katz & Hetherington 2006; Healy & Oltedal 2010). The focus on individual responsibility translates into attitudes of blame towards struggling parents and inadequate attention to structural stressors such as poverty. Lonne et al. (2009) argue that these features are responsible to some extent at least for what they consider to be systemic failures in child protection systems in Anglophone countries.

In the Concluding Observations on Australia of 2012, the Committee on the Rights of the Child ('the Committee') expressed concern that the 'availability and quality of childcare remains inadequate' (United Nations Committee on the Rights of the Child 2012, Para. 49) and recommended 'implementation of appropriate measures to strengthen current programmes of family support, including ensuring the availability and affordability of quality childcare facilities, the adequacy of family assistance payments and of the recently approved paid parental leave entitlement' (Para. 50). At Para. 56 it also recommended prioritization of 'early intervention approaches, including at the antenatal period, to provide support to families in situations of heightened vulnerability and prevent or mitigate abuse and neglect of children and violence in the home'. The Australian Government responded to these concerns in the fifth and sixth joint report (Government of Australia 2018) through reference to the Third Action Plan (2015–2018) created under the National Framework for Protecting Australia's Children 2009–2020 (Council of Australian Governments 2009). The National Framework's six supporting outcomes include: children live in safe and supportive families and communities; children and families access adequate support to promote safety and intervene early; risk factors for child abuse and neglect are addressed; and Indigenous children are supported and safe in their families and communities. As well as citing the Paid Parental Leave scheme, assistance with childcare costs, and the Child Care Safety Net scheme to support the most vulnerable children, the Government also pointed to its ParentsNext initiative as a programme designed to support parents. However, this programme, which aims to address child poverty and welfare dependency by supporting parents (expected to be overwhelmingly mothers) into work, conforms to a neoliberal 'welfare to work' model. It has been criticized by campaigners for adopting punitive measures to force some parents into work, devaluing parenting by expecting parents to return to work while their children are still very young and failing to address the structural barriers facing mothers who do wish to return to the workforce (McLaren 2017). In contrast to 'workfare' type initiatives primarily intended to get parents into work, Box 3.1 describes an evidence-based peer-led parenting intervention available in Australia which more directly addresses the goals of the National Framework.

The Committee in its Concluding Observations (United Nations Committee on the Rights of the Child 2012) also called upon the Australian Government to 'take urgent measures to address disparities in access to services by Aboriginal and Torres Strait Islander Children and their families' (Para. 30), in accordance with article 2–1 of the Convention, which reads:

> States parties shall respect and ensure the rights set forth in the present Convention to each child within their jurisdiction without discrimination of any kind, irrespective of the child's or his or her parent's or legal guardian's race, colour, sex, language, religion, political or other opinion, national, ethnic or social origin, property, disability, birth or other status.

There have been some further measures to address this issue through initiatives to promote family-led decision-making trials, in which the Family Group Conferencing model, originally developed from Maori cultural practices in New Zealand, is used to engage community leaders and wider family groups to solve child safety problems at the community level (Niddrie & Brosnan 2017). Petrie and Kruger (2014) argue that much greater use should be made of the Family Group Conference model in the Northern Territory to improve outcomes for children and to increase a sense of empowerment in indigenous communities. In the absence of longitudinal evaluations, it is difficult to assess the long-term success of such programmes in promoting child safety. However, the UN Committee appears not to have been convinced by the Australian Government's approach to provision and access to family support services, urging strong investment in preventative measures, particularly for indigenous families, in 2019 (United Nations Committee on the Rights of the Child 2019, para. 32).

Failures in government support to vulnerable families and lack of attention to structural and economic factors affecting the upbringing of children are likely to manifest in high numbers of children being removed from parental care and placed in the care of the state. In the Concluding Observations (United Nations Committee on the Rights of the Child 2012), the Committee expressed concern that the number of children in care in Australia was rising. In 2018, the Government acknowledged 'ongoing issues' in relation to high numbers of children in the child protection system and entering out of home care (Government of Australia 2108: 17). Government statistics (Australian Institute of Health and Welfare 2018) (AIHW) show that Aboriginal and Torres Strait Islander children were seven times more likely to receive child protection services and ten times as likely to enter out-of-home care than non-Indigenous children in 2016–17. Although the reasons for this are complex and include the legacy of historical policies, influential factors include the greater likelihood of indigenous children living in remote areas, suffering poor health and growing up in low socio-economic backgrounds compared with their non-indigenous peers. Particularly worrying is the fact that while the proportion of children receiving child protection services rose in indigenous and non-indigenous populations from 2012/13 to 2016/17, the increase was faster among indigenous children (AIHW 2018). This despite the fact that all states and territories have endorsed the Aboriginal and Torres Strait Islander Child Placement Principle since 1986 and a range of initiatives intended to reduce the gap between wellbeing outcomes for indigenous children and their non-indigenous peers have been implemented. In 2019 the Committee stated that it 'remains seriously concerned about' [*inter alia*] 'The continuing over-representation of Aboriginal and

Torres Strait Islander children in alternative care, often outside their communities' (United Nations Committee on the Rights of the Child 2019, para. 33).

Box 3.1 Supporting parents

Empowering Parents, Empowering Communities (EPEC) is an evidence-based, peer-led parenting intervention designed to improve access and reduce barriers to effective parenting support, particularly aimed at families from excluded communities and those experiencing disadvantage. Local parents, especially those who have benefited from the scheme themselves, are trained to deliver the programme in order to provide low-cost, high-quality parenting support that is readily accepted by families. The three core programmes focus on 'Our Baby and Us' (0–1 year), 'Being a Parent' (2–11 years) and 'Living with Teenagers' (11–16 years). EPEC has trained over 400 peer facilitators in the UK and Australia from a wide range of ethnic and cultural backgrounds. Evaluations have shown the programme to be extremely effective in improving parenting practices and children's behaviour.

Questions for reflection: What is or should be the relationship between programmes such as EPEC and formal child protection processes? What issues may arise as a consequence of the interaction between voluntary interventions and the statutory system?

The interaction of the guiding principles in decision making in the protective care continuum

One contributing factor to the over-representation of children from indigenous populations in Australia – and from minority communities across the world more generally – derives from the fact that norms and values in parenting practices vary across cultures. Article 3–1 of the UNCRC requires that '[i]n all actions concerning children, whether undertaken by public or private social welfare institutions, courts of law, administrative authorities or legislative bodies, the best interests of the child shall be a primary consideration'. In Australian law, although child protection legislation is enacted at state or territory level, the first principle of the National Framework for Protecting Australia's Children (Council of Australian Governments 2009) includes the statement that children's 'best interests are *paramount* in all matters affecting them'. But the concept of the 'best interests' of the child is ambiguous and subjective and liable to be interpreted according to the norms of the dominant culture, which may change over time. For example, male circumcision and female circumcision (known as female genital mutilation) are practices which have been regarded differently in different cultures and at different times and modern Western attitudes demonstrate some degree of inconsistency in societies' responses to cultural child-rearing practices.

There is no definition of what is meant by the child's best interests in the Convention. In its General Comment No. 14, the Committee on the Rights of the Child (UN Committee on the Rights of the Child 2013) indicated that determination of best interests is to be made on a case-by-case basis. The other general principles (i.e. non-discrimination, maximum survival and development and respect for the child's views) are all to be taken into account in the determination of a child's best interests (Hodgkin & Newell 2007). The requirement not to discriminate against children by reason of their ethnic or social background under article 2 implies the need for cultural competence and sensitivity in assessing parenting practices, but it is equally important that all children are entitled to the same level of protection and that respect for cultural difference is not used as an excuse not to intervene to protect children from minority ethnic backgrounds.

The Australian Family Law Act 1975 provides a lengthy and helpful list of factors that must be taken into account when a court is determining the best interests of a child in relation to parenting orders. These include 'any views expressed by the child and any factors (such as the child's maturity or level of understanding) that the court thinks are relevant to the weight it should give to the child's views'. This provision reflects article 12–1 of the UNCRC, which requires that

> States Parties shall assure to the child who is capable of forming his or her own views the right to express those views freely in all matters affecting the child, the views of the child being given due weight in accordance with the age and maturity of the child.

The second principle of the National Framework for Protecting Australia's Children similarly affirms that '[c]hildren and their families have a right to participate in all decisions affecting them'. Examination of serious case reviews (inquiries into the operation of the child protection system in cases in which children have died or suffered serious harm) reveals 'the invisible child', whose perspective is not gathered or not taken into account, to be a significant contributor to professionals' failure to take appropriate action (Sidebotham 2012 in the English context).

Listening to children's wishes and feelings is important at all stages of the protective care continuum, from identification of welfare concerns or maltreatment right through to placement in alternative care and leaving care arrangements. Article 12–2 of the UNCRC provides for children to be given 'the opportunity to be heard in any judicial and administrative proceedings affecting the child, either directly, or through a representative or appropriate body'. This is important for two key reasons. First, children's views and feelings are, as set out above, a crucial part of the assessment of their best interests in all decisions affecting them. Second, research involving 3,700 children in 25 European countries confirms that feeling that their voice has been heard and respected is integral to children's sense of justice (Kilkelly 2010). For older children in particular, understanding why a decision has been made and feeling that their views have been considered and taken seriously is likely to be influential in their ability to come to terms with and accept a decision which is contrary to their wishes. With the increasing use of out-of-court resolutions of family problems, such as Family Group Conferences, the United Nations Committee on the Rights of the Child (2019) has called on the Australian Government to ensure that all children have the opportunity to express their views in non-court-based fora (para 22(a)). Within formal proceedings, research in New South Wales (Ross 2013) suggests that notwithstanding provisions in legislation and guidance designed to facilitate children's participation in court through their legal representative, there is often no independent report of children's wishes and feelings and lawyers tend to adopt a protective approach to vulnerable child clients in relation to interviewing them for the purposes of care proceedings. In its Concluding Observations of 2019, the United Nations Committee on the Rights of the Child recommended training and support for children's lawyers to ensure that they make direct contact with the children they represent in family courts (para. 22(c)). Furthermore, children may struggle to understand the outcome of court proceedings and many do not feel they have been listened to in the process (Fernandez et al. 2013). A response to this dilemma from the English context is the provision of child-friendly versions of the judgement. An example taken from private law proceedings is set out in Box 3.2 (Re A (Letter to a Young Person) [2017] EWFC 48).

Box 3.2 Respecting children's participation rights in court proceedings

The Hon. Mr Justice Peter Jackson

13 July 2017

Dear Sam,

It was a pleasure to meet you on Monday and I hope your camp this week went well.

This case is about you and your future, so I am writing this letter as a way of giving my decision to you and to your parents.

When a case like this comes before the court, the judge has to apply the law as found in the Children Act 1989, and particularly in Section 1. You may have looked at this already, but if you Google it, you will see that when making my decision, your welfare is my paramount consideration – more important than anything else. If you look at s.1(3), there is also a list of factors I have to consider, to make sure that everything is taken into account.

...

Sam, I realise that this order is not the one that you said you wanted me to make, but I am confident that it is the right order for you in the long run. Whatever each of your parents might think about it, I hope they have the dignity not to impose their views on you, so that you can work things out for yourself. I know that as you get older, you will do this increasingly and I hope that you will come to see why I have made these decisions. I wish you every success with your future and if you want to reply to this letter, I know that your solicitor will make sure that your reply reaches me.

Lastly, I wanted to tell you that your dad and I enjoyed finding out that we both love the film My Cousin Vinny, even if it might be for different reasons. He mentioned it as an example of a miscarriage of justice, while I remember it for the best courtroom scenes in any film, and the fact that justice was done in the end.

Kind regards
Mr Justice Peter Jackson

The rights of children in and leaving care

Once children are taken into state care, their wishes and feelings should continue to be an important factor in decisions affecting them. Article 39 requires States Parties to address physical and psychological treatment for maltreated children, but care leavers are at much greater risk of mental health problems than their peers in the general population (Harris et al. 2010 in the US context). Young people leaving care continue to experience significantly poorer outcomes than their peers in a wide range of measures of disadvantage across the Western world (e.g. Jackson & Cameron 2010 in relation to Europe; Okpych & Courtney 2014 in the US). Liebenberg, Ungar and Ikeda (2015) drawing on research in Canada, conclude that neoliberal discourses of responsibilisation of the individual ignore the complexity of contextual factors in young people's lives and may operate to encourage the withdrawal of services from care leavers who are non-compliant. The 2019 Concluding Observations (United Nations Committee on the Rights of the Child 2019) specifically urged the Australian Government to ensure adequate access to mental health and therapeutic services for children in alternative care (para. 34(f)).

The 2012 Concluding Observations (United Nations Committee on the Rights of the Child, 2012) expressed 'serious' concern about the poor outcomes for care leavers in Australia, and contributing factors including inappropriate placements, poor support for carers, a shortage of options, abuse and neglect of children in care, inadequate preparation for leaving care, and placement of indigenous children outside their communities. The Committee's recommendations included ensuring compliance with article 25 of the UNCRC in relation to the periodical review of placements, establishing child-friendly arrangements for the report of maltreatment by carers, early involvement of young people in planning and preparation for leaving care, and intensification of collaboration with indigenous communities to increase available placements within indigenous families. These were recalled and enlarged in 2019, including serious concerns being cited as to 'badly trained and poorly supported staff' (para. 33(d)(i)) and recommendations for investment in support for indigenous children in care and for their reintegration into families and communities. The Government's report in 2018 stressed that all states and territories are committed to implementing the Aboriginal and Torres Strait Islander Child Placement Principle and this is reflected in statistics demonstrating that over half of Indigenous children in out-of-home care were placed in kinship care or with other Indigenous carers or in Indigenous residential care (Government of Australia 2018, para. 153). The Aboriginal and Torres Strait Islander Child Placement Principle includes a commitment to ensuring that Indigenous children in out-of-home care are supported to maintain connections with their family, community and culture. The right to enjoy their culture with others from that culture is also one of the factors that a court must consider in assessing the child's best interests under the Family Law Act 1975 and reflects article 30 of the UNCRC ('In those States in which ethnic, religious or linguistic minorities or persons of indigenous origins exist, a child belonging to such a minority or who is indigenous shall not be denied the right, in community with other members of his or her group, to enjoy his or her own culture, to profess and practise his or her own religion, or to use his or her own language'). Where minority cultures are significantly disadvantaged compared with mainstream communities, however, balancing the right to culture and community against the paramount need to ensure the safety of the child may be a very difficult exercise for professionals, and one which can only be addressed by attention to structural inequality and significant investment in support for carers, as discussed in relation to support for families (see pp. 56–57).

Policy implications

The current political environment in many Western democracies is one in which large and increasing populations of elderly people coupled with neoliberal economic policies have tended to result in the withdrawal of the state from some social care functions in favour of market-led responses, combined with a transfer of political attention from the young to the old. Reduction in support for families, discourses of responsibilisation and high levels of inequality place pressure on child welfare services, resulting in a shift from early help to child protection and higher numbers of children in care. Advocates for children's welfare should not be slow to remind policy-makers of the commitment to children's rights that ratification of the UNCRC represents, nor of the implications of article 4 of the UNCRC in prioritising budgetary allocations. Evidence strongly suggests that family support and child welfare services are an excellent investment in financial terms, not to mention the strong moral imperative to prevent maltreatment or to limit the ongoing emotional and physical impact of maltreatment. The UNCRC places clear duties on ratifying states to uphold children's rights and the reporting mechanism provides regular opportunities for governments to be held to account. It should also be borne in mind that the Convention applies to all children within the jurisdiction, regardless of their national identity and the rights must be accorded to all children without discrimination under article 2.

Practice Implications

For professionals, the primacy of children's voice as one of the guiding principles of the UNCRC is central to good practice in child welfare. In the Australian context, where services are delivered to a large extent by non-profit and for-profit organisations under contract, there is a risk, as described on p. 55 in relation to the corporativist model of social welfare policies, of widely varying models and standards of practice. A children's rights approach may help professionals hold fast to fundamental principles that place the child at the centre of decision-making processes and negotiate the quagmire of cultural diversity in assessing the best interests of the child. It is also at the heart of facilitating strong and trusting relationships with children, through recognition of children not merely as objects of professional concern but as experts in their own lives and individuals worthy of dignity and respect.

Discussion questions

1 The state's duty to support children's upbringing within their family: What are the implications of article 2 (non-discrimination) for family policies at national and local level? What practical steps can professionals working with children take to help parents and carers who are struggling to meet the needs of children?
2 Children's involvement in proceedings affecting them: How can child welfare professionals support children through child protection proceedings and help them understand and accept the decisions that are made?
3 Alternative care: Article 9–3 requires States Parties to respect the right of a child separated from his/her parents to maintain personal relations and direct contact with them, unless it is not in the child's best interests. Why is this important and when might it not be in the child's interests to have an ongoing relationship with his/her parents?

References

Archard, D., 2014, *Children: Rights and childhood* (3rd edn). London: Routledge.

Australian Human Rights Commission, 2018, Information relating to Australia's joint fifth and sixth report under the Convention on the Rights of the Child, second report on the Optional Protocol on the sale of children, child prostitution and child pornography, and second report on the Optional Protocol on the involvement of children in armed conflict. Submission to the Committee on the Rights of the Child. www.humanrights.gov.au/our-work/childrens-rights/publications/report-un-committee-rights-child-2018, accessed 15 October 2019.

Australian Institute of Health and Welfare, 2018, Child protection Australia 2016–17: Child welfare series no. 68. Cat. no. CWS 63. Canberra: AIHW.

Council of Australian Governments, 2009, Protecting children is everyone's business: National Framework for Protecting Australia's Children. Canberra: Commonwealth of Australia.

Davidson, H., 2014, 'Does the U.N. Convention on the Rights of the Child make a difference?', *Michigan State International Law Review, vol.* 22, no. 2, pp. 497–530.

Deeming, C., 2017, 'The lost and the new 'liberal world' of welfare capitalism: A critical assessment of Gøsta Esping-Andersen's *The three worlds of welfare capitalism a quarter century later*', *Social Policy and Society*, vol. 16, no. 3, pp. 405–422.

Deeming, C. & Smyth, P., 2015, 'Social investment after neoliberalism: Policy paradigms and political platforms', *Journal of Social Policy*, vol. 44, no. 2, pp. 297–318.

Esping-Andersen, G., 1990, 'The three political economies of the welfare state', *International Journal of Sociology*, vol. 20, no. 3, pp. 92–123.

Fernandez, E., Bolitho, J., Hansen, P. & Hudson, M., 2013, 'The children's court in New South Wales', in R. Sheehan, & A. Borowski (eds), *Australia's children's courts today and tomorrow*, Dordrecht: Springer.

Government of Australia, 2018, Australia's joint fifth and sixth report under the Convention on the Rights of the Child, second report on the Optional Protocol on the sale of children, child prostitution and child pornography and second report on the Optional Protocol on the involvement of children in armed conflict. For the reporting period June 2012–15 Jan 2018. Canberra: Government of Australia.

Harris, S., Jackson, L., O'Brien, K. & Pecora, P., 2010, 'Ethnic group comparisons in mental health outcomes of adult alumni of foster care', *Children & Youth Services Review*, vol. 32, no. 2, pp. 171–177.

Healy, K. & Oltedal, S., 2010, 'An institutional comparison of child protection systems in Australia and Norway focused on workforce retention', *Journal of Social Policy*, vol. 39, no. 2, pp. 255–274.

Hodgkin, R. & Newell, P., 2007, *Implementation Handbook for the Convention on the Rights of the Child* (3rd edn). Geneva: United Nations Children's Fund.

Holt, J., 1974, *Escape from childhood*, New York: E.P. Dutton.

Jackson, S. & Cameron, C., 2010, *Young people from a public care background: Establishing a baseline of attainment and progression beyond compulsory schooling in five EU countries.* London: Institute of Education, University of London.

Katz, I. & Hetherington, R., 2006, 'Co-operating and communicating: A European perspective on integrating services for children', *Child Abuse Review*, vol. 15, no. 6, pp. 429–439.

Kilkelly, U., 2010, Listening to children about justice: Report of the Council of Europe consultation with children on child-friendly justice. CJ-S-CH (2010) 14 rev. Strasbourg: Council of Europe.

Liebenberg, L., Ungar, M. & Ikeda, J., 2015, 'Neo-liberalism and responsibilisation on the discourse of social service workers', *British Journal of Social Work*, vol. 45, pp. 1006–1021.

Lonne, B., Parton, N., Thomson, J. & Harries, M., 2009, *Reforming child protection*, Abingdon: Routledge.

Lundy, L., Kilkelly, U. & Byrne, B., 2013, 'Incorporation of the UNCRC: A comparative review', *International Journal of Children's Rights*, vol. 21, pp. 442–463.

McLaren, J.M., 2017, Parents vexed? ParentsNext is poorly designed to support mothers into work, www.powertopersuade.org.au/blog/parents-vexed-parentsnext-is-poorly-designed-to-support-mothers-into-work/18/10/2017, accessed 18 October 2018.
Minow, M., 1986, 'Rights for the next generation: A feminist approach to children's rights', *Harvard Women's Law Journal*, vol. 9, pp. 1–24.
Niddrie, N. & Brosnan, K., 2017, *Evaluation: Aboriginal and Torres Strait Islander family led decision making trial.* Winangali/Ipsos, https://apo.org.au/node/174101.
Okpych, N. & Courtney, M., 2014, 'Does education pay for youth formerly in foster care? Comparison of employment outcomes with a national sample', *Children and Youth Services Review*, vol. 43, pp. 18–28.
Petrie, N. & Kruger, L., 2014, Child protection matters in the northern territory, http://ssrn.com/abstract=2473466, accessed 10 October 2019.
Ross, N., 2013, 'Different views? Children's lawyers and children's participation in protective proceedings in New South Wales, Australia', *International Journal of Law, Policy and the Family*, vol. 27, no. 3, pp. 332–358.
Scruggs, L. & Allan, J., 2008, 'Social stratification and welfare regimes for the twenty-first century: Revisiting the three worlds of welfare capitalism', *World Policy*, vol. 60, no. 4, pp. 642–664.
Sidebotham, P., 2012, 'What do serious case reviews achieve?', *Arch Dis Ch*, vol. 97, no. 3, pp. 189–192.
Spratt, T., Nett, J., Bromfield, L., Hietamäki, J. & Kindler, H.P., 2015, 'Child protection in Europe: Development of an international cross-comparison model to inform national policies and practices', *British Journal of Social Work*, vol. 45, no. 5, pp. 1508–1525.
United Nations Committee on the Rights of the Child, 1991, General Guidelines regarding the form and content of initial reports to be submitted by states Parties under article 44, paragraph 1(a) of the Convention. CRC/C/5. Geneva: United Nations.
United Nations Committee on the Rights of the Child, 2012, Consideration of reports submitted by States parties under article 44 of the Convention: Concluding observations: Australia. CRC/C/AUS/CO/4. Geneva: United Nations.
United Nations Committee on the Rights of the Child, 2013, General comment No. 14 on the right of the child to have his or her best interests taken as a primary consideration (art. 3, para. 1), CRC /C/GC/14, Geneva: United Nations.
United Nations Committee on the Rights of the Child, 2019, Advanced Unedited Version: Concluding observations on the combined fifth and sixth periodic reports of Australia. CRC/C/AUS/CO/5–6. Geneva: United Nations.
United Nations General Assembly, 1989, Convention on the Rights of the Child. United Nations, Treaty Series, vol. 1577, p. 3. www.unicef.org.uk/what-we-do/un-convention-child-rights/, accessed 10 October 2019.

Useful websites/links

Australian Children's Commissioner
www.humanrights.gov.au/about/commissioners/ms-megan-mitchell-national-childrens-commissioner.
Australian Human Rights Commission on Children's Rights in Australia
www.humanrights.gov.au/our-work/childrens-rights/about-childrens-rights.
UNICEF's information on the UNCRC
www.unicef.org/crc/index_30225.html.

Part 2

Child abuse and neglect

Chapter 4

Working with cases of neglect and emotional abuse

Alice Loving and David Shemmings

Overview/Introduction

In this chapter, we consider what contemporary research tells us about emotional abuse and neglect. We will consider the key pathways and mechanisms surrounding both forms of maltreatment, as well as some of the most recent evidence-based interventions to help families and children. We consider emotional abuse and neglect from a 'trauma-informed' perspective. We will also include in the chapter a discussion of how emotional abuse and neglect tend to occur both in families as well as in non-familial settings such as online abuse, and child sexual exploitation.

We have included a series of short, practice-related vignettes. They have been anonymized and are taken from the working notes of one of us (Alice) who has drawn out a number of relevant points on emotional abuse or neglect.

Definitions

Single definitions of neglect are rare, perhaps because neglect relates to an absence of a behaviour, unlike the other categories of abuse (physical, emotional, sexual) that focus on the presence of a specific behaviour. The parameters of neglect therefore appear more open and varied. Even within the four countries of the United Kingdom, the definitions of neglect are not identical. However, there are shared similarities (Gardner & Cuthbert 2016). The common areas referenced within the literature are:

1 Parents persistently not meeting their child's basic needs, physically and/or emotionally.
2 Not protecting a child from harm and/or providing inappropriate levels of supervision.
3 Not seeking medical advice or correctly administering medication.
4 Environmental neglect: the conditions in which the child is living.

Treisman (2017: 2), a clinical psychologist with expertise in trauma, notes that neglect can also be referred to as '*invisible trauma*', as it may not always have the same noticeable indicators as other forms of abuse, such as physical maltreatment. It may also be characterized by an '*absent presence*', meaning a lack of availability from caregivers. In addition, she also notes how neglect can encompass '*relational poverty*', due to the potential absence of a caregiver providing a sense of love, care and interconnectedness.

Emotional abuse is also noted within the literature to be difficult to define and, similar to neglect, this is due to the wide range of behaviours that it can encompass, and in some cases it may not be as easily observable. The National Institute for Clinical Excellence (NICE 2017) guidelines list the following behaviours under their definition of emotional abuse that specifically relate to the parent–child interaction.

1 Negativity or hostility towards a child or young person.
2 Rejection or scapegoating of a child or young person.
3 Developmentally inappropriate expectations of/or interactions with a child, including inappropriate threats or methods of disciplining.
4 Exposure to frightening or traumatic experiences.
5 Using the child for the fulfilment of the adult's needs (for example in marital disputes).
6 Failure to promote the child's appropriate socialization (for example involving children in unlawful activities, isolation, not providing stimulation or education).

The National Society for the Prevention of Cruelty to Children (NSPCC 2014) refers to emotional abuse as behaviour that causes the child to feel *worthless, unloved or inadequate*. They also note how emotional abuse can be connected with all of the domains of abuse but can also occur in isolation.

In terms of prevalence, the Department for Education published statistics stating that during 2016–2017, in the UK, 48% of child protection plans detailed neglect as the main concern. Emotional abuse is listed as the second most common form of known abuse, featured in 33.8% of cases. Therefore, focusing this chapter on both forms of abuse and the potential parental mechanisms that may contribute to its presence, as well as the potential useful forms of intervention, appears both relevant and meaningful for current social work practice. Others (for example, Bilson 2018; Tickle 2018) seriously question whether the notion of 'future risk of emotional harm' can be 'justified grounds to remove children' (Bilson 2018).

The charity Action for Children (2018) reported on the underpinning legislation connected to both neglect and emotional abuse. In relation to neglect, they note that the legal framework surrounding it dates back as far as the 19th-century Poor Law Amendment Act of 1868 when it became illegal not to provide a child with adequate clothes, food, medical support or a home. The current law used for the prosecution of neglect in the UK is the Children and Young Persons Act 1933. They note that our understanding of the impact of neglect has dramatically increased and emotional neglect is another dimension to consider. As mentioned previously, the fact that neglect relates to an absence of parental behaviour can cause some difficulty when it comes to the criminal conviction of an individual. This is predominantly due to the fact that The Children and Young person's act states that cruelty to a child must be 'wilful' in order to be regarded as a criminal offence.

In relation to emotional abuse, Action for Children played a significant role in campaigning for four years alongside British politicians in updating the child cruelty offence to include sustained emotional abuse. Police officers have informed the charity that they anticipate this new change will aid them in responding to emotional abuse and increase their own understanding of it.

When it comes to every day social work practice, the burgeoning of research focusing on neglect and its impact over the past 10 to 15 years is likely to have contributed to a positive movement away from what has been famously termed in the literature as 'the neglect of neglect' (Wolock & Harowitz 1984). Social work practitioners can draw upon a plethora of studies to demonstrate the potential likely outcome for a child who continues to experience neglect. However, an awareness of such research is unlikely to be enough to make a significant difference to practice. Many social workers find themselves in a stalemate situation with neglect cases, whereby they are waiting for a 'significant event' to help move things forward and in some cases provide greater evidence for removal.

Common issues documented in reviews of neglect cases are high caseloads within child protection contributing to social workers having sufficiently less time to spend on neglect allegations with priority being given to emergency cases, court cases and cases where the child is coming up to two years on a child protection plan. This can influence how social workers respond to immediate positive changes by removing services despite there being evidence to suggest that neglectful behaviour could return without this provision. This approach can contribute to a 'cyclical situation', and may also lead to an increase in re-referrals of neglect cases, which can be common practice. Findings reported by Troncoso (2017) suggest that the re-referral rate of cases in the UK is particularly high, with 54.5% of cases that were worked during 2010–2011 returning during 2015–2016.

The fact that neglectful parenting relates to the parent not doing something, rather than a deliberate act such as physical abuse, has most likely contributed to the difficulties that social workers can experience when working on neglect cases.

Case example 1

A few years ago, I worked with a mother with a baby who was eight months old. The concerns centred on chronic neglect and she had been diagnosed as 'failure to thrive'. During an unannounced evening visit at 9pm, the mother was found having a cigarette outside her flat. She greeted me and let me know the baby was inside and that I could go in. I went inside the flat and I walked through the living room and popped my head into the bedroom but couldn't see the baby there. I went back to ask the mother where she was and she told me she was in the living room in her high chair. I hadn't seen her when I went into the living room because she was in her highchair, which was facing the wall. She appeared distant and shut down, whilst staring blankly at the wall. The mother then joined us and explained that the baby had just had her dinner, which was why she was in there. When I left and got back into my car, I was struck by the fact that, had that baby had a visible injury, my response would likely to have been different; although there was no physical damage that could escalate this case into court, the internal effects of this continuous level of neglect were likely to be significant. Two additional siblings in the home also had significant developmental delay, with concerns raised throughout the years of physical and emotional neglect.

Daniel (2015) believes that the planning, assessment and intervention of neglect cases has become 'mired in bureaucracy'. He urges practitioners to first simply consider these questions:

- What does this child need?
- What does this child need me to think?
- What does this child need me to do?

Many practitioners speak to us about the sense of frustration they experience that the legislative and court processes in the UK do not necessarily reflect what has been emerging from the research. Gardner and Cuthbert (2016) note that despite the 'media glare' that surrounds high profile neglect cases featured within serious case reviews, policies surrounding neglect have not progressed to where they need to be. One of the consequences of this is that it is sometimes difficult to help the family if the presenting concerns don't 'tick the right boxes'. Where professionals are forced to operate within highly proceduralized and bureaucratic 'risk audit' systems – for example in the UK and elsewhere 'tariffs' and 'thresholds' often determine access to help and support – options to support the family to change can become limited as the next example illustrates.

Case example 2

A few years ago, I did a visit with an assistant team manager to a three-year-old boy who had been in and out of social care involvement since he was born. We were aware that in the mornings the mother would take her son out of the cot and let him roam around the flat while she went back to bed. On this particular visit, there was food, clothes and paper all over the floor, a tub of Sudocreme that he had spread across the living room and a number of nappies, one of which was heavily soiled. The family had recently got a puppy and the puppy had clearly been urinating and defecating around the flat. At one point, the little boy picked up a small clump of faeces and squished it into his palm. Proceedings for his removal from her care had been initiated, but social services had not been granted an Interim Care Order (ICO) at the initial hearing and so they had to wait for the final hearing to apply for this. In light of this and most likely with a mindset of needing the weight of significant events behind this case, the assistant team manager requested that the police conduct a joint visit and she was hopeful that given the conditions in the flat they may consider issuing a police protection order. Unfortunately, the police officer involved did not feel that the conditions of the flat reflected 'imminent risk of harm'. She agreed that he was clearly not being supervised but stated that she needed to have seen something like a coal fire burning in the corner for the level of risk to be significant enough for an order.

Despite the concerns surrounding policy and procedure, research has also highlighted certain practice-based issues that may be impacting on the success of neglect cases. Howarth and Tarr (2015) present four themes to emerge from research that explored 'child visibility in cases of chronic neglect'.

1 '*Generalised assessments and the neglect of identity*'. The lived experience of the child and the impact of these experiences appeared to be missing. When it came to identity, this tended to be focused around their nationality rather than their 'internal working model' of themselves and others. The internal working model of self and other refers to one's thoughts and feelings about who they are as a person and their understanding and expectations of others. This model starts to formulate in early childhood and derives from our relational interactions and experiences. The researchers question how it is possible to meet the child's individual needs without conveying a true sense of who they are.
2 '*Superficial engagement by social workers with children*'. They noted 'generalised comments' when it came to detailing the wishes and feelings of the child such as, 'X would like mother to stop drinking' and 'J wants dad to stop hitting mum'.

Therefore, there was limited evidence of what it was like for X to experience a mother who drank heavily.

3 *'A lack of awareness of the different needs of children in the family'*. They stated that when there was a number of children in the family, they could be viewed more as a 'sibling group'. Despite each child having a separate report for the child protection conference, often the same statements were used in relation to descriptions of the impact of parental behaviour on the child. The example given to demonstrate this was a statement such as 'child is dirty and unkempt' under the heading of 'social presentation'. The authors discuss how this term was regularly used with all siblings and that it was then seen as the responsibility of the conference panel to reflect on how this might affect a teenager differently from (say) a two-year-old.

4 *'Parenting in a vacuum'*. Of participants surveyed, 50% felt that some child protection plans consisted of lists of actions for the parent to address with an absence of 'child-focused outcomes'. They note that 'generalised statements' were being used to discuss the progress of the family such as, 'everything going well; drinking at an acceptable level; no issues arising; engaged with services'. Progress indicators were predominantly based on 'measurable actions', such as 'better home conditions, improved school attendance, keeping health appointments, parents engaging with services and attending parenting course'. Therefore, there was a lack of connection with the lived experience of the child.

It would appear that the broad nature of neglect and the complexity of many cases being intertwined with additional concerns has perhaps contributed to a lack of clear guidance on successfully assessing and intervening. When considering emotional abuse, the limited research in this area is likely to be responsible for the same level of uncertainty when it comes to how to intervene successfully. Gardener and Cuthbert (2016) attribute this uncertainty to a lack of longitudinal research that focuses on outcomes. They concluded that, 'we still know disappointingly little about what works with whom'.

Currently, we also are witnessing different forms of emotional abuse which are not usually perpetrated by family members. Strangers, in the form of sexual exploitation gangs, traffickers, online groomers and radicalization groups, nowadays deploy methods to entrap children and young people that are sinister, and ultimately long-lasting or even fatal.

In sexual exploitation gangs and during radicalization processes, children and young people are given a safe haven and secure base where they experience people who appear to care for them. This is especially true of online grooming, where adults pose as other children and then use their knowledge of the pressures of childhood – such as 'pushy, helicopter parents', jealousy within friendship groups, fashion consciousness, anxiety over academic performance, peer-to-peer sexual relationships etc. – to insinuate themselves into the core of their intended victim's personality and being. They gain their trust in order subsequently to abuse it. The adult intends over time to dominate the child for the purposes of direct sexual abuse or to force them into performing sexual acts with strangers.

There are now a growing number of examples of sexual exploitation gangs who have lured young people into their circle by offering clothes, alcohol, drugs and other temptations for young people; often, little or nothing is asked of the young person until later on. Gangs regularly deploy 'spotters' – individuals whose job is to 'recruit' new victims –

whose job is to gain the trust of a young person by flattery, seduction, acting as a 'role model', or by protecting them against a rival gang member (who is actually a member of the spotter's gang but unknown to the young person being groomed). Adults sometimes use threats or actual violence to force the child to obey them but often they use psychological techniques aimed at undermining the child's confidence in themselves, their right to an opinion, or even their right to exist, without the permission of the adults controlling them.

There is also growing evidence of gangs and individuals using brainwashing and mind-control techniques deliberately to create multiple personalities – 'alters' – each of which is unknown to the 'others' (Epstein, Schwartz & Schwartz 2011). The aim behind these methods is firstly to subjugate and then to force a young person to perform sexual acts or to commit offences, including acts of terrorism. The methods are pernicious and damaging precisely because they are aimed at undermining the child's confidence about their identity and worthiness. They are similar to the kinds of emotional abuse outlined earlier in this chapter but they are more likely to have long-lasting effects and the young people who fall victim may require expert help to recover.

In one recent example, a 15-year-old girl was enticed into a gang in the ways described above by a 17-year-old boy. They went out on a few dates and she soon became infatuated with him (which was his sole aim). He said he wanted to take a couple of (explicit) photos and a short (explicit) film. He told her that he loved and respected her and that, if she loved him, she would do this because 'it was cool to do it; and everyone he knew did it'. She never saw him again. The gang he belonged to told her she was going to have to meet different men in a local park once or twice a week for oral sex. She was told that if she did not comply, or if she told anyone, two things would happen: the film and photos would be posted on the internet and then her mother would be raped. It took a lot of skilled and well-timed police work along with help from friends, family and social workers experienced in child sexual explication gangs to help her survive this emotional abuse.

The following section of this chapter will detail why we believe that using an '*attachment and trauma lens*' is likely to be most beneficial when conducting assessments and intervening in cases of neglect and/or emotional abuse. The two key areas that need to be explored when using this lens is the parent's attachment trauma history and their capacity to mentalize.

It is now relatively well evidenced that traumatic childhood abuse where a key attachment figure is the main perpetrator can have a significant impact on all aspects of a child's development, sense of self and psychological wellbeing. It would be incorrect to assume, though, that all children who have been abused are likely to go on to abuse their own children. The transmission rate is in fact estimated to be around 18–30%. However, Widom et al. (2015) highlight a number of issues with transmission rate research, such as a lack of prospective longitudinal studies following children into adulthood, as well as inflated rates of transmission within studies with a population who had all been abused and had subsequently become abusive. Therefore, participants who have been abused and who *didn't* become abusive are often not represented in the data. They also note that the majority of cases have focussed on transmission rates relating to cases of physical abuse. Therefore, neglect and emotional abuse are underrepresented.

Within the last 30 years, the fields of attachment and trauma have produced theoretical concepts and evidence-based findings that suggest that one mechanism likely to impact on transmission rates of emotional abuse and neglect is the extent to which somebody has been able to make sense of, process and reflect on the abusive experiences they were exposed to during their childhood. The term '*unresolved*' is often attributed to the traumatic memories that have not been processed and as such these memories may not be sitting in the optimal place in the brain. This is because when the brain is engaged in trauma, it can do little but focus on surviving; its functioning quickly shifts to the use of our more primitive parts, such as the brain stem and limbic area which are responsible for our 'flight, fight or freeze' responses.

The fact that during a traumatic event the brain is diverted away from its higher order pre-frontal functioning most likely contributes to the fact that it has not been able to file and process these traumatic memories when they happen, as it is simply trying to ensure survival. This can result in these memories floating around in the mind, which increases someone's vulnerability to experiencing PTSD-type symptoms, such as flashbacks. These can be triggered by certain sights, sounds, and smells that the brain connects to the original traumatic incident. Van Der Kolk (2014), a leading trauma expert, notes that for some people, the trigger can be so powerful that the brain and body react and respond in the same way as if the original incident were happening to the person again. As he puts it, 'the body keeps the score'.

For those parents who have not processed and reflected on earlier abusive or neglectful emotional experiences, their own child, or a child they are taking care of, can soon become their trauma trigger. In young babies, it is often the vulnerability and dependability witnessed in them when they cry that can be enough to trigger, on an unconscious level, feelings of vulnerability that they themselves experienced during the abuse they suffered. This can result in the parent becoming overwhelmed by associated feelings of anger or fear, which may then lead to aggressive or emotionally abusive behaviour towards the child. When explosive outbursts like this occur, the parent's brain is likely to have switched to what is termed the '*low road*' – and not the '*high road*' – and that, furthermore, a more rational and appropriate response to the child displaying their needs is not possible due to the fact the pre-frontal cortex is '*offline*' (Siegel 2011).

The connection between their child and their childhood self as the victim can be so powerful that the parent may in fact 'see' the face of an emotionally abusive or neglectful parent in their child, a term referred to as experiencing '*Ghosts in the nursery*' (Fraiberg, Adelson & Shapiro 1975). One example of this is a mother whose own mother had been emotionally and physically abusive towards her, so when her baby would cry in the night, she would go to her but the mother quickly became overwhelmed by fear, as she saw her mother's eyes in those of her baby. It is understandably distressing and dysregulating for a baby to be met by a fearful response towards them at the point at which their attachment system is activated and signalling a need.

Case example 3

A young mother with whom I worked in a mother and baby assessment unit told me, whilst doing a session on why babies cry, that when her son cries, all she can see is her father's mouth, and she stated 'it's like I'm looking right at him'. Her own mother left her in the care of her father when she was two years old and she had been subjected to different kinds of abuse. She was removed from his care and placed in foster care when she was 11. This is a powerful example of how the '*ghosts*' can interfere significantly with the developing attachment relationship as, in essence, if at the point when he is communicating that he needs her the most in her mind she sees her abusive father, then this will likely determine the level of sensitivity she is able to muster in that moment. This is also then likely to affect the extent to which he views her as an available attachment figure.

It is important to consider how a parent's own defence mechanisms resulting from any attachment-based trauma could account for the types of abusive behaviour they are displaying. In cases of physical and emotional abuse, this response pattern is likely to be connected to a state of 'hyper arousal', a 'fight response'. However, the brain can also respond to traumatic triggers by assuming a 'hypo aroused' state, whereby the brain shuts down and disconnects, resulting in a 'freeze' response and potential momentary absences termed 'dissociation'. This disconnect may be more likely to lead to neglectful parental behaviour.

My (Alice's) PhD research found that, for those parents who had their child removed from them due to concerns around neglect (including emotional neglect), they appeared to be in constant state of 'hypo arousal'. Their defence mechanism to cope with the abuse they had experienced in their childhood had most likely been to shut down, which resulted in them becoming shut down to all aspects of connecting with emotions in themselves, those of others, but most importantly their child's (Loving 2018). This 'disconnect' unfortunately impacted on a range of aspects of their care, including feeding the baby on time, regulating feed temperatures, responses to their baby when crying, and the amount of interaction and stimulation they provided their babies. Although this description relates to the care of young babies, it's not hard to imagine how these types of potential neglectful behaviours could continue to play out for the developing toddler and child.

A complementary mechanism to account for this disconnect as well additional neglectful and emotionally abusive behaviour is the parent's capacity to mentalize. Mentalization refers to one's ability to reflect upon the 'intentional states' of others. It involves accurately making links between thoughts, feelings and behaviour. This includes being able to mentalize for oneself: e.g. 'I was thinking I hate my job, I was feeling so unhappy, and so I was really distant and quiet with my husband when I got home.' The emotional landscape and quality of our relationships are also dependant on our ability to mentalize others: i.e. 'My husband told me he had an equally bad day and seemed frustrated with a colleague, which is probably why he seemed to get more angry than usual when our dog wouldn't let him give her a bath.'

The capacity to mentalize for one's child is believed to be central to developing a secure attachment relationship. Parents who are able to view their children as an '*autonomous*' being, with their own set of interlinked thoughts, feelings and behaviours confer a number of developmental advantages to them. The ability to respond sensitively and appropriately to a child's behaviour, especially a young baby, is almost entirely dependent on the ability to connect with what is perceived to be in their mind: what are they signalling, what do they need/want? Therefore, when abusive and neglectful behaviour does occur, it is likely that the parent is struggling to mentalize; for example, in the case of a parent whose toddler is in a nappy that is visibly full from which urine has started to leak. What would drive us to want to change the nappy is our connection with how it may be feeling for him, the fact that it may be getting sore and that he might develop a rash.

Case example 4

One mother with whom I worked in a mother and baby unit found the intimacy of feeding her baby uncomfortable and often appeared bored and impatient as her baby was a slow feeder. This was thought to be as a result of her own trauma history in childhood. She was therefore keen for feeds to be quicker and as such she used her teeth to make larger holes in the teats of the bottles so that the milk would come out quicker. What she hadn't connected with was how this would feel for the baby who was, I imagine, feeling a sense of drowning in milk as it came out too fast for her to drink. The majority of the feed was also often spilling out and down her neck. This was most likely contributing to the baby not gaining as much weight as she needed to.

Case example 5

This example concerns emotional abuse towards the eldest child and neglect of all three children. The parent struggled to mentalize her nine-year-old who had been supervising his younger siblings in the morning. He attempted to make porridge and burnt himself. When his mother discovered what had happened, she started shouting and swearing at him, telling him he needed to be more careful.

Attachment-based trauma and the capacity to mentalize are interlinked because we become interested in the mind of another person when we experience our attachment figure doing this for us. However, when subjected to abuse and or neglect, this process may fail. Instead the child is exposed to a caregiver who demonstrably *doesn't* seem to understand what is in their mind; and what's more appears uninterested anyway. Peter Fonagy, a leading expert in mentalization, believes that not developing the capacity to mentalize can actually be viewed as a defence mechanism.

> The deactivation of mentalization is a defence available to the abused child or any individual suffering from trauma where the aim is the reduction of the psychic experience of pain, terror or other overwhelmingly negative affect.
>
> (Fonagy 2011)

A number of intervention programmes have been designed aimed at enhancing the parent's capacity to mentalize. These include programmes such as 'Circle of Security' (Powell et al. 2013). 'Minding the baby' (Sadler et al. 2013) and 'Attachment and Bio-behavioural Catch up' (ABC) (Dozier et al. 2018). Programmes that make use of video feedback such as 'Video Interaction Guidance' (VIG) (Kennedy, Landor & Todd 2010) and 'Video-feedback Intervention to Promote Positive Parenting' (VIPP) (Juffer et al. 2017) have been recommended by NICE (2017) to be used for cases of abuse and neglect in children under the age of five.

Case example 6

I am trained in VIPP and used it most recently when working with a single mother (Kate) and her eight-year-old daughter (Jodie). The concerns were based around emotional abuse and sensory neglect. Kate had experienced emotional abuse and physical abuse during her childhood and had been the victim of severe domestic abuse by Jodie's father while pregnant. Jodie had been excluded from school due to challenging behaviour and violence directed towards staff. She had been diagnosed with Autism and ADHD, which I believe may have been a misdiagnosis as her behaviour appeared more closely linked to the attachment-based trauma she was experiencing.

Our work together consisted of alternating between weekly recording sessions of them interacting together, which included completing a puzzle, playing a game, or baking together, and then weekly feedback sessions alone with Kate. During these feedback sessions, I focused on encouraging Kate to consider what might be in her daughter's mind when she was doing or saying certain things, especially things that provoked an extreme response in Kate or that caused her to view her daughter's intentions negatively, even when in many cases Jodie was behaving as you might expect from any nine-year-old child. A common pattern identified in their relationship was that Kate would misinterpret Jodie's behaviour by seeing it as containing deliberate attacks on her. She would then become angry with Jodie, which often left Jodie feeling confused and angry herself.

In the absence of being offered any sensory regulation such as cuddles, as Kate found any close contact with her daughter very uncomfortable, Jodie had failed to develop any self-regulatory mechanisms. This resulted in her going from 0–100 very quickly whenever she did feel any negative emotions and then lashing out at those around her. I worked intensely with Kate over a number of weeks. I was grateful that the local authority were willing to allow me this time to work with the family and in the end this piece of work played a significant part in a positive outcome for Kate and Jodie.

When we consider the critical role that the capacity to mentalize can have on parenting behaviour, it is not surprising that interventions consisting solely of group parenting classes using methods associated with social learning theory that teach the parent strategies for managing behaviour may be less likely to be successful and lead to more sustained positive change. In cases of neglect and emotional abuse when the capacity to mentalize is thought to be a contributing factor, this requires intervention that is more intensive and focused on helping parents tune in to the individual mind of their own child.

When it comes to therapeutic intervention, to target '*unresolved*' trauma, the first challenge can be getting a parent to be willing to engage in therapy. Second, it can be a struggle to find available services. In relation to childhood trauma, trauma-focused cognitive behavioural therapy (CBT) and eye movement desensitization and reprocessing (EMDR) therapy are both highly recommended trauma treatments (World Health Organization 2013). Parent–infant psychotherapy is both mentalization-based and trauma-focused but, certainly in the UK, it is not a service made widely enough available to parents working with social services for concerns relating to neglect or abuse, with a trauma history, who are struggling to mentalize.

This chapter aimed to highlight the potential difficulties arising in practice when working with cases of neglect and emotional abuse. It has been argued that using an 'attachment and trauma lens' is likely to help us to better understand the parental mechanisms that can lead to neglectful and emotionally abusive behaviour. However, we still have a substantial way to go in ensuring social care practitioners can feel confident in using this lens and in offering families the interventions most likely to lead to the best possible chance at eradicating or at least reducing abusive behaviour.

References

Action for Children, 2018, Neglect Law, www.actionforchildren.org.uk/how-to-help/support-our-campaigns/our-campaign-successes/neglect-law/, accessed 17 October 2019.

Bilson, A., 2018, Future emotional harm the statistics, paper presented at the Transparency Project's conference15 September 2018, https://bilson.org.uk/presentations/emotional-harm/?doing_wp_cron=1571277998.8071169853210449218750, accessed 10 October 2019.

Daniel, B., 2015, 'Why have we made neglect so complicated? Taking a fresh look at helping and noticing the neglected child', *Child Abuse Review*, vol. 24, pp. 82–94.

Dozier, M., Roben, C.K., Carone, E., Hoye, J. & Bernard, K., 2018, 'Attachment and biobehavioral catch-up: An evidence-based intervention for vulnerable infants and their families', *Psychotherapy Research*, vol. 28, no. 1, pp. 18–29.

Epstein, O.B., Schwartz, J. & Schwartz, R.W. (eds), 2011, *Ritual abuse and mind control: The manipulation of attachment needs*, London: Karnac Books.

Fonagy, P., 2011, 'Multiple voices versus meta-cognition: An attachment theory perspective', in V. Sinason (ed.), *Attachment, trauma and multiplicity: Working with dissociative identity disorder*, 2nd edn. Hove, UK: Brunner-Routledge, pp. 21–36.

Fraiberg, S., Adelson, E. & Shapiro, V., 1975, 'Ghosts in the nursery: A psychoanalytic approach to the problems of impaired infant–mother relationships', *Journal of the American Academy of Child Psychiatry*, vol. 14, no. 3, pp. 387–421.

Gardner, R. & Cuthbert, C., 2016, 'Special issues on child neglect: Research, policy and practice across a devolved United Kingdom – an overview of the field', *Research, Policy and Planning. The Journal of Social Services Research Group*, vol. 32 no. 1, pp. 3–10.

Horwath, J. & Tarr, S., 2015, 'Child visibility in cases of chronic neglect: Implications for social work practice', *The British Journal of Social Work*, vol. 45, no. 5, pp. 1379–1394.

Juffer, F., Struis, E., Werner, C. & Bakermans-Kranenburg, M.J., 2017, 'Effective preventive interventions to support parents of young children: Illustrations from the Video-feedback Intervention to promote Positive Parenting and Sensitive Discipline (VIPP-SD)', *Journal of Prevention & Intervention in the Community*, vol. 45, no. 3, pp. 202–214.

Kennedy, H., Landor, M. & Todd, L., 2010, 'Video Interaction Guidance as a method to promote secure attachment', *Educational and Child Psychology*, vol. 27, no. 3, p. 59.

Loving, A., 2018, Attachment, trauma and parenting in social work, unpublished doctoral dissertation, Royal Holloway, University of London.

NICE Guideline NG76, 2017, Child abuse and neglect: Recognizing, assessing and responding to abuse and neglect of children and young people, www.nice.org.uk/guidance/ng76, accessed 15 October 2019.

NSPCC, 2014, Core-info: Neglect or emotional abuse in children ages 5–14, www.nspcc.org.uk/services-and-resources/research-and-resources/2014/neglect-emotional-abuse-core-info/, accessed 15 October 2019.

Powell, B., Cooper, G., Hoffman, K. & Marvin, B., 2013, *The circle of security intervention: Enhancing attachment in early parent-child relationships*. New York and London: The Guilford Press.

Sadler, L.S., Slade, A., Close, N., Webb, D.L., Simpson, T., Fennie, K. & Mayes, L.C., 2013, 'Minding the baby: Enhancing reflectiveness to improve early health and relationship outcomes in an interdisciplinary home-visiting program', *Infant Mental Health Journal*, vol. 34, no. 5, pp. 391–405.

Siegel, D., 2011, The low road, www.youtube.com/watch?v=WkEcpBU3TpE, accessed 15 October 2019.

Tickle, L., 2018, Number of children in care for emotional abuse soars, www.theguardian.com/society/2018/sep/14/number-of-children-in-care-for-emotional-abuse-soars, accessed 15 October 2019.

Treisman, K., 2017, *Working with relational and developmental trauma in children and adolescents*, London: Routledge.

Troncoso, P., 2017, Children's services in England: Repeat referrals. London: Department for Education.

Van Der Kolk, B., 2014, *The body keeps the score*, New York: Viking.

Widom, C.S., Czaja, S.J. & DuMont, K.A., 2015, 'Intergenerational transmission of child abuse and neglect: Real or detection bias?' *Science*, vol. 347, no. 6229, pp. 1480–1485.

World Health Organization, 2013, WHO releases guidance on mental health care after trauma [Homepage of The World Health Organization] Available: www.who.int/mediacentre/news/releases/2013/trauma_mental_health_20130806/en/ accessed February 2015.

Wolock, I. & Harowitz B., 1984, 'Child maltreatment as a social problem: The neglect of neglect', *The American Journal of Orthopsychiatry*, vol. 54, no. 4, pp. 530–543.

Chapter 5

Child sexual abuse

Dale Tolliday

Introduction

Child sexual abuse evokes strong responses individually and socially. Over the past 40 years there has been increasing public awareness and official responses to child sexual abuse. In Australia significant levels of recognition and response to child sexual abuse occurred in the 1980s soon after adult and early child sexual assault services were established in the mid to late 1970s. This mirrored processes internationally across North America and much of Europe. Researchers and clinicians began mapping the scale of the issue and suggesting ways of responding (Finkelhor et al. 1986; Herman 1981, 1992; Sgroi 1982). Early Australian experience included an overwhelmingly successful NSW advertising campaign in the late 1980s 'No excuses, never, ever' resulting in unprecedented rates of reporting child sexual abuse.

Focus on child sexual abuse has however not been constant. Recognition has been met with resistance, ranging from public and institutional denial, sometimes displayed by legal systems slow to respond to the needs of child victims of sexual abuse, and public funding for reforms being tied to political cycles. For example it was not until 1985 that in NSW prosecution for the sexual assault of young children no longer required a 'reliable' older witness or physical evidence. NSW was one of the last common law jurisdictions internationally to remove this restriction on children being able to give evidence and be believed. Remote witness facilities began being used in the 1990s and in some instances their use remains vexed.

The most recent substantial response in Australia to focus public, political and legal attention on child sexual abuse was the Royal Commission into Institutional Responses to Child Sexual Abuse (Final Report 2017). The 17 volumes of the final report catalogue an enormous amount of material documenting decades of poor institutional responses and practices in relation to child sexual abuse. It substantially adds to contemporary understanding of institutional child sexual abuse while acknowledging most child sexual abuse occurs in private contexts. This Royal Commission is numerously referenced in this chapter as not only did it refocus attention on the issue of child sexual abuse, it did so in new and unique ways, identified major deficits in data, understanding and response. It also commissioned many pieces of research to both review best available evidence and conduct research where important gaps in the evidence base was established.

There are a number of headline issues in relation to the sexual safety of children. These include:

1 Children are not only most at risk of sexual abuse from people closely known or related to them, harm is more likely to come from another young person who is under the age of 18 years.
2 The impacts of sexual abuse are broad, generally long-lasting and harm by another child or young person is no less severe than harm by an adult.
3 Advances in technology in the online environment are substantially influencing sexual development and creating opportunities for new ways to harm.
4 Child Sexual Abuse (CSA) is gendered behaviour, something which at times is not noted in the literature including much of the contemporary trauma focus. The gendered nature of CSA is evidenced by over 90% of all sexual abuse being carried out by men and boys and studies of women and girls identify gendered experiences which are significant precursors to engaging in harmful sexual behaviour. Very little detail is provided in the literature of gender-informed responses to CSA.
5 Disclosure of child sexual abuse is a process and is often delayed for reasons related to the dynamics of CSA and specific to the context of individual children.
6 Government and non-government responses continue to struggle to be well co-ordinated, sensitive to the needs of children, demonstrably effective, though there are some encouraging signs of improvement.

Language and recognition of child sexual abuse

Child sexual assault and child sexual abuse are terms used interchangeably, the former more commonly having a legal definition of a (class of) sexual offence(s) and the latter referring more to a deliberate process in which the 'abuser' is acting in a strategic manner to achieve a sexually abusive act. Neither of these descriptors satisfactorily encompasses the breadth of behaviour being considered in this chapter. This is especially the case when it is a child or young person engaging in sexual behaviour which causes harm to another. The developmental capacity of children and young people is different to adults and diversity of children and young people who engage in this behaviour reveals that intention, indifference to, or ignorance of harm means applying a single framework of culpability is inadequate. The Australian Royal Commission into Institutional Responses to Child Sexual Abuse (the 'Royal Commission'), in relation to children and young people, adopted the language in use in the United Kingdom of 'harmful sexual behaviour' (NSPCC 2016) in preference to 'sexually harmful behaviour'. This descriptor achieves separating the behaviour from the child or young person, does not require an attribution of intention or culpability while recognising the harmful effect for the child upon whom the behaviour is imposed. Harmful sexual behaviour (HSB) is preferable to 'sexually harmful behaviour' as the harm is more than sexual: it is emotional, physical, psychological, relational and spiritual as well as sexual and can have profound developmental implications.

> This, it stole me, I lost myself. He took me away and I'm here today, a shadow of the person I could have been because he took it away from me and I can never get

> that person back. ... And society, to want to pretend that it doesn't happen, and this is where we are still victims and they're still making us victims.

This quote appears at the beginning of the 2006 New South Wales Aboriginal Child Sexual Assault Taskforce Report, 'Breaking the Silence: Creating the Future, Addressing child sexual assault in Aboriginal communities in NSW'(2006). For any child or adult survivor, the effects of child sexual assault may be profound, frequently long term and transgenerational (Cashmore & Shackel 2013).

Contemporary recognition of the nature and extent of CSA in Australia substantially developed as a result of feminist activism in the 1970s and beyond which generated awareness resulting in legislative and service reforms (Carmody & Carrington 2000). Nationally, a number of key government inquiries, taskforces and royal commissions have examined and re-examined the complex issues which surround child sexual abuse. These include: the nature and prevalence of CSA in Australia, the dynamics of CSA, impact of CSA, building improved responses to disclosure, enacting and amending laws and criminal procedures, examining the effectiveness of response for victimised children and those who have victimised them, identifying and targeting areas of higher risk and the ultimate goal, the prevention and elimination of CSA. In NSW the first significant report to Government was that of the NSW Child Sexual Assault Task Force (1985) and the most recent in the national context is the Final Report of the Royal Commission into the Institutional Responses to Child Sexual Abuse (Final Report 2017). In 2019, over 40 years since the first specialist responses to child sexual abuse were developed in child protection, health, police investigation and public prosecution, there remain significant challenges to recognise and respond effectively to CSA.

Defining child sexual abuse

Forty years of attention has not seen universal agreement on some fundamental issues including definition of child sexual abuse. The Royal Commission found there to be considerable variance between Australian States and Territories in responses to CSA. Associated with this it found gaps in data and inconsistencies across agencies in recognition and understanding what constitutes CSA. One significant dynamic issue is that the forms and types of behaviour constituting CSA are evolving, and no doubt will continue to do so (Australian Institute of Family Studies 2015). Not only have there been changes to social and legal standards over time, the advent of new technologies has facilitated a broader range of sexual behaviours establishing new norms as well as potential for harm.

The definition of child sexual abuse adopted by the Royal Commission is:

> Any act which exposes a child to, or involves a child in, sexual processes beyond his or her understanding or contrary to accepted community standards. Sexually abusive behaviours can include the fondling of genitals, masturbation, oral sex, vaginal or anal penetration by a penis, finger or any other object, fondling of breasts, voyeurism, exhibitionism, and exposing the child to or involving the child in pornography.

> It includes child grooming, which refers to actions deliberately undertaken with the aim of befriending and establishing an emotional connection with a child, to lower the child's inhibitions in preparation for sexual activity with the child.
>
> (Royal Commission Final Report, Volume 2, p. 30)

Prevalence

Data collection limitations as well as the changing landscape in sexual behaviour and ability of systems to respond to disclosures of child sexual abuse impact upon the ability to measure the prevalence of CSA. Frequently measured in retrospect post disclosure, prevalence estimates based upon cohorts of past victims are used at times to suggest they reflect current as yet unreported or undetected CSA. A recent Australian study notes 18% of women and 4.7% of men report that they experienced sexual abuse before they turned 15 years of age (Australian Institute of Health and Welfare 2018). Overall, systemic and meta-analytic reviews confirm reported rates for incidence of CSA are high, with one significant study noting Australia as having the highest reported rate for CSA of girls internationally at 21.5% (Stoltenborgh et al. 2011). It should also be noted that child sexual abuse is frequently experienced alongside other forms of child abuse and harm including children living in contexts of domestic and family violence (Finkelhor 2011, Hackett et al. 2013).

Australia is one of few developed countries where a nationally representative prevalence study on child maltreatment and CSA has not been conducted (Mathews et al. 2016), a matter now being remedied by a study under way in 2019 by Professor Daryl Higgins through the Institute of Child Protection Studies, Australian Catholic University, Melbourne.

Reported prevalence rates of CSA can vary greatly due to a range of factors, including how sexual abuse is defined in terms of the acts, characteristics of the person who is carrying out the acts, how 'child' is defined by age, the time and manner in which data is collected and how subjects of a survey are assembled (Costello and Backhouse 2019). For example, the Australian Personal Safety Study (PSS 2016) collected information on child sexual abuse defining CSA limited to persons under 15 years of age at time of the abuse and the 'perpetrator' as being 18 years or older. Consequently children imposing harmful sexual behaviour were excluded as were victimised children aged 15, 16 and 17 years (if we were to define children according to the law, it is people up to the age of 18 years). The age at which children can consent to sexual behaviour is 16 years and some research unhelpfully conflates age of consent with maturation from childhood to becoming an adult. The real issue is of sexual abuse of minors, being people under the age of 18 years. Despite the PSS 2016 limitations which present an underestimate of CSA owing to exclusions due to age criteria set out above, it produced valuable insights into CSA. For example, 9 in 10 women who reported experiencing CSA indicate this was by an adult known to them. For men it was adults known to them for 8 in 10.

Where is the risk?

Costello and Backhouse, while noting the strengths and limitations of the PSS 2016, cite other Australian research noting there are contexts which define vulnerable populations at risk of CSA.

Vulnerable populations (Costello and Backhouse 2019):

- ▶ Children and young people with intellectual disabilities, psychiatric disabilities or complex communication disabilities (Mitra-Kahn, Newbigin & Hardefeldt 2016).
- ▶ Young people in correctional or juvenile justice settings (Royal Commission into Institutional Responses to Child Sexual Abuse 2017).
- ▶ Both men and women report experiencing sexual abuse as a child by someone known to them. However, women are more likely to have reported being sexually abused in all other settings including by family members and in the community where the majority of child sexual abuse occurs, while the majority of victims of sexual abuse in institutions, particularly religious institutions, were male (Royal Commission into Institutional Responses to Child Sexual Abuse 2017).
- ▶ The sexual abuse of boys is far more common than generally believed and, in comparison to girls, boys are more likely to be assaulted by siblings or other boys (Cashmore & Shackel, 2013; Royal Commission into Institutional Responses to Child Sexual Abuse 2017).
- ▶ Sibling sexual abuse is more prevalent than other types of intra-familial sexual abuse (Caffaro 2014; Tapara 2012; Welfare 2008).
- ▶ 'Australian studies find that 30–60% of childhood sexual abuse is carried out by children and young people, and "most young people target younger children or peers, and know their victim" ... However, accurate statistics are difficult to obtain' (El-Murr 2017).

One further substantially vulnerable population is children and young people in out-of-home care (OOHC). Research commissioned by the Royal Commission suggests four dimensions of risk for children in out-of-home care (Parkinson & Cashmore 2017):

- Situational risk, which arises from the opportunities for abuse that the environment offers
- Vulnerability risk, which arises from the history and/or characteristics of the children cared for
- Propensity risk, which is the risk posed by the greater-than-average clustering of those with a propensity to abuse children
- Institutional risk stemming from the characteristics of an institution that may make abuse more likely to occur and less likely to be dealt with properly if disclosed.

The three main sources of risk for sexual abuse of children in OOHC is from

1. People engaged in some way to provide care for the children
2. Other children in OOHC or children of carers
3. People targeting children in OOHC seeking to sexually exploit them.

Vulnerability to risk of sexual abuse can be located in the trauma histories many children in OOHC carry, the most significant being prior experiences of being sexually abused and absence of proximate and protective care from a significant adult.

The principles of child safe organisations have been developed to prevent sexual abuse of children in all institutional settings including OOHC (National Principles of Child Safe Organisations 2018). Key to OOHC is the way in which care organisations are structured, whether children and their best interests are the highest priority at all points in the care system, how carers and staff are trained and selected and how direct care for children is delivered. Substantially related to the vulnerability of children in care is dislocation from family and community. Significantly, this is most evident for Aboriginal and Torres Strait Islander children in OOHC (Anderson et al. 2017). Frequently non-kinship OOHC struggles to sustain familial relationships, especially with parents regarded as failing to adequately protect or provide for children. Failure to connect children with family and culture only adds to a child's vulnerability, does little to support development of identity and diminishes opportunity to address past traumas, which undermines development of secure and protective relationships with siblings, parents, grandparents and extended family.

The OOHC sector recognises the need for well-trained carers and in the case of residential care, preferably this to include formal qualifications of some kind; which qualifications, content and standard of training in relation to child sexual abuse remains unresolved. There is no industry standard or accreditation for carers beyond receiving a Working With Children Check clearance in relation to supporting the sexual safety of children in care. Some care organisations have commenced undertaking significant work in this area (McKibbin 2017) but this is occurring with little direction from regulators or through funding agreements.

The risk for children from people closely related or known to them means CSA typically occurs in private spaces: the child's own home or the home of the person harming them (Smallbone & Wortley 2006). When a child is harmed in their own home it is most likely to be by a family member upon whom the child is dependant or subordinate to in the family or home context. Situational prevention is difficult to apply in domestic settings where the person harming is a member of the same household. Sexual abuse of a young child in their home often is enacted in the context of intimate personal care – normative family care such as play, bathing, dressing and bedtime activities. Family relationships have implicit trust and to build prevention around these activities in general raises difficulties of gender roles, suggesting, for example, for children to be safe, men should not be involved in their intimate care.

In relation to single parents (usually mothers) who together with their children may be targeted by extra-familial males, situational prevention suggests women need to carefully screen and limit interactions with male friends and potential partners. This understandable but misguided advice fails to recognise single mothers do assess the safety of their children around strangers and new friends and that the mothers themselves are being targeted and subjected to a range of tactics by the harming adult which aim to build her trust and overcome her suspicions or concerns. A gender-based observation of these circumstances recognises the targeted mothers are often caring for children without the children's fathers sharing parenting equitably and frequently have experienced past violence and abuse in intimate relationships. A poorly applied situational prevention strategy levels primary responsibility for children's safety with mothers and blames them for any harm that comes to the children by 'allowing' the person who harmed them access, all the while ignoring the underlying vulnerability of these mothers and the way they have been victimised in this process. A more informed situational prevention strategy would have community programmes for mothers rearing children on their own, providing practical and personal support including educational and social activities, breaking through isolation loneliness for the mothers and children. Confident and assertive children are less vulnerable to being engaged in dependency relationships with people who may seek to sexually abuse, in part because they do not provide the emotional response such people often seek as part of the process of sexual abuse (Smallbone & Wortley 2006).

Disclosure

Disclosures made in forensic settings such as police or child protection agencies do not go anywhere near matching or even approaching the population-based incidence numbers. Non-forensic disclosures made to others such as family or friends are often not reported to authorities at all, or are time-delayed due to, amongst other issues, family members not responding supportively, abuse by children and adolescents being seen as 'normative exploration' and victims reluctant to disclose the abuse due to shame, self-blame, fear, and coercion by others not to tell (Kaufman et al. 2006, Leach et al. 2017).

Practice issue

A recent systematic literature review by Alaggia, Collin-Vézina and Lateef (2019) identifies five themes which have emerged through the research literature:

1. Disclosure is an iterative, interactive process rather than a discrete event and is best done in a relational context,
2. The complex interplay of individual, family, contextual and cultural factors are best understood using social-ecological person-in-environment perspectives,
3. Age and gender significantly influence disclosure, with a sub-theme emerging that intrafamilial abuse or maintaining a family-like relationship of an abuser has an impact of disclosure delays or withholding,
4. There is a lack of a 'life-course' perspective in the research. Disclosure has been under-studied in terms of its place amongst 'life pathways' following child sexual abuse,
5. Barriers to disclosure continue to outweigh facilitators of disclosure.

Consider the implications of barriers to disclosure and nominate ways to enhance or add new facilitators to disclosure. (See also McElvaney & Culhane 2017.)

Factors at play inhibiting disclosure include the direct influence of the person who has abused the child. Adults may use threats against the child, loved ones or even pets. They may also use a broad range of tactics which are generally grouped together and described as 'grooming' (Pratt & Tolliday 2018).

Grooming

> The use of a variety of manipulative and controlling techniques; with a vulnerable subject; in a range of inter-personal and social settings; in order to establish trust or normalise sexually harmful behaviour; with the overall aim of facilitating exploitation and/or prohibiting exposure.
>
> (McAlinden 2012: 11)

Children sexually abused by adults and in some instances by other young people are selected based on a number of factors associated with the interest and perception of the person seeking to abuse, including but not limited to the perceived vulnerability of the child, opportunity and anticipation of avoiding detection; typically, a process which focusses on influencing ('grooming') the child as well as others in the child's environment, such as parents. In relation to sexual abuse by a parent or other family member or person to whom the child has a dependent relationship, the grooming of others around children is often invisible. Critically important in achieving sexual abuse is the separation of children from key supports. The deception of other's around targeted children is frequently mistaken for indifference or even collusion. Within families this is invariably the position of mothers, vilified as 'unprotective', with failure to be recognised as victimised through a grooming process (Tolliday, Laing & Spangaro 2018).

Examples of conditioning aka 'grooming'

- Position of advantage and/or trust
- Develop close relationship with the child
- Emotionally separate child from others
- Gradual violation adult–child boundaries
- Desensitise child to sexual behaviour
- Entrapping child:
  - Secrecy
  - Sense of culpability
  - Blame
  - Fear
  - Isolation
- Extortion (often referred to as bribery)
- Ploys: seemingly accidental touching/confusion
- Covert warning of silence
- Non-verbal cueing of abuse
- Words to place responsibility on victim
- Coercion/physical force

- Conditioning (grooming) child's carers/family
- Subverting relationships within the family
- Ensuring position of control and influence (immediate and extended family)
- Promoting a positive image of self
- Promoting a negative image of child's carers/family

(Tolliday, Laing & Spangaro 2018)

This list is not extensive and there are variations for every circumstance. Key to these is isolation of child and family, introduction of behaviours while avoiding alarm and preventing disclosure or discovery and planning defence should sexual abuse be suspected. If these conditioning strategies are internalised by the victimised child, disclosure and responsiveness to assistance can be severely impacted:

> Jane was 9 years old when her step-father Chris first touched her in sexual ways and over time directed her to touch him sexually. Chris has been very attentive to Jane and is regarded as a great Dad. Now, at age 12 Jane has indicated by silence and not wanting to always be with Chris that she has growing discomfort about Chris' sexual behaviours. He has progressed in his sexual behaviour to seek confirmation from Jane that his touch is not hurting her. He also has compelled her to describe to him what she experiences as part of his aim is to evoke a physical sexual response. He explains to her what she experiences is normal and part of something they share which is 'special' and 'they' would get into trouble if others found out.

It is hard to imagine how Jane could disclose. The layers of intrusion, physically, psychologically and emotionally are likely to have her carrying significant responsibility for her sexual abuse, and as time goes on, increasingly for *not* telling. Children like Jane generally just want the sexual abuse behaviour to stop. Chris' defence should Jane disclose is likely to be total denial and pointing to issues of character, citing times she has been unreliable or told lies, moody or distant from her mother – all believable if Chris has all the while been working to undermine Jane's relationship with her mother and build reputational damage of Jane within the family. If sexual behaviour is confirmed, by discovery, admission or forensically, Chris is likely to assert Jane was the initiator and at the very least an active participant, thereby playing on shame and guilt he has built for Jane around the sexual response he evoked in her body. And these scenarios around what may unfold if Jane discloses do not include how they relate to any threats Chris may have made which could include direct threats to harm Jane, other family members, a loved pet or that Jane would not be believed, she may be sent away or if he is taken away to jail, the family will suffer financially, lose their home … and that would all be her fault.

Responses to children by parents and carers

At the core of the response a child needs from parents or carers is belief and connection. While this is a simple statement, it is difficult and can take considerable time to achieve at a level where the child is not continuing to suffer significant negative impacts from the sexual abuse. If the child's relationship with the key primary carer has been undermined, a process of mutual recognition of their processes is needed. They may well have said or done things hurtful to each other and recognition of their context for doing so can facilitate this, but it may take time. The journey to recovery for the child is actually a journey of recovery and healing for significant others also victimised. The process is best led by the adults around the child and often this requires those adults to work this through on their own, as the child typically needs to have a discreet personal opportunity to process aspects of their experience without other family members present. It should be recognised that the tactics of CSA do not cease at disclosure, particularly presence of shame, self-doubt and self-blame.

It can be overwhelming to face the full picture of how a child has been sexually abused. It is common for parents to want it to be all over, for children to recover as quickly as possible and to contemplate the most contained picture of the abuse. This can include not recognising the full extent or nature of the abuse, not as a part of a desire to deny the abuse but to be able to accommodate as much as they can at any point in time. The closer and more intimate the relationship of a parent with the person who sexually abused their child, the more difficult it can be to hold a picture which includes both.

A simple model for relational recovery has the following four parts:

1 Knowing
2 Believing
3 Conveying belief
4 Communicating empathic belief.

Knowing means knowledge about what was done, when and how. It includes the tactics used to set up the abuse, carry it out and avoid detection.

Believing is recognition that the sexual abuse took place in the terms disclosed with no minimisation and being clear that the person carrying out the abuse is fully responsible for the abuse and its effects.

Conveying belief follows knowing and believing as it is essential for the child to be fully believed with no space for blame, whether that be for the abuse or not telling. If a parent holds a view the child should have told earlier, this places the child in the difficult position of being told they did the wrong thing. A poor message which will undermine recovery and indicates the parent does not know or understand how all the abuse was carried out.

Communicating empathic belief is important for recovery in the context of safe and secure connected relationships. It conveys an understanding of what the abuse experience entailed including the pressures and influences to not disclose. It also opens the way for the child and parent to recognise how their relationship was undermined and how the other was groomed.

People who have sexually abused children can facilitate recovery of children

Taking a position of responsibility to benefit the child without pursuing other agenda(s) can facilitate belief, contribute to validation of children's experiences and if done soon after disclosure can assist the child by not being required to give evidence at Court. It should also be noted that some children wish to give evidence at Court, to be able to give their own account of what was done to them. In well-constructed legal processes, both should be possible. The advantage of the harming person providing a detailed acknowledgement is that if done well it will include elements the child may not have been aware of such as planning and managing the environment around the child. These are practices of restorative justice which need to be carefully managed as they can be misapplied, as in the following example.

> A letter from a father to his daughter after he was convicted based on guilty pleas to all charges brought against him.
>
> Dear Carla,
>
> I have been trying to write this letter for three days now, nothing that I write can make the pain I have caused you go away. I hope and pray that one day you can maybe find it in your heart to forgive me and maybe you can never be able to.
> I am proud of you for standing up for your rights. You were always my favourite one even though you were a bit of a devil. I love you kids more than life itself. Make everyone that loves you proud of you and forget about me so that you can go through life with a clear conscience.
>
> With all my heart. Please believe I love you forever.
>
> Dad
> xxxx

This letter was not sent to Carla (not her real name). The content held no real surprises as rather than being an acknowledgement it was more a continuation of the messages and tactics used by this father. He had sexually abused Carla and her sister. Neither knew about the other until one disclosed. The letter invites Carla from the outset to feel for her father and she is asked to forgive him. It suggests complicity by Carla and concludes with ingenuine self-deprecation and a final invitation for Carla to focus on his plight. At a later stage Carla, her sister and mother jointly reviewed the letter with their counsellors and used it as part of a shared exploration of their experiences of and around the sexual abuse of the two sisters (Tolliday, Laing & Spangaro 2018).

Children and young people and harmful sexual behaviour

It is difficult for many to conceive of children engaging in sexual behaviour and more difficult again that this could be harmful. The Royal Commission did not anticipate the scale and scope of harmful sexual behaviour (HSB) of children towards other children. The significance of this is reflected throughout the Final Report with substantial attention to the issue in the volumes concerning OOHC and schools as well as a whole volume on the subject of children and HSB (Final Report, Volume 10).

It is now conservatively estimated that 30%–50% of all harmful sexual behaviour experienced by children is from other children under the age of 18 years. Most researchers and commentators indicate a view that the rates reported in various studies are likely to be under-representations as they relate generally to children for whom some level of criminality is established and that it may be incredibly difficult for children to complain or have their complaints for this behaviour acted upon in a way the incidence is recorded. Few studies indicate rates below 30% of reported CSA some exceeding 60% (Allardyce & Yates 2018; Print 2013). While there is not concurrence on actual rates there is concurrence that children and young people are responsible for a very significant proportion of all child sexual abuse.

As with adults, the children who engage in HSB are predominantly boys. Rates for girls vary between 3% (Hackett et al. 2013) and 10% (KPMG 2014). Children and young people come to engage in HSB for a number of reasons. The good news is that the vast majority, contrary to public belief, do not carry this behaviour into adulthood (Caldwell 2016). For some children and young people their harmful behaviour is strongly associated with online consumption of sexual material, though a causal link has not yet been established (Peter & Valkenburg 2016) and some studies have found accessing pornography early is associated with seeking earlier sexual experiences and accessing particular types of pornography, notably violent pornography is more associated with HSB (Ybarra & Thompson 2017).

Children and young people referred to treatment settings for this behaviour frequently have trauma histories and have disrupted developmental histories. These clinical populations have also been noted to have significant proportions of sibling HSB. The New Street Services in NSW report this at 50% of referrals and this figure has also been reported in a USA national survey (Kreinert & Walsh 2011). While it appears most children and young people mature out of this behaviour, the harm caused to others can have profound and long lasting effects. Little longitudinal work has been completed with adults who as children engaged in HSB. One substantial study noted low rates of later sexual offending as adults but sub-optimal outcomes on a range of social indicators (Hackett et al. 2013).

The evidence base for effective therapeutic intervention for children and young people who have engaged in HSB is not settled. However, key research-supported elements for effective programmes have been identified (Shlonsky et al. 2017):

- Holistic and ecosystemic
- Family/care and context focussed
- Developmentally appropriate
- Coordinated multi-agency in partnership with families
- Individually assessed and unique therapeutic processes (with specialist approach to the HSB).

Challenges and new norms in sexual development associated with online technologies

Social media, the internet, gaming, smart phones and personal devices have been-associated with generational changes in the way young people connect with each other and the world around them including sexual and broader personal development

(Quadara, El-Murr & Latham 2017). The fifth (and most recent) National Survey of Australian Secondary Students and Sexual Health (Mitchell et al. 2014) noted high and, compared with previous surveys, increasing rates of engaging through these technologies and media with sexual content. The sending and receiving of explicit intimate images of self or partner may be a new 'norm' which can expose users to harm, particularly children. Harm can range from reposting of intimate images to being directly engaged in sexual abuse online. Amongst the impacts for young people of engaging in explicit material online is significantly younger age of first sexual intercourse (Kraus & Russell 2008).

It has not been established that exposure to explicit online material is causally connected to harmful sexual behaviour but high levels of online viewing of this material has been noted in populations of young people who have sexually harmed others (El-Murr 2017).

It has been observed that for many young people sex education is substantially gained through accessing explicit material online which is not based in reality and rarely focusses upon respect for self and others, consent and relationships (Crabbe 2016). The issue is not able to be managed by use of web filters or prohibition. Internet providers are unlikely to limit online access except to comply with laws related to illegal content. The substantial answer is in education and close supportive and therefore safe parent/carer and peer relationships. Providing accessible resources to help remains a challenge as the online world including social media continues to evolve rapidly and ahead of resources and technical capability to respond, ideally before any harm takes place. The Australian Government has established an eSafety Commissioner to lead action in this area (www.esafety.gov.au).

Limitations of the Australian Royal Commission

The focus of the Royal Commission was on institutions and their responses. The Royal Commission has provided a generational opportunity to address many institutional failings. It has provided a focus on CSA which allowed thousands of survivors to come forward. It has led to public recognition of men and boys as survivors as well as women and girls and is driving systemic change in law, policies and practices across government and non-government agencies and service providers. Unfortunately, the Family Court of Australia was not included as an institution for the Royal Commission to examine. While the States and Territories are responsible for statutory child protection, Federal law prevails over State law when matters arise as a conflict of laws between State and federal jurisdictions. In matters before the Family Court new orders can be made which in effect overturn child protection action by State or Territory authorities. For example, access could be granted to a parent in contested matters where CSA is alleged and State authorities have put in place restrictions on contact, or on some occasions parents have been subject to orders to remove a child from sexual assault counselling. It will be for a future Inquiry or perhaps Royal Commission to examine whether the complex Australian Federal–State arrangements and powers do effectively protect children in matters involving statutory State child protections and the Family Court.

Promising developments in the Australian context

While the responses to CSA have varied across different States and Territories in what is done, when and to what degree, the elements of a move to a public health approach are increasingly evident. Overwhelmingly, initial efforts have been to respond to victimised children with tertiary services. Over time, vulnerable populations of children have been identified who are now targeted with secondary level intervention, for example children in OOHC and children with disabilities who are in some form of institutional care. The changes and risks associated with the arrival of online technologies: new ways in which children are being accessed and exploited as well as shifts in normative sexual development, as well as recognition of the high prevalence of harmful sexual behaviour by children and young people mean primary prevention is under way through programmes to all school age children and young people. The establishment of a national eSafety Commissioner is highly significant in this regard (https://esafety.gov.au/).

Following the Royal Commission the government of each Australian State and Territory has responded to the 409 recommendations in the Final Report. While the Royal Commission focussed upon CSA in institutional settings, it also noted the high prevalence of CSA in domestic and private settings and the majority of the recommendations have direct implications in both private and institutional settings. Unlike many other Royal Commissions and Government Inquiries, the Commonwealth Government has committed to the Royal Commission recommendation of a 10-year review of progress in implementing recommendations (Recommendation 17.4).

Perhaps the most significant structural development has been the establishment of The National Office for Child Safety, initially situated in the Department of Social Services and moved at the initiative of the Prime Minister into the Department of Prime Minister and Cabinet at the time of the national apology to the victims of institutional child sexual abuse and their families (https://pmc.gov.au/domestic-policy/national-office-child-safety).

Key actions of the National Office of Child Safety:

- Oversee and implement the National Strategy to prevent CSA which will be a broad-based public health framework to include cultural change, measures to provide victim services, build evidence of effective practice and drive coordination and collaboration between government sectors and the community.
- Sits within national arrangement of 'Child Safe Framework', a national process to overview activities of States and Territories, operation of strategies such as working with children clearances and application of principles of Child Safe Organisations.
- Facilitate public reporting (visibility and accountability) of major institutions involved in child-related work, focussing initially on those identified by the Royal Commission (religious, education, OOHC, sports, arts and recreation, health, child care and statutory children's authorities).

In 2027 it will be interesting to see whether the National Office has met its priorities and whether better data exists to demonstrate substantial decline in the sexual abuse of children, there is evidence of institutions embracing effective child safe practices and whether the focus upon institutions and CSA has improved the safety of children in private and domestic settings as well. It may need to be a simple measure of whether in 2027 children are seen, heard and believed.

Reflective practice questions

1 How do you distinguish child sexual abuse by an adult and harmful sexual behaviour by children and young people?

2 Identify three key strategies which could counter risks presented by availability of online sexual material and technology-based sexual behaviour.
3 What approach would you take to working with a parent of a child who has been sexually abused and the parent is struggling to recognise all of the child's experience of victimisation? Would your approach be different if the person who harmed the child was a sibling, a peer or an adult?
4 Identify an online strategy for the eSafety Commissioner as a public awareness campaign aimed to facilitate girls and boys disclosing sexual abuse.
5 Review the material online regarding the National Office of Child Safety. What steps could be taken to strengthen the ability of this office to meet its priorities and what risks to its work can you identify?

References

Alaggia, R., Collin-Vézina, D. & Lateef, R., 2019, 'Facilitators and barriers to child sexual abuse (CSA) disclosures: A research update', *Trauma, Violence & Abuse*, vol. 20, no. 2, pp. 260–283.

Allardyce, S. & Yates, P., 2018, *Working with children and young people who have displayed harmful sexual behaviour*, Edinburgh: Dunedin.

Anderson, P., Bamblett, M., Bessarab, D., Bromfield, L., Chan, S., Maddock, G., Menzies, K., O'Connell, M., Pearson, G., Walker, R. & Wright, M., 2017, Aboriginal and Torres Strait Islander children and child sexual abuse in institutional settings, Report for the Royal Commission into Institutional Responses to Child Sexual Abuse, Sydney.

Australian Institute of Family Studies, 2015, What is child abuse and neglect? CFCA resource sheet – September 2015, www.aifs.gov.au/cfca/publications/what-child-abuse-and-neglect>, accessed 1 September 2019.

Australian Institute of Health and Welfare, 2018, Family, domestic and sexual violence in Australia 2018. Cat. No. FDV 2, Canberra: AIHW, www.aihw.gov.au/getmedia/d1a8d479-a39a-48c1-bbe2–4b27c7a321e0/aihw-fdv-02.pdf.aspx?inline=true, accessed 1 Sept 2019.

Breaking the silence: Creating the future, addressing child sexual assault in Aboriginal communities in NSW (2006) Report of the Aboriginal Child Sexual Assault Taskforce, Attorney General's Department NSW.

Caffaro, J., 2014, *Sibling abuse trauma: Assessment and intervention strategies for children, families, and adults* (2nd edn), New York: Routledge.

Caldwell, M., 2016, 'Quantifying the decline in juvenile sexual recidivism rates', *Psychology, Public Policy and Law*, vol. 22, no. 4, pp. 414–426.

Carmody, M. & Carrington, K., 2000, 'Preventing sexual violence?', *Australian and New Zealand Journal of Criminology*, vol. 33, no. 3, pp. 341–361.

Cashmore, J. & Shackel, R., 2013, The long-term effects of child sexual abuse, Australian Institute of Family Studies, https://aifs.gov.au/cfca/publications/long-term-effects-child-sexual-abuse, accessed 01 September 2019.

Child Sexual Assault Task Force, 1985, Report of the NSW Child Sexual Assault Task Force, Sydney: Government Printer.

Costello, M. & Backhouse, C., 2019, Avoiding the 3 'Ms': Accurate use of violence, abuse and neglect statistics and research to avoid myths, mistakes and misinformation. A resource for NSW Health Workers, Education Centre Against Violence (ECAV) and Prevention and Response to Violence, Abuse and Neglect (PARVAN) Unit, Sydney: Ministry of Health, NSW Health.

Crabbe, M., 2016, The porn factor, in the picture and 2013, Love and sex in an age of pornography, www.itstimewetalked.com.au/about-us/reality-risk/, accessed 1 September 2019.

El-Murr, A., 2017, Problem sexual behaviours and sexually abusive behaviours in Australian children and young people, Australian Institute of Family Studies, CFCA Paper No. 46, https://apo.org.au/sites/default/files/resource-files/2017/12/apo-nid124376-1135166.pdf, accessed March 2019.

Final Report Royal Commission into Institutional Responses to Child Sexual Abuse, 2017, www.childabuseroyalcommission.gov.au/final-report, accessed March 2019.

Finkelhor, D., Araji, S., Baron, L., Browne, A., Peters, S. & Wyatt, G., 1986, *A sourcebook on child sexual abuse*, Newbury Park, CA: Sage.

Finkelhor, D., 2011, 'Prevalence of child victimization, abuse, crime and violence exposure', in J.W. White, M.P. Koss & A.E. Kazdin (eds), *Violence against women and children: Mapping the terrain*, Washington DC: American Psychologist Association, pp. 20–21.

Hackett, S., Phillips, J., Masson, H. & Balfe, M., 2013, 'Individual, family and abuse characteristics of 700 British child and adolescent sexual abusers', *Child Abuse Review*, vol. 22, pp. 232–245.

Herman, J., 1981, *Father–daughter incest*, Cambridge, MA: Harvard University Press.

Herman, J., 1992, *Trauma and recovery*, New York: Basic Books.

Kaufman, K.L., Mosher, H., Carter, M. & Estes, L., 2006, 'Empirically based situational prevention model for child sexual abuse', in R. Wortley & S. Smallbone (eds), *Situational prevention of child sexual abuse*, Monsey, NY: Criminal Justice Press/Willow Tree Press, pp. 101–144.

Kraus, S. & Russell, B., 2008, 'Early sexual experiences: The role of internet access and sexually explicit material', *CyberPsychology & Behavior*, vol. 11, no. 2, pp. 162–168.

KPMG, 2014, Evaluation of New Street Adolescent Services, Report for NSW Kids and Families, Sydney: NSW Health, www.health.nsw.gov.au/parvan/hsb/Documents/new-street-evaluation-report.pdf, accessed 1 September 2019.

Kreinert, J. & Walsh, J., 2011, 'Sibling sexual abuse: An empirical analysis of offender, victim, and event characteristics in national incident-based reporting system (NIBRS) data, 2000–2007', *Journal of Child Sexual Abuse*, vol. 20, pp. 353–372.

Leach, C., Powell, M. B., Sharman, S. J. & Anglim, J., 2017, 'The relationship between children's age and disclosures of sexual abuse during forensic interviews', *Child Maltreatment*, vol. 22, no. 1, pp. 79–88.

McAlinden, A., 2012, *'Grooming' and the sexual abuse of children: Institutional, internet and familial dimensions*, Oxford: Clarendon Studies in Criminology.

McElvaney, R. & Culhane, M., 2017, 'A Retrospective Analysis of Children's Assessment Reports: What Helps Children Tell?', *Child Abuse Review*, vol. 26, no. 2, pp.103–115.

McKibbin, G., 2017, 'Preventing harmful sexual behaviour and child sexual exploitation for children & young people living in residential care: A scoping review in the Australian context', *Children and Youth Services Review*, vol. 82, pp. 373–382.

Mathews, B., Walsh, K., Dunne, M., Katz, I., Arney, F., Higgins, D., Octoman, O., Parkinson, S. & Bates, S., 2016, Scoping study for research into the prevalence of child abuse in Australia, Sydney: Royal Commission into Institutional Responses to Child Sexual Abuse, p. 2, www.childabuseroyalcommission.gov.au/sites/default/files/research_report_-_scoping_study_for_research_into_prevalence_of_child_sexual_abuse_in_australia_-_causes.pdf, accessed 1 September 2019.

Mitchell A, Patrick K, Heywood W, Blackman P, & Pitts M., 2014, 5th National Survey of Australian Secondary Students and Sexual Health 2013, (ARCSHS Monograph Series No. 97), Australian Research Centre in Sex, Health and Society, Melbourne, Australia, La Trobe University.

Mitra-Kan, T., Newbigin, C. & Hardefeldt, S., 2016, Invisible women, invisible violence: Understanding and improving data on the experiences of domestic and family violence and sexual assault for diverse groups of women: State of knowledge paper, Sydney: ANROWS, http://media.aomx.com/anrows.org.au/DiversityData_151216.pdf, accessed 1 September 2019.

National Principles of Child Safe Organisations, 2018, Australian Human Rights Commission, https://childsafe.humanrights.gov.au/sites/default/files/2019-02/National_Principles_for_Child_Safe_Organisations2019.pdf.

NICE Guideline NG55, 2016, Harmful sexual behaviour among children and young people, www.nice.org.uk/guidance/ng55, accessed 10 October 2019.

NSPCC, 2016, Harmful sexual behavior framework: An evidence-informed operational framework for children and young people displaying sexual behaviours, www.nspcc.org.uk/services-and-resources/research-and-resources/2014/neglect-emotional-abuse-core-info/, accessed 25 August 2019.

Parkinson, P. & Cashmore, J., 2017, Assessing the different dimensions and degrees of risk of child sexual abuse in institutions, report prepared for the Royal Commission into Institutional Responses to Child Sexual Abuse, Sydney.

Personal Safety Survey, Australia 2016, www.abs.gov.au/ausstats/abs@.nsf/PrimaryMainFeatures/4906.0.55.003?OpenDocument.

Peter, J. & Valkenburg, P., 2016, 'Adolescents and pornography: A review of 20 years of research', *The Journal of Sex Research*, vol. 53, pp. 509–531.

Pratt, R. & Tolliday, D., 2018, Understanding the process of CSA disclosure: What does the research tell us? Commissioned report to The Office of the NSW Children's Guardian.

Print, B., 2013, *The good lives model for adolescents who sexually harm*, Brandon, VT: Safer Society Foundation.

Quadara, A., El-Murr, A. & Latham, J., 2017The effects of pornography on children and young people: An evidence scan. (Research Report). Melbourne: Australian Institute of Family Studies.

Sgroi, S., 1982, *Handbook of clinical intervention in child sexual abuse*, New York: The Free Press.

Shlonsky, A., Albers, B., Tolliday, D., Wilson, S., Norvell, J. & Kissinger, L., 2017, Rapid evidence assessment: Current best evidence in the therapeutic treatment of children with problem or harmful sexual behaviours, and children who have sexually offended, Sydney: Royal Commission into Institutional Responses to Child Sexual Abuse.

Smallbone, S. & Wortley, R., 2006, 'Applying situational principles to sexual offenses against children', *Crime Prevention Studies*, vol. 19, pp. 7–35.

Stoltenborgh, M., van Ijzendoorn, M.H., Euser, E.M. & Bakermans-Kranenburg, M., 2011, 'A global perspective on child sexual abuse: Meta-analysis of prevalence around the world', *Child Maltreatment*, vol. 16, no. 2, pp. 79–101.

Tapara, A., 2012, 'Best practice guidelines for health service professionals who receive initial disclosures of sibling sexual abuse', *Kōtuitui: New Zealand Journal of Social Sciences Online*, vol. 7, no. 2, pp. 83–97, https://doi.org/10.1080/1177083X.2012.729513.

Tolliday, D., Laing, L. & Spangaro, J., 2018, *Therapy with harming fathers, victimized children and their mothers after parental sexual assault: Forging enduring safety*, London: Routledge.

Welfare, A., 2008, 'How qualitative research can inform clinical interventions for families recovering from sibling sexual abuse', *Australian and New Zealand Journal of Family Therapy*, vol. 29, no. 3, pp. 139–147.

Ybarra, M. & Thompson, R., 2017, 'Predicting the emergence of sexual violence in adolescence', *Prevention Science*, vol. 192, pp. 1–13.

Chapter 6

Assessment in child protection

Elizabeth Fernandez

Child protection operates in the context of a statutory welfare mandate. In this chapter the landscape of child protection is profiled and the distinctive practice of assessment in protective services is examined. In Australia, State and Territory governments are responsible for protection of children who are abused or at risk of being harmed. Although State governments are involved in the investigation of child protection cases, they usually work in collaboration with a network of non-government organizations in protecting children and young people and providing services to families.

Engagement with this system usually begins with reports or notifications of alleged abuse or neglect that are made to the respective State Department by professionals, members of the community, organizations, parents, relatives or children themselves. Such notifications are assessed to determine whether investigation of the degree of harm and the child's protective needs is warranted (AIHW 2019). The services that follow are then based on the nature of the report; the focus is on whether risk of harm is present, whether the child is in need of protection, whether the family is in need of services and whether specialist assessments are needed to make decisions. If there is no concern about harm but unmet needs are identified, assessment will focus on the nature of need and the help and support services required by the family.

Overall, interventions in child protection can be categorised into four major areas: (a) preventative and supportive services to strengthen family functioning; (b) protective services directed at safeguarding children through a system of notification, (c) investigation and intervention; and (d) out-of-home care through placement in foster care, kin care or adoption. This chapter will outline the nature and scope of assessment at specific decision-making points in the child welfare continuum; provide an overview of the content and context of assessment; describe some of the frameworks and tools used to support consistent and accurate decisions; and, discuss some of the tensions that confront practitioners in this contested area of practice.

As will be discussed, a range of assessments are conducted with children and families who come to the attention of child welfare systems. These include risk and safety assessments to guide child protection decision making and predict recurrence of harm; assessments of child wellbeing while children are in protective care; and, assessments of family needs, strengths and resources to inform service planning for children and families. In many of these contexts the assessment occurs in an involuntary context within a statutory framework. While a major focus will be the assessments within child protection, different types and contexts of assessment in the field of child welfare practice will be discussed.

Nature of assessment

The concept of assessment is defined in various ways and there are different approaches to assessment. Hepworth et al. (2013) define assessment as both a process and a product. Assessment is conceptualised as a

> process occurring between a social worker and client in which information is gathered, analysed and synthesised to provide a complete picture of the client and his or her needs and strengths … a fluid and dynamic process that involves receiving, and analysing and synthesising new information as it emerges during the entire course of a given case.
>
> (Hepworth et al. 2013: 186)

The process of assessment involves weighing up the information/data, identifying critical facts, finding theoretical ideas that illuminate and help to interpret the facts, testing interpretations and making recommendations (Milner, Myers & O'Byrne 2015). Assessment is not an outcome in itself but is intended to inform a case plan and subsequent interventions. Assessment needs to move beyond the assembling of facts. It requires analysis of the information to reach decisions about how to proceed. Assessment entails an analytic process of categorising and synthesising data to develop an informed understanding that progresses to action. Thus, assessment is designed to create a composite picture of the case based on analysis of facts and impressions gleaned from different sources to establish whether the child and family need a specific intervention or service and the formation of a case plan. The term assessment is also used to refer to the written product resulting from the assessment activity. It entails a statement comprising analysis and synthesis of relevant information assembled into a working definition of the difficulties, problems and the factors that create, sustain and mitigate the problem, and encompasses a working hypothesis based on the most current data available (Hepworth et al. 2013).

When a case is screened into the system following a report, an assessment process is set in motion. Pertinent data is gathered through interviews, previous reports and accounts from different sources to determine whether maltreatment has occurred and how serious the risk is for future maltreatment. The focus of the assessment is based on the auspices and mandate of the agency in which the practitioner works and the theoretical orientation and clinical focus of the worker and the team. A worker who is investigating an allegation of maltreatment will pursue a line of inquiry related to risk and safety and potential for recurrence.

Child protective services are directed at the overarching goal of child safety. Working towards the outcome of child safety requires an understanding of the concepts of safety and risk and this includes the best approaches to the assessment of risk at all stages of case management. Within this context, assessment is an interactive process and involves a series of sequential assessments focused on specific objectives of a case and different stages of case management. The process is undertaken in the knowledge that a child's safety needs may change over time (Munro 2008). As a result, caseworkers are often required to revise their assessment at different points in time and for different contexts of decision making. This is because factors that are predictive of maltreatment at the time of investigation and prior to intervention may not be the same as those that are predictive of maltreatment at another point in time, or in another context such as reunification following service.

Milner et al. (2015) suggest major stages of the assessment process in a linear model, recognising that sequential steps may overlap as new information comes to light and re-evaluation occurs.

- Preparation:
  a Identify key informants and sources of information/data
  b Prepare a statement of intent or purpose
  c Prepare a template/schedule for collecting information
  d Document tentative/early explanations
- Collection of information/data
  a Access documents and file data sources, memos, working charts, reports and key informants
  b Identify key informants
  c Check verbal and written data for factual accuracy, unsubstantiated opinion, incongruities
  d Widen data sources if accuracy is doubtful or if there are gaps
- Weighing the information/data
  a Estimate the seriousness and urgency of the situation
  b Identify pervasive themes in the information and prioritise them
  c Weigh risks involved
  d Consult relevant individuals for their input
- Consider how child and family is functioning in the current situation
- Analysing the information/data
  a Identify theoretical perspectives and use them to gain depth of analysis
  b Reach tentative explanations of the situation and consider how they can be tested
  c Develop tentative goals for intervention
  d Check/validate with key informants
- Utilising data analysis
  a List outcomes to be achieved or avoided, and mechanism to monitor outcomes
  b Prepare intervention plan
  c Prepare draft assessment report detailing insights reached, sources of information, recommendation
  d Obtain feedback and revise.

(Milner et al. 2015: 56–58)

While recognising assessment is a staged process, it is important to maintain a reflexive approach. By this, it is meant that practitioners should continually evaluate each of the assessment decisions they make along the way to adjust their approach and consider whether they have approached the case objectively, and not in light of pre-existing assumptions.

Approaches to assessment

Practitioners draw on a range of conceptual approaches to assessment depending on the purpose and context of assessments. Smale and Tuson's (1993) conceptualisation of three approaches to assessment is instructive:

- *The Questioning Model* – the assessor is viewed as the expert with limited input or interpretation from service users
- *The Procedural Model* – assessment focuses on whether the threshold for intervention or service is reached
- *The Exchange Model* – clients are viewed as experts in their strengths and potential. The emphasis here is on exchanging information and facilitating a needs-led assessment driven by goals identified by the client. This model encapsulates principles of partnership and empowerment, emphasising working collaboratively to promote a sense of personal agency (Smale & Tuson 1993 cited in Milner & O'Byrne 2002).

The extent to which power shared between practitioners and clients varies in the different models is outlined. Research evidence suggests working in partnership with families leads to better outcomes for children (Cleaver, Walker & Meadows 2004; Thoburn, Lewis & Shemmings 1995) while Brandon, Bailey and Belderson (2010) remind us about the need to remain alert to the child's perspective and be open to re-evaluating information as new evidence emerges.

Additionally, legislation and agency policies incorporate the notion of interagency partnership into assessment practice. Depending on the purpose and focus assessments this requires portrayals of the situation from the perspective of different actors and agencies ensuring the child is the primary focus (Devaney 2008; Horwarth & Morrison 2011). Assessment needs to be interactive, underpinned by relevant and professional knowledge, and responsive to the service user (Welbourne 2012). Co-operation and collaboration between different agencies dealing with the protective situation is crucial. To this end multidimensional centres/teams are established to provide assessment services under one roof so that children are not required to attend different locations and see different people in the process of validating the abuse.

A range of methods – qualitative and quantitative – are used to approach the assessment task. Qualitative assessment is used as one method to gather information to formulate a comprehensive assessment. A qualitative approach to assessment enables gaining the depth and breadth of information that cannot be achieved by a quantitative approach. It emphasises context and process through collection of detailed information with individuals and families, capturing their meanings, realities and interpretation of events and the contexts in which problems or needs exist. To maximise objectivity, qualitative assessment requires a high level of self-awareness from practitioners to ensure personal beliefs and biases do not influence their clinical judgement and their ability to discern their interpretations from that of the family. Qualitative assessment uses words, ecomaps, genograms and narrative rather than numbers and scores to convey the complexity of the family situation. By contrast, quantitative methods involve the administration of pre-designed measures or surveys that have previously been validated for use in child or family contexts. Important examples in the child context include the Child Behaviour Checklist or Strengths and Difficulties Questionnaire.

The need for best practice in assessment

Assessing children at risk of significant harm requires considerable skill in assembling, analysing, weighing and synthesising relevant information to underpin child protection decisions. The context in which child protection decisions are made may be fraught with uncertainty. Important information may not be readily available, time frames may be compressed, risk may not be immediately apparent, and resources may be limited or rationed. Studies analysing protective care decision making have found wide discrepancies and inconsistency among practitioners on what constitutes abuse and the circumstances warranting removal to protective care. For example, Rossi et al. concluded that the likelihood of a child being removed from its home depended on the individual managing the case (Rossi et al. 1996 cited in Rycus & Hughes 2008). The importance of carefully designed assessment frameworks to enhance the quality and consistency of decisions becomes evident. To respond to these challenges and, to facilitate sound decision making, child welfare agencies have drawn on a range of decision-making frameworks and associated instruments to assess and guide critical decisions related to children who have been maltreated or are at high risk of being maltreated (D'Andrade, Austin & Benton 2008; Gambrill & Shlonsky 2001).

The use of formalised risk assessments systems by child protection agencies is on the increase. Risk assessments are used to make critical decisions during the investigation including whether the child is at immediate risk of maltreatment, what actions might be needed to protect the child during investigation, whether the child needs to be removed to protective care, and in the preparation of an initial case plan to address current needs or concerns. Such considerations of risk and safety are used frequently in child protection. Risk factors are commonly defined as the conditions that threaten the child's safety and safety factors are those that mitigate on offset risk. One type of risk assessment undertaken concerns the determination of imminent risk of harm to a child from maltreatment (Rycus & Hughes 2008). It involves assessing the seriousness of the concern, the duration, the vulnerability of the child, the imminence of harm.

While safety assessments are concerned with determining risk of imminent harm to children, risk assessment focuses on estimating the likelihood of harm from maltreatment in the future as part of the continuum of safety assurance strategies (Hughes & Rycus 2007). Risk assessment is defined as the 'systematic collection of information to determine the degree to which a child is likely to be abused or neglected at some future point in time' (Doueck et al. 1993: 442). Risk assessment is future oriented in that it estimates a child will be maltreated at a later time. It is often used to prioritise cases to determine the level of intervention and the types of services the family receives.

Approaching assessment in child protection

Assessment is an integral part of child protection case management. Meyer (1993: 3) characterises assessment as 'the thinking process that seeks out the meaning of case situations, puts the particulars of the case into some order, and leads to appropriate interventions'. The assessment is designed to identify needs that require intervention to alleviate the problem. Webb (2006) proposes a tripartite conceptualisation of assessment, highlighting the potential interaction of biological, social and psychological factors with respect to the child and family:

- factors related to the individual (e.g. age, developmental stage, cognitive level, home, school, interests, abuse history, resilience)
- factors related to the problem situation (e.g. presence of trauma, life threat, onset and duration of abuse, involvement of significant others)
- factors in support system (nuclear family, extended family, school, peers, neighbourhood, formal service systems).

A crucial question that arises is determining 'who' or 'what' is to be assessed. A series of helpful questions are to be considered by case managers in undertaking the assessment:

- who is the focus of the assessment (child, parents, family unit, neighbourhood)?
- In what sequence should these assessments occur and what protocols are to be followed?
- What assessment tools/standardised measures are be used to support the assessment (genogram, ecomap, decision-making tool ...)?
- How might parents/children/young people be engaged in the assessment?
- How is the assessment to be documented (for case conferences, courts, agency records)?
- What information should be sought from collateral sources (school, medical, legal, other agencies)?
- What knowledge/concepts might be drawn on to analyse the information generated from the assessment (e.g. developmental theory, trauma, loss, ecological systems)? (Fernandez 2016).

The assessment of 'risk' is central to the work of practitioners in child protection. Assessment of risk frequently involves identifying the probability of immediate and long-term harm. In responding to reports of maltreatment, practitioners are required to undertake an assessment of risk. Such an assessment may focus on 'specific harms' or 'imminence' of further harm or potential for 'cumulative harm' in the future (Munro 2008). The complexity of isolating and interpreting risk factors in assessing child physical, sexual and emotional abuse and neglect is the subject of a wide literature (Cooper & Ball 1987; Corby, Shemmings & Wilkins 2012; Crosson-Tower 2008; Doyle & Timms 2014; Lawrence 2004; O'Hagan 2006).

Brearly proposes core questions to be posed in the context of uncertainty and risk:

- What are the various possibilities?
  - How probable are they?
  - How serious are they?
  - How imminent are they?

(Brearly 1982 cited in Cooper & Ball 1987: 77)

Cooper and Ball (1987) apply the work of Brearly to illuminate themes that underpin the analysis of risk in the field of child abuse. They cite specific factors which are said to predispose children to abuse by parents including: a lack of affectional bonds; gross distortion of parenting models; absence of or maladaptive interaction between parents; absent or distorted communication network within the family and between the family and the outside world; dysfunctional styles of coping with stress and disproportionate aggression; absent or exaggerated disciplinary techniques; and, the absence of developmentally appropriate life experience to satisfy children's needs. In addition to these existing 'hazards', extra familial factors are identified that exacerbate risk. These include: deficits in support services; failures of inter-professional communication; deficiencies in monitoring and supervision; and, ambiguous case conference decision making. Exploring the notion of risk further, they highlight the complex mix of 'predisposing' and 'situational hazards' operating within families as well as within agency and worker networks. 'Predisposing' factors include hazards associated with practitioners, managers and the network of agencies that influence case outcomes. Over-sensitivity to the needs and feelings of parents, over-optimism about cooperative work with parents and about the rehabilitation of children with their families, and paucity of alternate care placements are among 'predisposing' attitudes and actions of practitioners considered to impact on appraisal of risk. Identified 'situational hazards' located within the network of agencies, professionals and case managers are also worthy of note:

- Inadequate supervision of the family
- Minimising risks to the child
- Failure to detect warning signs
- Over-optimism about particular families
- Confusion about case responsibility and accountability
- Lack of supervision or excessive supervision
- Knowledge and skill deficits: skills in assessment, skills in communicating and engaging with families and children, knowledge of the impacts of adverse environments on families and children
- Poor inter-professional communication
- Lack of community resources and services.

Families have strengths and competencies that also can be mobilised to mitigate risk and enhance wellbeing. Against the above analysis of existing or anticipated hazards, strengths and protective factors are to be catalogued to underpin child protection assessment and case planning decisions and justify strategies for intervention.

Approaches to risk assessment

Several major approaches to risk assessment are differentiated. The first of these is consensus-based approaches. Consensus-based approaches emphasize a comprehensive assessment of risk based on theories of maltreatment, empirical literature on maltreatment and input from practitioners. A consensus-based approach to risk assessment tends to be multidimensional and draws on several domains. These domains provide a structure for workers' process of information gathering for the purpose of assessment of risk. Some consensus-based instruments use qualitative and/or quantitative approaches to consider relevant areas to be assessed and may code information under categories of high, moderate or low risk based on clinical judgement.

Consensus models rely on the expertise of professionals to identify the level of risk based on the body of knowledge on individual, family and environmental conditions considered to be associated with maltreatment. Consensus models draw on the knowledge base of practitioners and their experience and practice wisdom and are often used in the context of team decision making. Attention is drawn to the potential factors that can negatively impact the objectivity and accuracy of decisions such as personal values and beliefs, preconceptions, selective attention, history and organisational pressure to negotiate compromise (Gambrill & Shlonsky 2000; Munro 1999). Consensus-based frameworks are perceived by some as poorly conceptualised, global and subjective (Rycus & Hughes 2008), and that they are insufficient for differentiating between different dynamics and types of abuse and tend to be overly focused on the characteristics associated with maltreatment rather than what predicts its recurrence (Doyle & Dolan 2002; Wald & Wolverton 1990).

By contrast, actuarial approaches to assessment focus risk assessments on a limited set of case characteristics and use statistical procedures to weigh factors that are predictive of future maltreatment which are then incorporated into a checklist. Practitioners score each factor and scores are summed into overall risk scores for particular types of maltreatment categorising families/parents into low, moderate and high-risk groups. This classification approach often results from the application of an algorithm that combines the information in a mathematically optimal way so as to indicate the probability of different events, e.g., the risk of further abuse. Such methods can often yield predictions that are at least as accurate as professional judgement, but they have to be used with caution because there can be a danger that many cases with certain pre-coded 'risk factors' will be repeatedly classified as higher risk, without scrutiny, e.g., people from certain ethnic, indigenous, geographic or lower socio-economic backgrounds. Questions can, therefore, arise as to the fairness or 'natural justice' associated with purely algorithm-based decision making and this is likely to become an increasing concern as AI technology and big data analyses become more commonplace in child-protection contexts.

Actuarial methods have also come under criticism for their focus on a limited range of factors overlooking case-specific factors, and for the tendency to focus on static factors resulting in passive predictions. Other limitations identified include: the tendency for clients to present themselves in a favourable light (social desirability); failure to capture fluctuating client characteristics and interactions with the environment; their over-emphasis on problems and deficits overlooking individual differences in coping styles and client strengths; inability to make linkages between needs, problems and interventions, and errors and pitfalls in administration (Jordan & Franklin 1995). Actuarial instruments are also criticised for being value driven (Ryan et al. 2005) for limiting wholistic clinical judgement of practitioners and for constraining practice (Gillingham & Humphreys 2010; Hollows 2008).

A third approach involves the use of psychometric instruments or risk assessment tools. Risk assessment tools offer a reliable and systematic approach to assessing risk (Doueck et al. 1993) establishing the severity of abuse (English & Graham 2000) providing a structure for documentation and for determining the type of intervention or services needed (Wald & Wolverton 1990). However, as in research contexts, the quality of any assessment tool is determined by its validity and reliability. Validity refers to the extent to which the measure captures what it is supposed to measure and reliability refers to the consistency of the measure (i.e., does it capture the construct or quality the same way each time?) There are several different indicators of validity and reliability, but Hughes and Rycus (2007) suggest that two essential psychometric qualities are needed in risk assessment involving children and families. The first of these is predictive validity (how well the instrument can predict a particular outcome) and test-re-test reliability which refers to the degree to which the use of the instrument results in consistent decisions by the worker for similar cases over time. Reliable and valid risk assessment tools have been demonstrated to enhance child safety by ensuring resources and strengthening case monitoring for those families at risk of maltreatment recurrence (Baird & Wagner 2000).

Limitations of risk assessment methods

While risk assessment instruments are intended to reduce worker idiosyncrasies, there are a number of shortcomings. A critique of both actuarial and consensus-based approaches is that they focus on interpersonal characteristics of parents to exclusion of community and societal factors that may explain maltreatment. Rycus and Hughes (2008) caution that, while actuarial risk assessment instruments categorise families into probabilities of high and low risk, they may not accurately predict occurrence of maltreatment. A large percentage of families classified as high risk do not go on to re-abuse or neglect their children. Nonetheless, identifying such families enables agencies to effectively allocate resources and services to prevent recurrence of maltreatment and also make relevant case disposition decisions, including alternative responses. They elaborate on how safety and risk assessment instruments can be used in conjunction with clinical judgement to inform child protection decisions.

The reason for this caution is that there are costs for families in being labelled as being at risk but who will not abuse their children. The experience of investigation can be traumatic and may not result in services or having to be labelled as being at risk of maltreatment in order to access services when risk assessments are skewed towards thresholds for service and carry the potential to exacerbate the social exclusion experienced by families in child protection systems (Dare 2015). Recognising the limited ability to predict severe injury or death Reder, Duncan and Lucey (2003) advocate resources be directed towards preventive services for families rather than targeted interventions.

Recognising practitioners are concerned with the clinical responsibility for assessment and case management, and to a lesser extent of prediction Doyle and Dolan (2002), propose an approach which combines the merits of the actuarial approach and the priorities of clinical assessment and management of the case, suggesting that evidence-based frameworks are used flexibly to accommodate case-specific and contextual factors. On a similar note, it is suggested that risk assessments should be combined with assessments of family strengths and needs and information from both assessments integrated into decisions about service interventions (Shlonsky & Wagner 2005).

The items incorporated in an actuarial risk assessment tool are often drawn from professionals in the field and from research evidence and thereafter tested for reliability and validity before being approved as a risk assessment tool. Despite the inclusion of professional perspectives in the construction of instruments, questions are raised as to whether they reflect the full range of information to evaluate situations. In this context, a combination of formal risk assessment tools and professional judgement is advocated (Hollows 2008; Holosko & Ojo 2016).

Ethical considerations in using standardised measures are also to be noted, not the least of which are ensuring practitioners are trained in the use of scoring of the measure and interpretation of results. Multiple methods of assessment are advocated rather than single indicators to ensure the measure is complemented with other sources of information. Consistent with social work values, confidentiality of scores should be maintained to ensure they are not used to negatively label clients and not misused in legal contexts or for purposes for which they were not intended. Client strengths and assets should be captured.

Given the cultural and ethnic diversity of families and children practitioners work with, they need to be attuned to the possibility that instruments may be biased against certain cultural groups and geographies if they are not 'normed' with these populations, leading to mislabelling the attributes of culturally diverse clients (Broadhurst et al. 2010; Fernandez 1991; Jordan & Franklin 1995).

Structured decision-making tools

Another approach to assessment, and widely used, are structured decision-making tools. One example is the Structured Decision-making Tool (SDM) developed by the Children's Research Centre, Wisconsin. Designed to improve decision-making capabilities of child protection practitioners and outcomes for children, the SDM comprises a set of assessment tools to assist in deciding how best to assess families reported to child protection services through to engagement with services. The compendium of instruments comprising the SDM includes the California Family Risk Assessment (CFRA), a 20-item instrument eliciting information on child and family characteristics to estimate the likelihood of recurrence of maltreatment within two years if they do not receive any intervention, classifying assessed families into 'low', 'moderate' and 'high' risk. Other instruments include the SDM Safety Assessment (SA), and the Family Strengths and Needs Assessment (FSNA). The SA involves a 20-item tool which identifies immediate threats to the child with a view to developing a safety plan enabling the child to remain with parents pending fuller investigation, or one requiring the child's placement in protective out-of-home care placement. The FSNA, a consensus-based instrument, prioritises the three most pressing areas of need to be addressed by services based on an assessment of 11 domains of family functioning using a four-point scale from 'strength' to 'severe need'. Other associated SDM tools are the Family Risk Assessment and the Family Strengths and Needs Reassessment, and the Reunification Safety Assessment (Johnson 2004).

The SDM has been implemented in several states in the USA and has been adopted in selected States in Australia (Queensland, South Australia and New South Wales). Drawing on the Queensland experience of its implementation Gillingham and Humphreys (2010) observe that the tools undermined practitioner's development of knowledge and skills in child protection and lacked the capacity to deal with the complexities of family situations.

Assessing child wellbeing and key assessment points

Children and young people who come to the attention of child welfare systems reflect lower levels of wellbeing than their counterparts in the community (Wulczyn et al. 2005; Zimmer & Panko 2007). For example, these disparities are illustrated in the National Survey of Child and Adolescent Wellbeing (NSCAW) of the US Department of Health and Human Services. The importance of holistic ecological assessments of children that incorporate both deficits, strengths and overall wellbeing is stressed (Leslie et al. 2003) as is the importance of multidimensional and multi-system perspectives that capture the interface of the child and the environment as portrayed in the resilience literature (Jenson

& Fraser 2006; Ungar 2004; Wulczyn et al. 2005) and the developing literature on children's subjective wellbeing (Ben-Arieh et al. 2001). Measures of child wellbeing attempt to balance risk and protective factors. However, the approach to assessment should take into account developmental stages and processes and the complexities of socio-emotional aspects of wellbeing, perspectives of multiple informants including children and young people's subjective wellbeing. The broad nature of wellbeing is evident from the range of multidimensional instruments developed and in use (Ben Arieh et al. 2014).

Austin's (2010) overview of selected well validated, widely used instruments to assess child wellbeing in the context of child welfare interventions is instructive. These instruments are identified as reflecting comprehensiveness and are strength based. Among them are the Ages and Stages Questionnaire (ASQ) to assess social and emotional development of young children (Squires, Bricker & Potter 1997); the Social Adjustment Inventory for Children and Adolescents (SAICA) (John, Gammon & Kruger 1999) which focuses on adaptive functioning in the areas of peer relations, activities, academic achievement and family relations. Also included is the Behavioural and Emotional Scale (BERS) (Epstein 2004) which assesses emotional and behavioural strengths, allowing for independent perspectives of child, parent and teacher. Credited with strong psychometric properties, it is found to be useful in pre-referral assessments and in evaluating outcomes of interventions over time. Other widely used instruments to assess children and young people are the Achenbach Child Behaviour Checklist (Achenbach 1991) and the Strengths and Difficulties Questionnaire (Goodman 2001).

An especially useful strength-based and multidimensional tool for child welfare workers engaged with youth transitioning from care is the Ansell-Casey Life Skills Assessment (ACLSA) (Casey Family Programs 2005; Nollan et al. 2000). All four versions tailored to specific ages assess life skills in physical, social and moral development, educational/ vocational development, money, housing and transportation and may be completed by youth and caregivers.

A child wellbeing assessment may be undertaken at particular decision points: removal to protective care; monitoring and review while in placement; in permanence decisions involving reunification or guardianship and adoption, and transition from care. At a macro level, individual wellbeing assessment can enable aggregation of outcome to inform program and policy development. For example, there are multiple assessments needed to underpin decisions that follow from court's determination to place a child in out-of-home care. These include such questions as: What is the most appropriate placement: with relatives, non-relatives, or residential care? What considerations apply in matching children's needs to attributes of the carer and foster home? How will issues of contact with the birth family be managed? Is reunification with the birth family to be considered?

Children's trajectories in care may be punctuated with a number of feelings, reactions and disappointments arising from separation and entry to care and adjusting to new and sometimes multiple care environments. Further challenges arise from maintaining a child's sense of identity, security and continuity in the context of his/her care being shared between foster carers and birth parents, and managing various forms of change inherent in placement breakdowns, school changes, transitions effected through reunification, or leaving care (Driscoll 2018; Fernandez 2019; Sebba et al. 2016; Tarren-Sweeny & Hazell 2006). Whatever the nature of change, effective communication, assessment and planning are needed in responding to the needs of children and carers, while engaging professionals and agencies, involved effectively as integral members of the therapeutic team.

The implementation of a permanency framework imposes a particular set of case planning expectations that have implications for assessment in the context of protective care. There are also pressures to fine tune out-of-home care to respond to the needs of particular children such as children who are exposed to substance abuse, children who are HIV-positive, children with disabilities, children of incarcerated parents, children of refugees and youth who are gay or lesbian.

The UK Looking After Children Initiative designed to facilitate assessment and track outcomes in the domains of health, education, emotional and behavioural development, identity, family and social relationships, self-care and self-presentation (Ward 1996) offers a potential framework for guiding assessment and care planning in out-of-home care. Through the establishment of the Looking After Children project, a collaboration of Barnardo's Australia and University of New South Wales, a guided practice case management system, MyStory, is implemented in out-of-home care programs of Barnardo's and selected non-government agencies to provide practitioners, carers and families a streamlined and guided practice approach to assessing outcomes through all stages of the child's care trajectory, ensuring the child's voice is at the centre of decisions that affect their lives.

Family assessment

A prime purpose of a risk assessment is to implement a process for determining which cases receive which interventions and services, serving as a strategy to target limited resources to the neediest (Rycus & Hughes 2008). In clarifying the purpose of assessing risk and safety, a distinction is made between risk assessment and family assessment. Rycus and Hughes offer this clarification 'while risk assessment is designed to accurately estimate the likelihood of future incidents of maltreatment, the purpose of family assessment is to explore, in considerable depth, the unique complex of developmental and ecological factors in each family and their environment that may contribute to or mitigate maltreatment" (Rycus & Hughes 2003: 11 cited in Austin 2010).

Families who are served by agencies present with a range of needs, resources and strengths. Many agencies have developed or adapted frameworks or protocols to carry out comprehensive family assessment to formulate a case plan. The focus and depth of the assessment is determined by purpose and context of decisions. A major challenge in initial assessments involves determinations about child removal and placement in out-of-home care in order to ensure their safety. Awareness of the traumatic impact of separation strategies to maintain the child safely in their own families is prioritised in the continuum of child welfare interventions.

It is recognised the child maltreatment reflects complex personal, familial, environmental and social factors that interact to undermine families' ability to care for their children. It is being increasingly recognised that the large number of reports coming to the attention of Statutory Child Welfare Departments are about wider child and family needs and that investigative and child rescue approaches are less optimal responses (Garbarino & Barry 1997; Scott 2009). Several commentators highlight the relationship between poverty, abuse and neglect and the disproportionate numbers of families from disadvantaged socio-economic backgrounds who become mired in the child protection system (Parton, Thorpe & Wattam 1997; Pelton 2015; Welbourne 2012). Gil (1979) draws attention to the pervasive pressures inherent in the deprivations of poverty that generate stress for economically disadvantaged families, creating the triggering context in which violence occurs. The structure of many disadvantaged families characterised by sole parenthood, female-headed households, and isolation from social supports and social networks that potentially offer respite and parenting support, further compound children's vulnerability to neglect and abuse (Ghate & Hazel 2002).

Initiatives that emphasise prevention of abuse and enhancement of parenting potential to improve the wellbeing of vulnerable children have emerged. In the United Kingdom emphasis on the principle of partnership with parents and emergence of the conceptualization of children in need (Little, Axford & Morphet 2004; Ward & Rose 2002), and development of family preservation services in the United States have prompted a shift from the exclusive focus on child removal to greater emphasis on family support and shared care. Parallel developments are evident in Australian Child Welfare reflected in models of family-based services (Wise 2017). The clientele of family support services involve children and families who are child protection referrals, as well as families whose children who are judged to be 'in need', requiring services to be addressed before their situation deteriorates to the level of a child protection concern. Families who are served by agencies present with a range of needs, resources and strengths.

In order to safeguard children in their own homes, practitioners must identify the resources, strengths and protective capacities in their immediate family, extended family and community that can be mobilised to mitigate threats to safety and stabilise the family situation. Many agencies have developed or adapted frameworks or protocols to carry out comprehensive family assessments to formulate a case plan. The focus and depth of the assessment is determined by purpose and context of decisions.

In family assessment, the focus is on assembling, analysing and weighing of information to capture key factors affecting a child's safety and wellbeing and parental needs, difficulties and protective capacities that impinge on children's wellbeing. The purpose of assessment is to represent the family in its needs, difficulties and struggles for resources, including a justification for treating the situation as a problem and the extent to which it falls within the agency's remit to deal with it. There are a number of contexts and key points in the life of a case when family assessments are undertaken: at initial contact with the family support agencies; and at several decision-making stages when protective care is needed such as visitation and contact during placement, reunification or adoption, and transition to independent living. Other assessment points might include reviews or changes in case plan.

Families typically come to the attention of agencies when problems or difficulties are experienced or identified. Resultantly, assessments tend to focus on problems and deficits leading to an overemphasis on pathology and dysfunction at the expense of strengths, abilities and achievements. Families have strengths and competencies that also can be mobilised to mitigate risk and enhance wellbeing. Against anticipated hazards, strengths and protective factors are to be catalogued to underpin assessment and case planning decisions and strategies for intervention. Emphasising strengths and empowerment in the assessment process, Cowger (1992) advocates

- prioritising the family's understanding of the situation and eliciting client goals and their perception of obstacles and challenges.
- assessing personal and environmental strengths at multiple levels.

Several approaches are used in conducting family assessments, including interviews, observation and self-report. The assessment may elicit or integrate perspectives of multiple actors – perspectives from children and family members, school and other practitioners involved in the case. The assessment process may involve sequential stages and functions: initial screening at intake; identification of need or problem and level of severity; planning and matching services with needs or problems; and monitoring progress and evaluating outcomes (Austin 2010).

A number of tools may be used as a means of understanding the family situation. For example, ecomaps can be used to gain information about the family's relationship with the environment. It enables focus on the social context of families and interactions between the family and society. This mapping technique is frequently used with families with language barriers and is visually oriented. The Genogram is used to map family structure, family history and relationships. The Social Support Networks map explores the structure and quality of the family's interconnected relationships and social support.

There has been an expanding empirical and clinical literature on family assessment with the advent of child protection policies and family preservation and family support initiatives in the US, UK and Australia. Concomitantly, there have been initiatives in the development of family assessment frameworks for use in these child welfare contexts. In response to the shortcomings of deficit-based assessment models, child welfare systems have undergone a paradigm shift in the direction of incorporating strengths and assets in the holistic assessment of children and families. Grounded in family systems theories and the developmental literature, they focus on relevant components of family functioning, parenting and social support.

Family assessment frameworks that comprehensively address major domains of family functioning validated for specific stage of assessment and relevant for use in child welfare settings are reviewed by Austin (2010). Austin's review of family assessment frameworks identifies selected instruments developed in the US for child welfare systems:

- The North Carolina Family Assessment Scale (NCFAS) and the NCFAS-R for reunification.
- The Family Assessment Form (FAF)
- The Darlington Family Assessment System
- The Clinical Assessment Package for Assessing Clients' Risks and Strengths (CASPARS).

The *NCFAS* (Reed-Ashcraft, Kirk & Fraser 2001) is a 39-item instrument designed to assist preservation services to assess family functioning at intake and case closure and capture measurable change demonstrated during the service period. The NCFAS makes provision for rating on a 6-point scale ranging from 'clear strength' to 'serious problems' on five domains: (1) environment, (2) parental capabilities, (3) family interactions, (4) family safety and (5) child wellbeing. Internal consistency and construct validity have been established for the instrument. To facilitate reunification decision making in programs using family preservation services to reunify children placed in out-of-home care with their families, the NCFAS for Reunification (NCFAS-R) (Reed-Ashcraft et al. 2001) has been developed. The instrument assesses family functioning on seven domains adding two new domains to the original five domains of NCFAS, namely Caregiver/Child Ambivalence and Readiness for Reunification using the same 6-point scale. Change scores are indicative of the degree of change achieved during the service period from the intake to the point of reunification or case closure. Internal consistency and construct validity have been established for this measure with respect to success or failure of reunification. The NCFAS and NCFAS-R are favoured for their strength-based orientation and extensive testing and validation with child welfare populations.

For many children in care, reunification is a goal. However, decisions about reunification are based on a comprehensive family assessment and reassessment of risk and the families' protective capacities to ensure any safety threats are reduced. Reunification entails several challenges for families arising from the disruptions and discontinuities from the child's placement in care and the re-establishment of relationships. There is the dual focus of assessing readiness for reunification and the supports and services needed by the family to sustain child safety.

The *Family Assessment Form (FAF)* has an ecological focus offering a structured method for identifying the strengths and concerns of families in five substantive areas (1) Environment, (2) Caregivers, (3) Interactions, (4) Developmental stimulation to children, (5) Support available to the family. It captures caregiver characteristics interactions within family subsystems and transactions of the family with the larger environment and is particularly useful in contexts where workers do not have a lengthy assessment period and when families need help for pressing problems. The FAF has been developed as a practice tool to enhance assessment procedures. It is designed to help caseworkers to develop service plans for families and monitor service outcomes systematically. It requires workers to undertake and structure family assessments in the complex atmosphere of the family home. The five-point rating scale and summary facilitates identification of family strengths from which to build problem solving and coping abilities while paying attention to areas of concern. Internal consistency and interrater reliability have been established (Austin 2010; McCrosky & Meezan 1997).

The Clinical Assessment Package for Assessing Clients' Risks and Strengths (CASPARS) (Gilgun 1999) is also seen as promising for its applicability to child welfare populations. It assesses strengths and risks in five domains: emotional expressiveness, family relationships, family embeddedness in the community, peer relationships and sexuality. Internal consistency, interrater reliability and construct validity are considered strong.

To complement the various family assessment frameworks, specialised instruments or standardised measures to assess parenting practices and behaviours are used in assessments of parenting of families who come to the attention of child welfare systems. Developed as a tool for child protective service practitioners, the Child Abuse Potential Inventory (CAPI) is one of them. It is designed as a self-report tool to identify parents who are most likely to be at risk for child maltreatment by assessing parenting practices and social interactions and has been subject to substantial psychometric evaluation. Programs have used the measure in pre- and post-interventions to measure change (Milner 1994).

Another measure, the Parenting Stress Index (PSI) (Abidin 1995), incorporates comprehensive self-report items which assess parenting in parent- and child-related domains. For rapid assessment, a 36-item short form is also available. Psychometric evaluations ascribe high internal consistency, construct validity and good test–retest reliability. A psychometrically validated measure designed to comprehensively assess a family's basic needs in addition to patterns of social interaction and parenting is the Home Observation for Measurement of Environment (HOME). Versions of the HOME tailored to age-specific populations (e.g. families with infants and toddlers; children in middle childhood) and versions adapted to minority and special needs populations are available.

In general, these instruments are intended to complement rather than replace professional judgement and enhance the assessment process by providing a structure for gathering and assembling information and ensuring specific aspects of family assessment are addressed. The results of such assessments can be used in different contexts including referral to services, court reports, monitoring clients and documenting child and family outcomes for supervision and agencies (Austin 2010).

In the UK, the Framework for the Assessment of Children in Need and their Families (FACN) (Department of Health 2000), has been designed to provide a systematic and consistent approach to assessment of families of all children in need. Its distinctive feature is its holistic focus on the complex interrelationships between three domains of the assessment 'triangle': children's developmental outcomes; the capacity of parents to respond appropriately to their needs; and the impact of factors within their family and broader environment, as well as the delicate balance of risk and protective factors in each of these domains. Implicit in this framework is a broadening of focus from a narrow concentration on risk and incidents of harm to a holistic and comprehensive assessment of the manner in which parenting capacity and factors in the wider environment affect children's developmental needs. The UK Framework for Assessment for Children in need and their families shifts the focus of assessment away from identifying deficits to assessing both strengths and difficulties to counter the tendency towards pathologizing families. It promotes a broad-based approach to assessment of need to facilitate responsive service and better sharing of information between agencies. Encompassing three domains, it focuses on children's needs (health, emotional development, relationships, selfcare, safety), parenting capacity (ability to provide basic care, emotional warmth, stimulation, guidance and boundaries) and environment (family history, housing, employment, income, community resources) (Seden, 2002; Ward & Rose 2002). The case management system Supporting Children and Responding to Families (SCARF), an Australian adaptation of the UK Assessment framework currently used in family support services of Barnardo's Australia and selected non-government agencies (Wise 2001), provides a strength-based, ecologically orientated, participatory approach with built-in mechanisms to engage parents and older children in the assessment process.

The UK Common Assessment Framework (CAF), introduced later, advances on the earlier Framework to facilitate linkage of families to a continuum of services based on level and complexity of needs. However, these frameworks are not without challenges. While the FACN provides adequate prompts to ensure comprehensive coverage of issues, it offers little guidance on how individual factors on each domain or dimension of the triangle should be weighted and integrated into an analytical account of the child's wellbeing and the standard of caregiving (Milner et al. 2015; Welbourne 2012). Calder and Hackett (2003), in particular, express concerns about the viability of assessing risk of physical and sexual abuse using the FACN, given its emphasis on identifying needs and strengths, the concern being that focus on strengths may obscure the workers' identification of risk. Other critical reviews of these frameworks and the guidance accompanying them have emphasised the need to balance procedural demands with professional judgement and flexibility (Munro 2011).

A further framework, *Signs of Safety*, was based on the work of Turnell and Edwards (1999) who propose a safety assessment process that captures concerns and safety issues incorporating perspectives of professionals and family members. The focus is on assessment of measurable indicators for the family to stay together and in this regard has both an assessment and interventive focus.

Issues for practice

An ecological approach to assessment

While many parental and family characteristics are associated with abuse and neglect including mental illness, substance use, domestic violence, social isolation and previous history of maltreatment (although not all adults who have been maltreated go on to abuse their children), the correlates of maltreatment are complex and are best understood from an ecological perspective. Social conditions such as poverty, deprivation, dangerous neighbourhoods, lack of support and social services, and societal tolerance of interpersonal violence are closely associated with maltreatment and constitute risk factors. As a result, there is some concern that many assessments focus narrowly on providing evidence of abuse and neglect, with little attention to ongoing needs of children and families.

For this reason, an ecological approach (Bronfenbrenner 1979) offers an effective framework for understanding ways in which risk and protective factors interact. Such an approach would require assessment of multiple domains including the child, parents and family unit at the micro level; the interactions between the family and systems including school, health and welfare agencies, and the capturing of environmental dimensions of housing, income security and social support that directly or indirectly influence parents and children. At the macro level, prevailing societal values, social policies, statutory systems and cultural contexts that impact micro and meso systems need to be factored in. Conducting assessments that utilise an ecological framework facilitates holistic assessment that captures the interaction of child, family and the outside world. Ecological assessments engage with the complexity of family situations and prompt the practitioner to draw on theories relevant to each of the systems involved – micro, meso and macro. Implied here is a broadening of focus from a narrow concentration on risk and incidents of harm to a holistic and comprehensive assessment of the manner in which parenting capacity and factors in the wider environment impact on children's developmental needs and wellbeing. The dual focus on parenting capacity and environmental determinants enhances the potential to draw on a wider repertoire of interventions in responding to the needs of parents and children.

Environment of risk assessment

Assessment in child protection involves operating in an environment of uncertainty where information is limited. For this reason, there have been critical discourses surrounding the almost default referral to risk assessment in child protection (Gillingham & Humphreys 2010; Kemshall 2002; Parton 2014; Webb 2006) as well as risk assessment tools, with concerns being raised about their ability to resolve issues of ambiguity and uncertainty and address risk elimination. Munro (2011) elaborates on the uncertainty inherent in the work arising from the ambiguity of the signs and symptoms of abuse and neglect and the possibility of alternative 'benign' explanations, and the challenges of making predictions of children's future safety. In this context she comments:

> The big problem for society (and consequently professionals) is establishing a realistic expectation of professionals' ability to predict the future and manage risk of harm to children and young people. Even when it is ascertained that abuse and neglect has occurred, there are difficult decisions to make about whether the parents can be helped to keep children safe from harm or whether the child needs to be removed. Such decisions involve making predictions about likely future harm and are so fallible. It may be judged highly unlikely that the child will be re abused but low probability events happen. This does not in itself indicate flaws in the professional reasoning. The ideal would be if risk management could eradicate risk but this is not possible; it can only reduce the probability of harm. It is important to be aware how much hindsight distorts our judgement about predictability of an adverse outcome. Once we know an outcome was tragic, we look backwards from it and it seems clear which assessments were critical in leading to that outcome.
>
> (Munro 2011: 18)

Further constraints of risk assessment as a predictor of maltreatment recurrence arises from the state of knowledge about the predictors of child maltreatment. Such factors continue to remain a focus of research, so that there may be value in practitioners and managers maintaining awareness of these developments through ongoing professional development activities. What is also needed is less reliance on selective uses of research evidence as well as over-reliance on expert assessments to validate preferred decisions, and the narrow focus of such assessments to the exclusion of relevant social factors (Milner et al. 2015).

In support of these concerns, researchers have identified a number of pitfalls and common errors in practitioners' decision making. These include disregarding important information, over-optimism in their ability to predict events, and valuing and prioritising certain sources of evidence over others. Scepticism over new information when it conflicts with their initial view of a family and being slow to reassess their judgements (Munro 1999), and difficulties in weighing different factors relevant to the decision (Helm 2010) are further concerns noted. Other errors of reasoning such as the tendency to reach explanations hurriedly and seeking evidence to confirm their preferred views and to ignore or not seek information that challenges early views, referred to as 'confirmatory bias' are also highlighted (Munro 2008; Plous 1993; Brandon, Bailey & Belderson 2010). For example, the work of Brandon et al. (2010) highlights ways in which confirmation bias can result in practitioners concluding a case does meet the threshold for child protection intervention, or conversely may result in families being subject to investigation and coercive intervention through failure to take on board evidence that challenges initial beliefs.

When conducting risk assessment, a range of different types of information may emerge. Some information will indicate deficits in the family and there will also be evidence of areas of strength or resilience. In many cases, evidence concerning family deficits may overshadow the positive aspects of the family and so it is important that assessments take a considered and balanced approach that tries to capture both of these aspects (Helm 2010). A tendency to over-emphasise the negative aspects of the family (negative halo effect) and to impute blame to individuals rather than their circumstances are recognised biases in psychological research (the fundamental attribution error). At all stages, practitioners should endeavour to take a reflective and systematic approach that is thorough in its appraisal of information, and also be mindful of their own potential biases or preconceptions.

Responding to diversity

The assessment process needs to be sensitive to variations in client characteristics that may influence how assessments are conducted and what recommendations might follow. Important issues to consider are economic class, race, culture, gender and sexual orientation or identity. These characteristics share the common quality of locating some clients outside the mainstream society where services, communication and policies may operate on the assumption that people do not possess the characteristics that are central to their identity. Such factors can render them vulnerable to social exclusion, prejudice and oppressive and discriminatory practice. Examples can include services that are not attuned to cultural sensitivities, which have no language services, or which exclude people from certain opportunities or decisions because of the structure of their family or sexual identity. In a diverse multicultural society, the importance of taking into account cultural differences in norms and power differentials should be emphasised. Already, there is an extensive empirically derived literature on poverty and its impact on children and families in child welfare systems that should sensitise practitioners to ways of understanding families who parent in poor environments and their experience of child welfare systems (Bywaters et al. 2015; Ghate & Hazel 2002; Jack & Gill 2010; Pelton 2015). A less extensive, but informative literature is also available concerning practice involving culturally diverse groups, including people from refugee backgrounds, particular religious groups, and those from Indigenous backgrounds (Laird & Tedam 2019).

Considerations based on client gender are also important. In child protection contexts, the clients are statistically more likely to be women and many of these will be single parents; victims of domestic violence; those who have misused drugs or alcohol and are experiencing poverty and who are living in marginal housing and disadvantaged neighbourhoods. There is a tendency in assessments to locate the source of problems of neglect and abuse within the behaviour of individual mothers because fathers, often the perpetrators of domestic violence, are absent and not involved within the assessment (Ferguson 2011). For this reason, opportunities to include men and fathers in assessment processes should be sought wherever possible. It is thought that father inclusive assessment will be an important step in the direction of moving beyond the focus on holding mothers solely responsible for children's outcomes (Campbell et al. 2015; Douglas & Walsh 2010; Featherstone 2009; Scourfield 2001).

There are also significant issues of culturally appropriate assessment and case management in the context of modern multicultural societies. The clientele of child welfare are often multicultural and these people will differ in their family structure, child rearing patterns, communication, and parenting goals. Culturally competent assessment therefore requires seeking out information and understanding of ways that cultural differences might surface in the assessment process and whether there are any biases evident in the process. Awareness that our culture shapes our world views and interactions with people and our perception of the world is important and so, in some child protection contexts, culture awareness training may play a significant role in minimising the intrusion of practitioners' cultural orientation and biases into the assessment process.

In countries such as Australia and Canada, cultural awareness is particularly important in relation to work involving Aboriginal or Indigenous people. In such contexts, assessment and case management needs to be more culturally sensitive to understand the values of Aboriginal societies, particularly in relation to their family structure and child-rearing practices and to recognise the entrenched problems of poverty, racism and social exclusion that contribute to their continuing over-representation in child protection and out-of-home care systems. In Australia, one of the central considerations is compliance with the Aboriginal Child Placement Principle that is enshrined in State legislation. This requires practitioners to identify and support placements with the child's extended family in the interests of their wellbeing and identity needs. For example, in the context of reunification assessments there is a need to take into account realities of domestic violence, substance abuse, poverty intergenerational trauma, and other factors that capture the challenges of Aboriginal living as a minority in a larger culture. It is important that practitioners recognise these complex circumstances that relate to systemic issues that cannot be addressed through individual behavioural change. As noted by Megan Davis:

> When mums and dads are given unrealistic, unachievable goals in order to have their children or grandchildren restored to them, this has historical resonance. Some of the restoration goals are incontrovertibly impossible to be achieved. Some of these practices demonstrate concrete examples of institutional racism. The system is replete with practice that renders our people voiceless and powerless.
>
> (Davis 2019)

Using knowledge in assessment

In carrying out assessments in child protection, practitioners are required to draw on and apply a wide range of knowledge to complex situations which are fraught with emotion and risk. In such situations, a core skill integral to the assessment process is analysis (Dalzell & Sawyer 2007), which has been found to be frequently lacking in assessments. Analytical assessments require:

- A sound knowledge of child development, parenting capacity and the impact of trauma and adversity in the social environment
- An ability to apply knowledge critically to understand each situation
- An organisational environment that supports such activity with resources.(Helm 2010)

The expectation that assessments will be evidence based highlights the significant role that knowledge, theory and research play in assessments in shaping the questions asked, the information sought and the hypothesis formulated. For example, as other chapters in this volume indicate, the field of child welfare needs to be cognisant of the concepts of developmental theory of attachment, loss, trauma, coping, interpersonal relationships, risk, and resilience and these concepts are to be used judiciously rather than selectively. Walsh (2006) cautions that theories used selectively and rigidly can oversimplify the problem and objectify the client and be less mindful of the subjective (and often) complex experiences that have shaped the client's situation. A danger is that theories and frameworks may be applied inappropriately to individual families that are different from the populations on which they were tested. Concentration on particular concepts or frameworks may obscure other important factors in the case and deter the practitioner from drawing on emerging new knowledge and interventions (Taylor 2004; Taylor & White 2006). It is sometimes assumed that all problems that arise in children are due to poor attachment relationships when there are other more complex issues relating to trauma that more validly account for the young person's experiences and outcomes (Whitt-Whoosley, Eslinger & Sprang 2018).

As previously discussed, child welfare and associated court decision making can often take a very individualistic orientation that obscures the structural factors and the economic, social and political contexts in which problems of inadequate parenting and childcare are identified and defined. In such contexts, there is a need to incorporate perspectives that challenge injustice and inequalities (Callahan & Lumb 1995; Healy 2014; Welbourne 2012) to show how individual action and circumstances are embedded in broader socio-political systems. Examples include people's socio-economic status, their cultural background, geography and access to transport and services. Moreover, at an individual level, there is a need to apply caution when applying developmental theories because these often have a strong Eurocentric bias and are derived from research often based on middle-class and often Caucasian populations. Although such knowledge may be applicable to other modern cultures (e.g., family structures in many Asian or Middle Eastern countries), they may be less applicable for children raised in families whose structure, parenting practices and expectations are different and which involve different parenting practices (Fernandez 1991; Laird & Tedam 2019; Lee & Fernandez 2019; Robinson 2007). A particular example of relevance to Australia is the strong role of relatives in the care of Indigenous children, which may be judged by some Western observers to have reduced the responsibility of parents or impacted attachment.

In other words, without a cross-cultural perspective, family assessments are likely to be biased towards deficits overlooking strengths as practitioners assess those who do not fit into the dominant developmental norms. In relation to indigenous children in particular, it is important to apply greater cultural sensitivity needed to understand the values of Aboriginal societies with respect to family structure and child-rearing practices and recognise the entrenched problems of poverty, racism and social exclusion that contribute to their continuing over-representation in child protection and out-of-home care systems. In particular, the Aboriginal Child Placement Principle entrenched in legislation will require case managers to identify and support placements with the child's extended family. There are also broader issues of culture-appropriate case management in the context of a multicultural society.

Adopting a child-centred approach

It is also important that children's views are taken into account, especially given that many decisions affect children's future and well-being. Practitioners are criticised for the weight attached to parental characteristics and the limited emphasis on the child's perspective. In the context of both risk or need assessments or care planning, the centrality of the child must be recognised. The importance of providing children with clear explanations of events in child protection situations that impact on them, eliciting their views in the assessment process, and providing opportunities for them to express their wishes is underlined (Alderson 2000; Holland 2000; Turney et al. 2011). The rights of children to participate in assessment is enshrined in Article 12 of the UNCROC (1989) which enjoins States Parties to

> assure to the child who is capable of forming his or her own views the right to express those views freely in all matters affecting the child, the views of the child being given due weight in accordance with the age and maturity of the child.

These principles/injunctions are translated into practice in specific legislation and assessment frameworks. For example, the UK Common Assessment Framework (CAF) (Department of Health 2000) in its guidance requires practitioners to involve children and families in assessments (Department of Education and Skills 2006). The extent to which this is implemented, however, is questioned (Cleaver, Walker & Meadows 2004; Gilligan & Manby 2008; Reder & Duncan 2003) acknowledging the need for organisational support and resources to achieve this.

In carrying out assessments involving children, a trusting relationship with the caregiver will be vital to accessing and engaging with the child. Depending on the child's level of development, he/she may be limited in communicating their needs, concerns, strengths and coping methods (Aldgate et al. 2006). Interviews with collateral contacts such as parents, family members, teachers may be needed to develop a comprehensive assessment, though these can be subject to distortions and biases. Ascertaining wishes and feelings of the child to assess their understanding of the situation with minimum distress is thus crucial (Holland 2001), as is also eliciting information from caregivers to determine wider social and environmental factors that impact on them.

Engaging parents

Engaging parents is an important part of parenting assessments. Parents may be wary of engaging with child welfare practitioners because of prior experiences of the child welfare system. Parents' reluctance to cooperate with the assessment process and disclose their difficulties is sometimes construed as an indicator of risk. Shemmings and Shemmings (1996) draw on their research to advocate the benefits of parental participation for the family and professionals involved, arguing that parents are more likely to be committed to implementing case plans they have contributed to, and value being trusted and given the opportunity to express their views. With mounting pressure to respond to child protection referrals, family support services have become a pathway for families to access needed services, though at times in an involuntary relationship. The process of engagement and working with families can often be influenced by the context of referral, posing challenges in relationship building (Forrester et al. 2008). Research has shown that parental engagement is realised when approaches are less coercive and when power is shared with them, and when they experience power and choice (Dumbrill 2006; Platt 2012; Thorpe 2008). Platt's (2012) model for understanding the behavioural, attitudinal and relational components of parental engagement derived from an ecological approach is useful here.

References

Abidin, R.R., 1995, *Parenting Stress Index* – Manual (3rd edn), Odessa, FL: Psychological Assessment Resources.

Achenbach, T.M., 1991, 'Manual for the youth self-report and 1991 profile, Burlington, VT', *Department of Psychiatry and Human Development*, vol. 20, pp. 135–147.

Australian Institute of Health and Welfare, 2019, Child protection Australia: 2017–18. Child welfare series no. 70. Cat. no. CWS 65. Canberra: AIHW.

Alderson, P., 2000, *Young children's rights*, London: Jessica Kingsley.

Aldgate, J., Jones, D.P.H., Rose, W. & Jeffrey, D., 2006, *The developing world of the child*, London: Jessica Kingsley.

Austin, M.J. (ed.), 2010, *Evidence for child welfare practice*, London and New York: Routledge.
Baird, C. & Wagner, D., 2000, 'The relative validity of actuarial and consensus-based risk assessment systems', *Children & Youth Services Review*, vol. 1, no. 1, pp. 85–116.
Ben-Arieh, A., Kaufman, N.H., Andrews, A.B., Goerge, R.M., Lee, B.J. & Aber, J.L., 2001, *Measuring and monitoring children's well-being*, Dordrecht: Kluwer Academic.
Brandon, M., Bailey, S. & Belderson, P., 2010, Building on the Learning from Serious Case Reviews: A Two-Year Analysis of Child Protection Database Notifications 2007–2009, DFE-RR-040, London: Department for Education, University of East Anglia.
Broadhurst, K., Hall, C., Wastell, D., White, S. & Pithouse, A., 2010, 'Risk instrumentalism and the human project in social work: Identifying the informal logics of risk assessment in children's statutory services', *British Journal of Social Work*, vol. 40, pp. 1046–1064.
Bronfenbrenner, U., 1979, *The ecology of human development*. Cambridge, MA: Harvard University Press.
Bywaters, P., Brady, G., Sparks, T., Bos, E., Bunting, L., Daniel, B., Featherstone, B., Morris, K. & Scourfield, J., 2015, 'Exploring inequities in child welfare and child protection services: explaining the "inverse intervention law"', *Children & Youth Services Review*, vol. 57, pp. 98–105.
Calder, M.C. & Hackett, S. (eds), 2003, *Assessment in childcare: Using and developing frameworks for practice*, Lyme Regis, UK: Russell House.
Callahan, M. & Lumb, C., 1995, 'My cheque and my children: The long way to empowerment', *Child Welfare*, vol. LXXIV, no. 3, pp 795–817.
Campbell, C., Howard. D., Rayford, B. & Gordon, D., 2015, 'Fathers matter: Involving and engaging fathers in the child welfare system process', *Children & Youth Services Review*, vol. 53, pp. 84–91.
Casey Family Programs, 2005, *Ansell-Casey Life Skills Assessments (ACLSA)*.
Cleaver, H., Walker, S. & Meadows, P., 2004, *Assessing Children's Needs and Circumstances: The Impact of the Assessment Framework*, London: Jessica Kingsley.
Cooper, D.M. & Ball, D., 1987, *Social Work and Child Abuse*, Macmillan Education
Corby, B., Shemmings, D. & Wilkins, D., 2012, *Child abuse: An evidence base for confident practice*, Maidenhead, UK: Open University Press.
Cowger, C.D., 1992, 'Assessment of client strengths', in D. Saleeby (ed.), *The strengths perspective*, New York: Longman.
Crosson-Tower, C., 2008, *Understanding child abuse and neglect*, Boston, MA: Pearson Education.
D'Andrade, A., Austin, M.J. & Benton, A., 2008, 'Risk and safety assessment in child welfare', *Journal of Evidence-Based Social Work*, vol. 5, no. 1–2, pp. 31–56.
Dalzell, R. & Sawyer, E., 2007, *Putting analysis into assessment: Undertaking assessments of need*, London: National Children's Bureau.
Dare, T., 2015, 'The ethics of predictive risk modelling', in L. Waterhouse & J. McGhee (eds), *Challenging child protection: New directions in safeguarding*, London: Jessica Kingsley.
Davis, M., 2019, Family is culture: Independent review of Aboriginal children in OOHC, Sydney, NSW Government.
Department for Education and Skills, 2006, *The common assessment framework for children and young people: Practitioners' guide*, London, TSO.
Department of Health, 2000, *Framework for the assessment of children in need and their families*, London: HMSO.
Devaney, J., 2008, 'Inter-professional working in child protection with families with long-term and complex needs', *Child Abuse Review*, vol. 17, pp. 242–261.
Doueck, H.J., English, D.J., DePanfilis, D. & Moote G.T., 1993, 'Decision-making in child protective services: A comparison of selected risk assessment systems', *Child Welfare*, vol. 72, no. 5, pp. 441–452.
Douglas, H. & Walsh, T., 2010, 'Mothers and the child protection system', *International Journal of Law Policy and the Family*, vol. 23, no. 2, pp. 211–229.

Doyle, C. & Timms, C., 2014, *Child neglect and emotional abuse: Understanding assessment and response*, London: Sage.

Doyle, M. & Dolan, M., 2002, 'Violence risk assessment and clinical information to structure clinical judgements for the formulation and management of risk', *Journal of Psychiatric and Mental Health Nursing*, vol. 9, pp. 649–657.

Driscoll, J., 2018, *Transitions from care to independence: Supporting young people leaving state care to fulfil potential*, London: Routledge.

Dumbrill, G.C., 2006, 'Parental experience of child protection intervention: A qualitative study', *Child Abuse & Neglect*, vol. 30, pp. 27–37.

English, D.J. & Graham, J.C., 2000, 'An examination of relationship between children's protective services social worker assessment of risk and independent LONGSCAN measures of risk constructs', *Children & Youth Services Review*, vol. 22, no. 11–12, pp. 897–933.

Epstein, M.H., 2004, 'Assessing the emotional and behavioural strengths of children', *Reclaiming Children & Youth: Journal of Emotional and Behavioural Problems*, vol. 6, no. 4, pp. 250–252.

Featherstone, B., 2009, *Contemporary fathering*, Bristol, UK: Policy Press.

Fernandez, E., 1991, 'The cultural basis of childrearing', in *B. Ferguson & M.E. Brown* (eds), *Health care and immigrants: A guide for the helping professions*, Sydney: MacLennan & Petty, pp. 97–121.

Fernandez, E.A., 2016, 'Case management in child protection: Challenges, complexities and possibilities', in E. Moore (ed.), *Case management inclusive community practice*, Oxford: Oxford University Press.

Fernandez, E., 2019, 'Working towards better education for children in care: Longitudinal analysis of the educational outcomes of a cohort of children in care in Australia', *Oxford Review of Education*, vol. 45, no. 4, pp. 481–501.

Ferguson, H., 2011, *Child protection practice*, Basingstoke, UK: Macmillan.

Forrester, D., McCambridge, J., Waissbein, C. & Rollnick, S., 2008, 'How do child and family social workers talk to parents about child welfare concerns?', *Child Abuse Review*, vol. 17, no. 1, pp. 23–35.

Gambrill, E. & Shlonsky, A., 2000, 'Risk assessment in context', *Children & Youth Services Review*, vol. 22, no. 11–12, 813–837.

Gambrill, E. & Shlonsky, A., 2001, 'The need for comprehensive risk management systems in child welfare', *Children & Youth Services Review*, vol. 23, no. 1, pp. 79–107.

Garbarino, J. & Barry, F., 1997, 'The community context of child abuse and neglect', in J. Garbarino, & J. Eckenrode (eds), *Understanding abusive families: An ecological approach to theory and practice*, San Francisco, CA: Jossey-Bass.

Ghate, D. & Hazel, N., 2002, *Parenting in poor environments: Stress, support and coping*, London: Jessica Kingsley.

Gil, D.G., 1979, *Child abuse and violence*, New York: AMS Press.

Gilgun, J.F., 1999, 'CASPARS: New tools for assessing client risks and strengths, families in society', *The Journal of Contemporary Human Services*, vol. 80, no. 5, pp. 450–459.

Gilligan, P. & Manby, M., 2008, 'The Common Assessment Framework: Does the reality match the rhetoric?', *Child & Family Social Work*, vol. 13, pp. 177–187.

Gillingham, P. & Humphreys, C., 2010, 'Child protection practitioners and decision-making tools: Observations and reflections from the front line', *British Journal of Social Work*, vol. 40, no. 8, pp. 2598–2616.

Goodman, R., 2001, 'Psychometric properties of the Strengths and Difficulties Questionnaire', *Journal of the American Academy of Child & Adolescent Psychiatry*, vol. 40, no. 11, pp. 1337–1345.

Healy, K., 2014, *Social work theories in context: Creating frameworks for practice*, Basingstoke, UK: Palgrave Macmillan.

Helm, D., 2010, *Making sense of child and family assessment*, London and Philadelphia, PA: Jessica Kingsley.

Hepworth, D.H., Rooney, R.H., Rooney, G.D., Strom-Gottfried, K. & Larsen, J., 2013, *Direct social work: Theory and skills*, Belmont, CA, Brooks Cole.

Holland, S., 2000, 'The assessment relationship: interactions between social workers and parents', *British Journal of Social Work*, vol. 30, pp. 149–163.

Holland, S., 2001, 'Representing children in child protection assessments', *Childhood*, vol. 8, no. 3 pp. 322–339.

Hollows, A., 2008, 'Professional judgement and the risk assessment process', in M. Calder (ed.), *Contemporary risk assessment in safeguarding children*, Lyme Regis, UK: Russell House Publishing.

Holosko, M.J. & Ojo, J., 2016, 'Risk assessment: Issues and implementation in child protective services', in J.S. Wodarski, M.J. Holoska & M.D. Feit (eds), *Evidence-informed assessment and practice in child welfare*, Cham, Heidelberg: Springer, pp. 85–98.

Horwath, J. & Morrison, T., 2011, 'Effective inter-agency collaboration to safeguard children: rising to the challenge through collective development', *Children & Youth*, vol. 33, no. 2, pp. 368–375.

Hughes, R. & Rycus, J., 2007, 'Issues in risk assessment in child protective services', *Journal of Public Child Welfare*, vol. 1, no. 1, pp. 85–116.

Jack, G. & Gill, O., 2010, 'The impact of economic factors on parents or caregivers and children', in J. Horwath (ed.), *The child's world: The comprehensive guide to assessing children in need*, 2nd edn, London: Jessica Kingsley.

Jenson, J.M. & Fraser, M.W., 2006, 'A risk and resilience framework for child, youth, and family policy', in J.M. Jenson & M.W. Fraser (eds), *Social policy for children & families: A risk and resilience perspective*, Thousand Oaks, CA: Sage, pp. 1–18.

John, K, Gammon, G.D. & Kruger, J., 1999, 'The social adjustment inventory for children and adolescents (SAICA)', *Journal of the American Academy of Child and Adolescent Psychiatry*, vol. 36, no. 7, pp. 980–988.

Johnson, W., 2004, *Effectiveness of California's child welfare structured decision-making (SDM) model: A prospective study of the validity of the California Family Risk Assessment*, Oakland, CA: Alameda County Social Services Agency.

Jordan, C. & Franklin, C., 1995, *Clinical assessment for social workers: Quantitative and qualitative methods*, Chicago, IL: Lyceum Books.

Kemshall, H., 2002, *Risk, social policy and welfare*, Buckingham, UK: Open University Press.

Laird, S.E. & Tedam, P., 2019, *Cultural diversity in child protection*, London: Springer Nature.

Lawrence, A., 2004, *Principles of child protection management and practice*, New York: Open University Press.

Lee, J-S. & Fernandez, E., 2019, 'Critical Multicultural Practice with ethnic minority children and their families', in S. Nippress & C. Williams (eds), *Critical multicultural practice in social work: New perspectives and practices*, Sydney: Allen & Unwin.

Leslie, L.K., Hurburt, M.S., Landsverk, J., Rolls, J.A., Wood, P.A. & Kelleher, K.J., 2003, 'Comprehensive assessment of children entering foster care: A national perspective', *Paediatrics*, vol. 112, no. 1, pp. 134–142.

Little, M., Axford, N. & Morpeth, L., 2004, 'Risk and protection in the context of services for children in need', *Child & Family Social Work*, vol. 9, no. 1, pp. 105–118.

McCroskeym, J. & Meezan, W., 1997, *Family preservation and family functioning*, Washington DC: CWLA Press.

Meyer, C., 1993, *Assessment in Social Work Practice*, New York, Columbia University Press.

Milner, J. & O'Byrne, P., 2002, *Assessment in social work*, 2nd edn. Basingstoke, UK: Palgrave Macmillan.

Milner, J., Myers, S. & O'Byrne, P., 2015, *Assessment in social work*, 4th edn, Basingstoke, UK: Palgrave Macmillan.

Milner, J.S., 1994, 'Assessing physical child abuse risk: The Child Abuse Potential Inventory', *Clinical Psychology Review*, vol. 14, no. 6, pp. 547–583.

Munro, E., 1999, 'Common errors or reasoning in child protection work', *Child Abuse & Neglect*, vol. 23, pp. 745–758.

Munro, E., 2008, 'Assessing risks throughout the life of a child welfare case', in D. Lindsey & A. Shlonsky (eds), *Child welfare research: Advances for practice & policy*, New York: Oxford University Press.

Munro, E., 2011, *The Munro review of child protection: Final report. A child-centred system*, London: Department of Health.

Nollan, K.A., Wolf, M., Ansell, D., Burns, J., Barr, L., Copeland, W. & Paddock, G., 2000, 'Ready or not: Assessing youth' preparedness for independent living', *Child Welfare*, vol. 79, no. 2, pp. 159–176.

O'Hagan, K., 2006, *Identifying emotional and psychological abuse. A guide for childcare professionals*, Maidenhead, UK: Open University Press.

Parton, N., 2014, *The politics of child protection: Contemporary developments and future directions*, Basingstoke, UK: Palgrave Macmillan.

Parton, N., Thorpe, D. & Wattam, C., 1997, *Child protection: Risk and the moral order*, Basingstoke, UK: Macmillan.

Pelton, L.H., 2015, 'The continuing role of material factors in child maltreatment and placement', *Child Abuse & Neglect*, vol. 41, pp. 30–39.

Platt, D., 2012, 'Understanding parental engagement with child welfare services: An integrated model', *Child & Family Social Work*, vol. 17, pp. 138–140.

Plous, S., 1993, *The psychology of judgement and decision making*, New York, McGraw-Hill.

Reder, P. & Duncan, S., 2003, 'How much should children's views count?', in P. Reder, S. Duncan & C. Lucey (eds), *Studies in the assessment of parenting*, London: Routledge.

Reder, P., Duncan, S. & Lucey, C., 2003, '*What principles guide parenting assessments?*', in P. Reder, S. Duncan & C. Lucey (eds), *Studies in the assessment of parenting*, London: Routledge.

Reed-Ashcraft, K., Kirk, R.S. & Fraser, M.W., 2001, 'The reliability and validity of the North Carolina Family Assessment Scale', *Research on Social Work Practice*, vol. 11, no. 4, 503–520.

Robinson, L., 2007, *Cross-cultural child development for social workers: An introduction*, Basingstoke, UK: Palgrave Macmillan.

Ryan, S., Wales, D., Cash, S. & Siebert, C., 2005, 'Risk assessment: Empirically supported or values driven', *Children & Youth Services Review*, vol. 27, pp. 213–225.

Rycus, J.S. & Hughes, R.C., 2008, 'Assessing risk throughout the life of a case', in D. Lindsey & A. Shlonsky (eds), *Child Welfare Research, Advances for Practice and Policy*, Oxford and New York: Oxford University Press, pp. 201–213.

Scourfield, B., 2001, 'Constructing women in child protection work', *Child & Family Social Work*, vol. 6, pp. 77–87.

Scott, D., 2009, 'Think child think family: How adult services can children at risk of abuse and neglect', *Family Matters*, vol. 81, pp. 37–42.

Sebba, J., Luke, N., Rees, A., Plumridge, G., Rodgers, L., Hafesji, K. & Rowsome-Smith, C., 2016, *Evaluation of the London Fostering Achievement Programme*, Oxford: The Rees Centre.

Seden, J., 2002, 'Underpinning theories for the assessment of children's needs', in H. Ward & W. Rose (eds), *Approaches to needs assessment in children's services*, London: Jessica Kingsley.

Shemmings, D. & Shemmings, Y., 1996, 'Building trust with families when making enquiries', in D. Platt & D. Shemmings (eds), *Making enquiries into alleged child abuse and neglect: Partnership with families*, Chichester, UK: John Wiley, pp. 67–85.

Shlonsky, A. & Wagner, D., 2005, 'The next step: Integrating actuarial risk assessment and clinical judgement into an evidence-based practice framework in CPS case management', *Child & Youth Services Review*, vol. 27, no. 4, pp. 409–427.

Smale, G. & Tuson, G., 1993, *Empowerment, assessment, care management and the skilled worker*, London: NISW House.

Squires, J., Bricker, D. & Potter, L., 1997, 'Revision of a parent-completed developmental screening tool: Ages and Stages Questionnaires', *Journal of Pediatric Psychology*, vol. 22, no. 3, pp. 313–328.

Tarren-Sweeney, M. & Hazell, P., 2006, 'Mental health of children in foster and kinship care in New South Wales, Australia', *Journal of Paediatrics and Child Health*, vol. 42, pp. 89–97.

Taylor, C., 2004, 'Underpinning Knowledge of child care practice: reconsidering child development theory', *Child & Family Social Work*, no. 9, pp. 225–235.

Taylor, C. & White, S., 2006, 'Knowledge, truth and reflexivity: The problem of judgement in social work', *Journal of Social Work*, vol. 1, pp. 37–59.

Thoburn, J., Lewis, A. & Shemmings, D., 1995, *Paternalism or partnership? Family involvement in the child protection process*, London: HMSO.

Thorpe, R., 2008, 'Family inclusion in child protection practice: Building bridges in working with (not against) families', *Communities, Families and Children Australia*, vol. 3, pp. 4–18.

Turnell, A. & Edwards, S., 1999, *Signs of safety: A solution and safety oriented approach to child protection casework*, New York: W.W. Norton.

Turney, D., Platt, D., Selwyn, J. & Farmer, E., 2011, *Improving child and family assessments: Turning research into practice*, London and Philadelphia, PA: Jessica Kingsley.

UN Convention on the Rights of the Child, 1989, Geneva, United Nations.

Ungar, M., 2004, 'The importance of parents and other agencies to the resilience of high risk adolescents', *Family Process*, vol. 43, no. 1, pp. 23–41.

Wald, M.S. & Wolverton, M., 1990, 'Risk assessment: The emperor's new clothes?', *Child Welfare*, vol. 64, pp. 431–450.

Walsh, J., 2006, *Theories for direct social work practice*, Belmont, CA: Thompson Brook.

Ward, H., 1996, 'Constructing and implementing measures to assess the outcomes of looking after children away from home', in M. Hill & J. Aldgate (eds), *Child welfare services: Developments in law, policy, practice and research*, London: Jessica Kingsley.

Ward, H. & Rose, W. (eds), 2002, *Approaches to needs assessment in children's services*, London: Jessica Kingsley.

Webb, S., 2006, *Social work in a risk society: Social and political perspectives*, Basingstoke, UK: Palgrave Macmillan.

Welbourne, P., 2012, *Social work with children and families: Developing advanced practice*, London and New York: Routledge.

Whitt-Woosley, A., Eslinger, J. & Sprang, G., 2018, 'Partners in child protection: A trauma informed approach to assessment in child welfare', in V.C. Strand & G. Sprang (eds), *Trauma responsive child welfare systems*, Cham: Springer International.

Wise, S., 2001, *The UK children in need approach in Australia*, Victoria: Australian Institute of Family Studies, Anglicare Victoria & University of Melbourne Department of Social Work.

Wise, S., 2017, *Developments to Strengthen Systems for Child Protection across Australia*, Victoria: Australian Institute of Family Studies, Anglicare Victoria & University of Melbourne Department of Social Work.

Wulczyn, F. Barth, R.P., Yuan, Y.T., Harden, B.J. & Landsberk, J., 2005, *Beyond common sense: Child welfare, child well-being, and the evidence for policy reform*, New Brunswick, NJ: Aldine Transactions.

Zimmer, M.H. & Panko, L.M., 2007, 'Developmental status and service use among children in the child welfare system: A national survey', *Archives of Paediatrics & Adolescent Medicine*, vol. 16, no. 2, pp. 183–188.

Chapter 7

Child protection and the role of the Children's Court

Rosemary Sheehan

The legal system exerts considerable influence on the child protection system in Australia and legislation and legal process specifically direct system and service responses. Each of Australia's eight States and two Territories has its own child welfare legislation and specialist Children's Courts to hear both child abuse and neglect and youth offending matters (AIFS 2014; Bromfield & Higgins 2005; Sheehan & Borowski 2013). The legislation sets out the legal framework for child protection investigations and interventions and whilst each State and Territory legislation varies in its crafting, it is this legislation that supplies the legal framework for child protection investigations and interventions.

The Children's Court: a specialist role

Children's Courts are a specialist jurisdiction in Australia. They hear criminal matters and also child abuse and neglect cases where they have the authority to determine matters relating to the child's care and protection. They are not courts of public record. Thus, no body of case law has been built to guide judicial officers' decision making in relation to either criminal or child welfare matters. Australia's legal system, like that of Canada, England, Wales, Ireland and New Zealand, is a common law adversarial one in which the judicial officer presides over matters brought to court, it is up to legal practitioners to present the issues in dispute, and the magistrate or judge adjudicates and decides the outcome of the case (Borowski 2013). It is very different from the European 'inquisitorial' approach in which judicial officers can be actively involved in the investigation and analysis of cases and the courts are perceived as 'truth seeking rather than proof-making' (Freiberg 2011: 83).

There are Children's Courts in the Australian Capital Territory (ACT), New South Wales (NSW), Queensland, Victoria, and Western Australia. South Australia has a Youth Court; in the Northern Territory both the Youth Justice Court and the Local Court deal with children and young people. Tasmania has no dedicated Children's Court, dealing with children and young people by a division of the adult Magistrate's Court (Borowski 2013). An additional complication is the overlapping roles of the Children's Court and the federal Family Court of Australia (now part of the Federal Circuit Court of Australia) where cases in the latter court involve child abuse. A wider system of courts and tribunals is also involved, in both Victoria and Queensland, for example, appeals in child welfare matters (most often by parents regarding court-ordered care arrangements) are directed to the Civil and Administrative Tribunals (CATs).

Statutory child protection agencies (e.g., Community Services Directorate in the ACT, Department of Children and Families in the Northern Territory and the Department of Human Services' Child Protection Service in Victoria) have the key child welfare responsibilities (Borowski 2013). There are mandatory reporting requirements across all jurisdictions although they vary in which professions are mandated to report suspected child abuse or neglect (AIHW 2012: 1). There are differences of emphasis in mandatory reporting. In Western Australia, it is for child sexual abuse only; Victoria and the ACT have mandatory reporting for suspected cases of child sexual abuse and physical abuse; the remaining jurisdictions have mandatory reporting of all forms of child abuse (physical, emotional and sexual abuse) and child neglect (Commission for Children and Young People 2012: 63).

Child protection legislation

There are common aims across Australian child protection legislation, that a child must be at risk of, or have experienced, 'significant harm' from physical, sexual or emotional harm, or harm to the child's physical development or health (see for example, Victoria's Children, Youth and Families Act 2005, S. 162 (2)), and it is in the child's 'best interests' that the court make a child protection order. Such an order obliges parents to meet certain obligations in the care of the child if the child is to either remain in, or return to, parental care; or the order provides for out-of-home care for the child, which may be long term. How 'significant harm' or 'best interests' are to be understood is not set out in legislation, nor is there any guidance, as there is in England and Wales (Sheehan 2018), about how these concerns might be materially understood.

Australian child protection legislation sets out that intervention is to be at the minimum necessary to secure the child's welfare and safety (see CYFA 2005, s.10 (2) (a)); its aim is the protection of the child from harm, rather than as a gateway to child and family services. The legislation confines child protection activity to identifying and responding to critical incidents of child abuse and neglect, with 'risk' as the key benchmark for deciding harm or likelihood of harm to a child. It is the statutory child protection authority in each Australian State and Territory which brings child abuse matters before the Children's Court, presenting evidence there is an unacceptable risk of harm to the child (see CYFA s.87 (1)(j)) to justify the need for intervention by the child protection service. Even though 'proof' in child protection matters is 'on the balance of probabilities' (Sheehan 2001), child protection services often struggle to present the child's circumstances in a way that fits the legal principles which dominate how child maltreatment is understood.

Legal vs welfare approaches

Court proceedings are part of the core business of the child protection service and child protection workers spend considerable time gathering evidence that is acceptable to the Court (Victorian Ombudsman 2009: 12; Allen Consulting Group 2003) to permit statutory intervention. The task of assessing whether or a not a child is sufficiently at risk of child abuse to justify child protection intervention is made more difficult because legal decisions made about children brought to court often differ from child protection recommendations about the need for formal intervention (Braye & Preston-Shoot 2006). Moreover, the legal approach to seek out discrete episodes of maltreatment fails to recognise that the majority of child protection cases are generally of a more chronic nature and about cumulative harm rather than 'specific dangerous parental behaviours' (Allen Consulting Group 2003: 29). Legal and welfare professionals use different frames of reference to deal with child abuse cases and what the child protection service views as harm and risk to the child can differ markedly from that of legal professionals (Sheehan 2006). How magistrates and judicial officers decide whether or not a child is in need of protection (see, for example, CYFA s.162) and how they assess a parent's failure to protect, is left to their discretion and the individual criteria they use to explain child abuse.

Australia's child protection systems frame formal child protection intervention as a legal enterprise, where entry into the child welfare system typically occurs via a single point, linked to a report or notification by a third party and is involuntary. The child protection system then investigates the notification and provides support to families, usually as child safety plans. The child protection intervention is thus invested with statutory legal powers, and where legal intervention is sought it is defined by adversarial, standardised and evidence-based procedures (Borowski & Sheehan 2013). It is a system that is separate from wider family support services, and focuses on families where there is a high or immediate, rather than residual, need (Allen Consulting Group 2003; Price-Robertson et al. 2013; Sammut & O'Brien 2009).

This approach to child protection is in marked contrast to Australia's overarching child protection framework: the *National Framework for Protecting Australia's Children 2009–2020* which advocates a 'whole of community' approach where child protection is 'everyone's responsibility' (Council of Australian Governments 2009). There is a rising demand for child protection services (AIHW 2017), bedevilled by systemic issues, such as the lack of 'fit' between legal process, court outcomes, child protection recommendations and child welfare needs, together with resource limitations that hinder suitable placements for children in care, early and timely family intervention, along with fragmented interagency collaboration (Bromfield, Arney & Higgins 2014; Price-Robertson et al. 2013; Sheehan & Borowski 2013). The number of children on care and protection orders in Australia continues to rise despite significant attempts by many jurisdictions to divert children and families away from statutory intervention and increasing family supports to maintain children in their family's care (AIHW 2017).

In Victoria, on 30 June, 2009, five in 1,000 Victorian children were the subject of a care and protection order, the largest proportion of whom were aged between birth and four years of age. The rate of Indigenous children on care and protection orders was more than seven times as high as for other children and the rate of Indigenous children in out-of-home care was almost nine times the rate of other children (VLRC 2010: 34). Additionally, in Victoria, most child protection notifications are about child neglect or emotional harm; the latter formed 44% of the notifications made, in 2000–01, to the Victorian child protection service, followed by physical abuse (38%) and child sexual abuse (6%) (Sheehan 2006).

Defining child maltreatment

A key challenge to child protection practice is the constraints around how child maltreatment is framed in legislation. Four Australian States and Territories – Victoria, New South Wales, the Australian Capital Territory and Queensland – have a legislative basis for cumulative harm, in an attempt to move away from the 'event' model and singular instances of harm to a child. Victoria's Children, Youth and Families Act 2005 (s.162 (1) (2)) sets out that 'harm may be constituted by a single act, omission or circumstance or accumulate through a series of acts, omissions or circumstances'. The ACT's Children and Young People Act 2008 directs that significant harm includes 'a single instance of significant harm or multiple instances of harm that together make up significant harm' (s.341 (2)). Queensland's Child Protection Act 1999 (s.9 (4)(b)) consolidates this by stating harm can be caused by 'a series or combination of acts, omissions or circumstances'. However, whilst it appears the parameters for deciding when a child is in need of protection have been redirected to understand harm as prolonged or repeated experiences of harm as well as episodic instances of harm (Sheehan 2012; Bromfield & Miller 2012), the lack of clear definition on what is considered 'harm to a child' continues the disconnect between framing welfare concerns as legal facts to put before a court (VLRC 2010).

Bromfield and Arney (2008) suggest one explanatory factor for the overall increase in child protection concerns is the complex family situations of these children, previously noted: the strong connection between child abuse and neglect, domestic violence, parental substance abuse and parental mental health. Certainly there is a clear relationship between socio-economic disadvantage and contact with child protection services (VLRC 2010: 35), characterised by housing instability, poverty, low education, social isolation and neighbourhood disadvantage (Bromfield & Arney 2008).

Yet, child protection legislation and Children's Courts struggle to accommodate the chronic problems of child abuse that are increasingly characteristic of the child protection jurisdiction. The *Protecting Children: The Child Protection Outcomes Project* (prepared and published in 2003 by the Allen Consulting Group for the Victorian Government) found that the legislation was not structured to respond to consequences of major social changes, such as deinstitutionalisation for people with intellectual disability or serious mental illness and the increase in parental substance abuse. These findings resonate still across the child protection jurisdiction. Whilst there are Children's Court innovations in a number of courts around the use of problem solving and therapeutic jurisprudence approaches, most notably with Indigenous matters and Family Drug Treatment Courts, the adversarial paradigm still predominates and continues to create tension between the child protection and legal systems. (Sheehan 2016a). This distracts from concentrating on the nature and merit of child protection concerns and how a child's best interests are best determined. The Victorian Law Reform Commission, in their Report on the child protection system (2010: 204) described how magistrates described their role as that of hearing and determining issues raised by parties, and it was not for the magistrate to decide what ought to be discussed. Both the VLRC (2010) and the Office of the Victorian Ombudsman (2009) noted that attention needed to be turned away from the Court to allow the child protection service to work with families apart from the legal system, recognising that a child's best interests are better understood when all facets of concerns are assessed rather than just those which meet legal criteria.

Reviewing the child welfare jurisdiction

Reviews of child protection systems across Australia call for legislation that shifts legal decision makers to a more holistic evaluation of children's health and wellbeing. The Victorian Law Reform Commission (2010) proposed that the Children's Court move away from an adversarial approach to a more problem-solving approach in reaching agreement on what is in the best interests of the child. The focus then is less about proving maltreatment and more about addressing harm to the child (Borowski & Sheehan 2013; VLRC 2010), and draws on inter-professional collaboration to respond to the broader context of child maltreatment, often occurring in a context of parental disadvantage and marginalisation.

The Wood (2008) *Report of the Special Commission of Inquiry into Child Protective Services in NSW* reported that current legal models of decision making which focus on specific incidents of maltreatment make it difficult to develop a holistic assessment of the needs of the child within their family and community context, commenting 'the systemic response is reactive not proactive' (Wood 2008: 373). Queensland (Queensland Child Protection Commission of Inquiry 2013), Northern Territory (NT) (Bamblett, Bath & Roseby 2010) and Tasmania (DHHS 2008; Select Committee on Child Protection 2011) reports on the operation of the child protection systems all recommend the need for legislative and policy frameworks to shift attention to the child's longer-term needs, rather than the immediate episodes of abuse.

The critiques of Victoria's child protection system: the Office of the Victorian Ombudsman's *Own Motion Investigation into the Department of Human Services Child Protection Program* (Victorian Ombudsman 2009) and the VLRC inquiry into the *Protection Applications in the Children's Court* advocated for a problem-solving approach to underpin practice in the Children's Court (see also Cummins, Scott and Scales 2012, *Protecting Victoria's Vulnerable Children Inquiry*). The Victorian Ombudsman's (2009) identified the need to move away from an event-oriented focus of maltreatment, towards a more longer-term impact-orientated focus. It was noted that risk frameworks need to better focus on likelihood of harm and predicting future behaviour rather than looking for a discrete event to explain harm to a child. However, Borowski and Sheehan's (2013) examination of practice within the Victorian Children's Court found that magistrates and practitioners said the current legislation was 'too large, too complex, too technical and lacking clarity about key constructs such as "cumulative" and "significant" harm, and "parental responsibility"' (Borowski & Sheehan 2013: 138). Child protection workers described the difficulty they had in conveying in a judicial setting their assessments about harm to a child when there are no legislative parameters to define this (Borowski & Sheehan 2013).

Certainly, child protection workers perceived that court outcomes are often a compromise, legally driven and based on an accommodation of parents' and children's instructions to their legal representatives, and on what they will agree to do rather than based on the child's developmental and welfare needs (Sheehan 2016a). Such outcomes are often difficult to implement, viewed by families as too intrusive and by child protection workers as insufficient for the child's safety.

Difficulty in deciding child abuse matters

Child protection legislation struggles to accommodate the chronic problems of child abuse that are increasingly characteristic of the child protection jurisdiction. Statutory intervention emphasises the importance of family preservation and minimum intervention whilst also directing that 'best interests of the child are paramount' (see CYFA s.10 (1)). The adversarial and highly legalised court processes surrounding child protection matters are described as confusing and, at times, hostile and traumatic (DHS 2002: 53) for children, families and professionals (See: National Commission of Inquiry into the Prevention of Child Abuse, 1997–8, in Walby 1998). Neither existing child protection legislation nor legal and court approaches are structured to respond to consequences of major social changes, such as deinstitutionalisation for people with intellectual disability or serious mental illness and the increase in parental substance abuse (Allen Consulting Group 2003).

The key legal criterion of significant harm raises particular challenges (Masson 2010) and Dickens (2007: 78) notes, especially in cases of child neglect. Although legislation in England and Wales does not require a 'decisive event' to satisfy the courts when making a child protection order, he found the focus of both social work and legal practice remained very much on incidents. He found the tensions about incidents and reasonable parenting epitomised the dilemmas of intervening in child neglect cases. They are cases, he notes, frequently characterised by parents 'facing great challenges of deprivation or vulnerability' (2007: 79).

This is especially evident in how cumulative harm is dealt with by legislation. Tasmania's Report into child protection by the Select Committee on Child Protection (2011) found child protection practice to be crisis driven, with negligible consideration given to the issue of cumulative harm. They recommended 'a complete overhaul of the legislative framework within which child protection in Tasmania is practiced' (Select Committee on Child Protection 2011: 188), 'with legislation amended to change the focus on episodic interventions to cumulative harm and new provisions introduced to enable child protection services to intervene with children who, over the long-term, have experienced cumulative trauma and harm' (Select Committee on Child Protection 2011: 191). Whilst there is no clear legislative basis in the Northern Territory (NT) to address cumulative harm, Bamblett, Bath and Roseby's (2010) *Growing them Strong, Together* Inquiry into the NT child protection system found that cumulative harm is a critical issue in the assessment of child protection concerns. The focus is on immediate and urgent harm rather than understanding that cumulative harm is also 'significant'. Despite the acknowledged concerns, cumulative harm is not mentioned in the legislative framework.

Victoria's *Protecting Victoria's Vulnerable Children Inquiry* (Cummins, Scott & Scales 2012) found that whilst cumulative harm was recognised for its impact on the child, child protection workers found it difficult to present evidence relating to it in a manner that is accepted by the court, given the legal and legislative ambiguity around how cumulative harm is to be interpreted. Risk assessment models that favour an event (or crisis) orientation further the court's response to child protection concerns (Cummins, Scott & Scales 2012). Whilst Victoria's CYFA acknowledges the 'effects of cumulative patterns of harm on children's safety and development' (s.10 (3)(d)), how the 'best interests' of the child (s.10 (1)) are applied is not clearly defined in the Act, nor is guidance provided on how these principles are to be materially understood in practice (Bromfield & Miller 2012; Sheehan 2012).

Cumulative harm is often associated with neglect (Bromfield & Miller 2012). The challenge is that compared to physical and sexual abuse, neglect – especially chronic neglect – often requires complex responses. It is very often less visible than physical or sexual abuse, often more pervasive and harder to resolve and embedded within complex family issues (CWIG 2013). Neither Victorian legislation nor NSW legislation include neglect as a ground for child protection; legislation for the other six Australian states and two territories does specifically mention neglect on the grounds for when a child is in need of protection. The specific link between cumulative harm and neglect needs to be more effectively flagged in legislation. Although legal practitioners acknowledged there was legal provision for neglect, and that a child's best interests might be better served by child protection involvement, they still looked for a specific event or a change of circumstances that justified legal action. The child's 'best interests' is often determined at court not solely by child welfare concerns but by a 'trade-off' between how such concerns can be accommodated by legal frameworks. Child welfare legislation in Australia continues to maintain adversarial and highly legalised processes to deal with child abuse which diminish the significance and utility of welfare contributions. There is little accommodation of the kind of multidisciplinary contributions that are necessary to both make sense of, and effectively respond to, the increasingly complex problems characteristic of child maltreatment.

National assessment of Australia's Children's Courts

A national assessment of Australia's Children's Courts (2009–2011) by Sheehan and Borowski (2013) examined the operation of these courts and the challenges to this, from the perspective of judicial officers and other stakeholders, and what reforms might enhance the work of the court. The national study covered Australia's six States and two Territories. The study participants varied in how they believed the court was viewed; in NSW, South Australia and the ACT, it was believed the child protection arm of the children's courts was generally held in high regard, which was a view not shared in Victoria or Western Australia.

Children's Court judicial officers comprise about 80 specialist judicial officers (mainly magistrates but also some judges) based in specialist Children's Court matters (SCRGSP 2012: 7.28). There is a larger number of 'generalist' judicial officers (in adult Magistrate's or Local Courts) based in regional and remote locations, who convene a specialist Children's Court when required, to deal with both youth offending and child welfare matters. This mix of specialist and generalist judicial officers delivers major variation in knowledge and skill in case management and decision making in, for example, child protection outcomes, given there is negligible professional development to prepare the court offers for dealing with child maltreatment matters.

Child protection workers experienced the Children's Court as a very difficult work environment. There was considerable criticism of them by study participants, despite acknowledgement of the pressures of child protection work (e.g., little support, high caseloads, tight timelines). Their professional expertise was often called into question in terms of the quality of their evidence or case planning, and they faced often hostile cross-examination in the adversarial court proceedings. They were frustrated that they, with child welfare training, were not treated with respect by legal practitioners or magistrates. Lawyers working in Australia's Children's Courts do not require any special accreditation, and have no formal training in how to identify or frame the best interests of the child (Blackman 2002). Legal practitioners act on the instructions of the child (direct representation), with no formal requirement for assessment of the child's best interests, unless they are appointed by the court as an independent children's lawyer, where a child because of age or disability is unable to give instructions.

The need for training, by those professionals working in the court, was raised especially by child protection workers, who said judicial officers and legal practitioners needed knowledge in developmental psychology and childhood trauma arising from abuse and/or neglect, mental health, intellectual disability, communication skills and in jurisdictions with large Indigenous (and, indeed, cultural and linguistic differences (CALD)) communities, training in cross-cultural professional practice.

Children's Courts serve a challenging clientele. The workload of the children's court has increased significantly (AIC 2012; SCRGSP 2012), and magistrates, legal practitioners and child protection workers commented on the pressure of this increase on effective responses to children in need of care and protection. The children, young people and families who appear before Children's Courts are highly socio-economically disadvantaged and marginalised. They have problems with alcohol and drug abuse, domestic violence, mental health, and a history of involvement with the child protection system. Child protection matters brought before the Court increasingly involve long-term factors impacting on the lives of the children and their families: low income, sole parenthood, parental mental illness, substance abuse and domestic violence (Allen Consulting Group 2003: 12). They typically are more difficult to prove legally, there is little agreement between legal and welfare systems about definition and recognition of the impact of these factors on children, and the child protection service struggles to present the type of evidence of demonstrated behaviour and events that the Court seeks and fits readily into legislative parameters about proof of harm and the need for care and protection. Sheehan (2016b) confirmed that difficulties in demonstrating significant harm for children affected, for example, by parental addiction or significant mental illness, when the child welfare concerns did not readily fit into legislative grounds for the making of a child protection order (Dawe, Harnett & Frye 2008).

Hearing children's matters at court was problematic in terms of the facilities available; whilst Children's Courts in some capital cities are located in purpose-built buildings (e.g., Brisbane, Adelaide, Melbourne and Canberra) which permit a completely separate hearing of matters, other cities (e.g., Darwin and Hobart), however, and in regional and remote locations, there is no physical separation between Children's Courts and adult courts, resulting in children's matters often being heard alongside adult ones. Whatever the setting, Children's Courts were described as overcrowded, tense, chaotic and often unsafe, with few interview rooms for lawyers to meet privately with clients.

A major finding of the national assessment was that in most (but not all) States and Territories there was strong support for a shift away from the critical incident-based, accusatorial approach in dealing with cases of child abuse and neglect. It was suggested by the key stakeholders interviewed for the study that an approach which focused less on disputation and more on dealing with the often long-term and complex problems of the children, young people and families who appear in court, was preferable – such as that characteristic of a collaborative problem-solving therapeutic jurisprudence approach (Sheehan & Borowski 2013; Sheehan 2016b). Problem-solving courts feature judicial monitoring of cases and close collaboration with statutory and non-government service providers (Berman & Feinblatt 2001); these approaches are found in the drug and alcohol, mental health and domestic violence courts already operating in Australia (Borowski 2013). Not all judicial officers concurred with this. The court is to have an impartial role, and the adversarial appraisal of evidence in child welfare matters is essential to upholding children's and families' rights (Borowski 2013). Yet, it was generally agreed that increasing complexity of cases coming before Children's Courts needed additional measures to manage and decide them.

Child welfare legislation is challenged by the difficult and uncertain nature of the social and individual problems that child protection workers respond to on a daily basis (Braye & Preston-Shoot 2006). Moreover, child protection legislation in Victoria – and this is typical of Australian child protection legislation in general – sets out overlapping interests that are not easily reconciled: the family's interest to live as it chooses without external interference; the State's interest in the protection of vulnerable children; and, the child's interest in exercising their own rights, which might differ from those of family and State especially when their wellbeing is being determined. How the child welfare, legal and adult service systems (mental health, substance abuse, family violence, for example) define child abuse and neglect may overlap, but will differ because they each serve a different purpose. In the absence of shared frameworks, legal and child protection systems find it almost impossible to develop agreed approaches about the risks and consequences of maltreatment.

Children's Courts: the need for a shared enterprise

The Victorian Law Reform commission (2010) proposed that approaches to deciding child maltreatment matters need to be more agreement focussed and more child centred (2010: 214), with legislative principles developed to encourage early resolution of child protection matters. The legal process should be problem solving in its approach and accommodate the kind of inter-professional contributions decision makers need to decide about a child's development and wellbeing. The incorporation of child welfare guidance for the court and child protection case conferences into statutory processes provides a way to assess the relevant information about a child and family and develop an agreed child protection plan to be put to the Court. Importantly, legal decision makers must have formal knowledge and education in child development, the effect of trauma on children, and the impact of parental mental illness and exposure to drugs and family violence on children (submission by the Director of Victorian Paediatric Forensic Medical Service to the VLRC 2010: 365). Families with multiple problems are the primary client group in child protection services, and their isolation and disadvantage places their children at greater risk of abuse and neglect. A more holistic and collaborative approach offers a more effective response to families where children are referred to the Children's Court because of concerns about child abuse and neglect.

The Council of Australian Governments (2009) believes that applying a public health model, rather than focussing solely on legal and rights-based approaches to child protection, may help to reduce the burden on child protection services and children's courts and deliver better outcomes for children and families. A public health model offers a service continuum, from primary services available to all families, such as health and education, to having secondary interventions available to families who are seen as at risk of child maltreatment, to tertiary child protection services which are a last resort for families when child abuse and neglect has occurred (Horsfall, Bromfield & McDonald 2010; Scott 2013). It is an approach that brings a broader understanding to deciding a child's best interests. Families turn to governments to help them deal with social concerns and the specific issues they face (Sheehan 2012). Child protection legislation and the legal process need to be better grounded in understanding the factors that influence children's outcomes, and work collaboratively to improve the living circumstances of vulnerable children.

References

Allen Consulting Group, 2003, *Protecting children: The Child Protection Outcomes Project*, Melbourne: Victorian Department of Human Services.

AIC, 2012, *Australian Crime: Facts and Figures 2011*, Canberra: Australian Institute of Criminology.

AIFS, 2014, *Australian child protection legislation*, Melbourne: Australian Institute of Family Studies.

AIHW, 2012, *Child Protection Australia, 2010–11*, Canberra: Australian Institute of Health and Welfare.

AIHW, 2017, *Child Protection Australia 2015–16*, Canberra: Australian Institute of Health and Welfare.

Bamblett, M., Bath, H. & Roseby, R., 2010, *Growing them strong, together: Promoting the safety and wellbeing of the Northern Territory's children*, Northern Territory, Australia: Northern Territory Government.

Berman, G. & Feinblatt, J., 2001, 'Problem-solving courts: A brief primer', *Law and Policy*, vol. 23, no. 2, pp. 125–140.

Blackman, L., 2002, *Representing children and young people: A lawyer's guide*, Melbourne: Victoria Law Foundation.

Borowski, A., 2013, 'A portrait of Australia's Children's Courts: Findings of a national assessment', in R. Sheehan, & A. Borowski (eds), *Australia's Children's Courts today and tomorrow*, New York: Springer.

Borowski, A. & Sheehan, R., 2013, 'The Children's Court of Victoria', in R. Sheehan & A. Borowski (eds), *Australia's Children's Courts today and tomorrow*, Dordrecht: Springer, pp. 123–142.

Braye, S. & Preston-Shoot, M., 2006, *Teaching, learning and assessment of law in social work education*, Bristol, UK: The Policy Press.

Bromfield, L.M. & Arney, F., 2008, *Developing a road map for research: Identifying the priorities for a national child protection research agenda*, Melbourne: National Child Protection Clearinghouse.

Bromfield, L., Arney, F. & Higgins, D., 2014, 'Contemporary issues in child protection, intake, referral and family support', in A. Hayes & D. Higgins (eds), *Families, policy and the law: Selected essays on contemporary issues for Australia*, Melbourne: Australian Institute of Family Studies.

Bromfield, L. & Miller, R., 2012, *Cumulative harm – Best interests case practice model: Specialist practice resource*, Melbourne: Department of Human Services.

Bromfield, L. & Higgins, D., 2005, *National comparison of child protection systems*, Melbourne: Australian Institute of Family Studies.

Child Welfare Information Gateway (CWIG), 2013, *Chronic child neglect*, Washington, DC: Department of Health and Human Services.

Children, Youth and Families Act 2005, Victoria.

Commission for Children and Young People, 2012, *The state of Western Australia's children and young people: Edition one*, Subiaco, Western Australia: The Commission for Children and Young People.

Council of Australian Governments, 2009, *Protecting children is everyone's business: National Framework for Protecting Australia's Children 2009–2020* (the National Framework), Annual Report, Canberra: The Council of Australian Governments.

Cummins, P., Scott, D. & Scales, D., 2012, *Report of the protecting Victoria's Vulnerable Children Inquiry*, Melbourne: Department of Premier and Cabinet.

Dawe, S., Harnett, P. & Frye, S., 2008, *Improving outcomes for children living in families with parental substance misuse: What do we know and what should we do*, Melbourne: Australian Institute of Family Studies.

DHHS, 2008, *New directions for child protection in Tasmania: An integrated strategic framework*, Tasmania: Department of Health and Human Services.

Department of Human Services, 2002, *Annual Report 2002–03*. Victoria: Victorian Government Department of Human Service.

Dickens, J., 2007, 'When a child care case is taken to court in England and Wales, Child Neglect and the Law: Catapults, Thresholds and Delay', *Child Abuse Review*, vol. 16, pp. 77–92.

Freiberg, A., 2011, 'Post-adversarial and post-inquisitorial justice: Transcending traditional penological paradigms', *European Journal of Criminology*, vol. 8, no. 1, pp. 82–101.

Horsfall, B., Bromfield, L. & McDonald, M., 2010, *Are social marketing campaigns effective in preventing child abuse and neglect?*, Melbourne: Australian Institute of Family Studies.

Masson, J., 2010, '(Mis)understandings of significant harm', *Child Abuse Review*, vol. 19, pp. 291–298.

Price-Robertson, R., Rush, P., Wall, L. & Higgins, D., 2013, Rarely an isolated incident: Acknowledging the interrelatedness of child maltreatment, victimisation and trauma (CFCA Paper No. 15). Melbourne: Child Family Community Australia, Australian Institute of Family Studies, www.aifs.gov.au/cfca/pubs/papers/a144788/index.html.

Queensland Child Protection Commission of Inquiry, 2013, *Taking responsibility: A roadmap for Queensland child protection*, Queensland: Queensland Child Protection Commission of Inquiry.

Sammut, J. & O' Brien, T., 2009, *Fatally flawed: The child protection crisis in Australia*, Sydney: Centre for Independent Studies.

Scott, D., 2013, *Meeting children's needs when the family environment isn't always 'good enough': A systems approach*, Melbourne: Australian Institute of Family Studies.

Select Committee on Child Protection, 2011, *Select committee on child protection: Final report*, Tasmania: Parliament of Tasmania.

Sheehan, R., 2001, *Magistrates' decision-making in matters of child protection*, Aldershot, UK: Ashgate.

Sheehan, R., 2006, 'Emotional abuse and neglect: The legal response', *Child Abuse Review*, vol.15, no. 1, pp. 38–54.

Sheehan, R., 2012, 'Deciding the best interest of the child: Legal responses to child protection concerns', in R. Sheehan, H. Rhoades & N. Stanley (eds), *Vulnerable children and the law: International perspectives on challenges to child welfare, child protection, and children's rights*, London: Jessica Kingsley.

Sheehan, R., 2016a, 'Legal responses to child sexual abuse cases in the Children's Court of Victoria: study findings on a case-management approach', *Journal of Social Welfare and Family Law*, vol. 38, no. 3, pp. 287–301.

Sheehan, R., 2016b, 'Child sexual abuse cases: Implementing a specialist judicial list', *Australian Social Work*, vol. 69, no. 4, pp. 403–416.

Sheehan, R., 2018, 'Child abuse and neglect and the judicial system: The limits of legal enterprise', in Y. Robinson, W. Petherick & I. Bryce (eds), *Child abuse and neglect: Forensic issues in evidence, impact and management*, San Diego, CA: Elsevier.

Sheehan, R. & Borowski, A., 2013, *Australia's Children's Courts today and tomorrow*, New York: Springer.

Steering Committee for the Review of Government Service Provision (SCRGSP), 2012, *Report on Government Services 2012*, Canberra: Productivity Commission.

VLRC, 2010, *Protection applications in the Children's Court: Final report*, Melbourne: Victorian Law Reform Commission.

Victorian Ombudsman, 2009, *Own motion investigation into the Department of Human Services Child Protection Program*, Melbourne: Office of the Victorian Ombudsman.

Walby, C., 1998, 'The national commission of inquiry into the prevention of child abuse: Will it make a difference?', *Child Abuse Review*, vol. 7, pp. 77–86.

Wood, J., 2008, *The report of the special commission of inquiry into child protection services*, Sydney: New South Wales Government.

Chapter 8

Therapeutic approaches to children and families in child protection contexts

Paul Delfabbro and Alexandra Osborn

Introduction and policy context

Children in child protection (CP) have usually been exposed to abuse and trauma (Bruce et al. 2018; Dorsey et al. 2013). Most come from families affected by multiple complex factors, including poverty, domestic violence, substance abuse and mental health problems. Such children have often suffered neurological harm and this places them at risk of future psychological, developmental and social problems (Applegate & Shapiro 2005; Perry 2002, 2009). As a result, child protection and social work practitioners are usually faced with clients who need intensive support and often from multidisciplinary teams. Decisions will therefore have to be made about the nature and timing of additional therapeutic services in the knowledge that a failure to deal with these problems can influence placement outcomes, the choice of cares, family relationships and whether children can live successfully with their biological families.

The aim of this chapter is to provide a broad overview of the types of therapeutic programs and approaches that are used to assist these families. The term 'therapeutic' refers to interventions which try to address the presence of conditions that are harmful for child wellbeing, their families and those who work with them. Such approaches generally try to encourage healthier psychological and social functioning in children, while also helping to foster the development of skills in parents that enhance parental ability to have productive and healthy interactions with their children. Although interventions of this nature are highly diverse and cannot be fully encapsulated in this brief chapter, the aim is to provide an indicative summary of some of the most empirically supported methods often advanced to address the most common problems faced by children and their families in the CP system. To this end, four principal areas of need are considered: (a) *Behavioural problems*: how to deal with externalised or conduct-related issues; (b) *Resilience*: building social competency and resilience in children; (c) *Early developmental harm*: dealing with trauma and attachment-related problems, particularly in out-of-home care and (d) *Parenting*: building parental skills and enhancing family functioning.

Context: Mental health problems in child protection populations

Much of the evidence for the challenges faced by children has emerged from studies involving children in out-of-home care. Studies have consistently shown that the prevalence of a range of clinical problems is higher for children in care than in the general population. Children are significantly more likely to display clinical level behavioural/

externalising problems than those in the general population (Delfabbro 2018; Sawyer et al. 2007) and are more likely to display internalising problems such as depression or anxiety (Sawyer et al. 2007; Tarren-Sweeney 2008, 2013). They are also likely to experience difficulties in forming adaptive and healthy attachments with other people (Bruce et al. 2018). The term ‘attachment disorder’ refers to problems associated with the bonds between young children and their parents (usually the mother) in early development and this can take several forms. CP practitioners may observe that the child’s attachments are disordered (e.g., the child will try to form bonds with both strangers and well as proximal carers); insecure (e.g., the child clings to the carer and is unwilling to engage with others or negotiate the environment confidently) or reactive (e.g., the child is unresponsive and does not seem to respond to attempts to provide affection or seek assistance when upset). They may also observe that children display symptoms consistent with disorders such as PTSD (e.g., anxiety, reliving traumatic experiences, nightmares, poor concentration) which often arises from exposure to early traumatic events including domestic violence, parental death, imprisonment or mental health issues (Dubner & Motta 1999).

Research: Informed practice

The following section highlights some of the principal areas that have received some of the most attention because of their significant policy importance. It will be noted that many of these approaches are multidisciplinary. They typically involve the interplay of different areas of expertise including professional practitioners in social work, psychology and psychiatry.

I. Approaches to behavioural problems

PRACTICE ISSUE: Children in care often have complex behaviours and this increases the risk of them coming into care and increases the changes of poorer outcomes in the care system. CP practitioners may find it difficult to find stable family placements and that it is more difficult for children to return to their families.

Behavioural therapy

These approaches do not try to address deeper underlying causes of behavioural problems (e.g., early trauma). Instead, these methods provide practitioners with practical strategies to deal with immediate challenges such as aggressive, disrespectful and challenging behaviour to enable children to adapt better to placements and to have greater success at school. Most are based on the principles of applied behaviour analysis and focus on a regime of punishments, rewards and contingencies, whereas others might also include cognitive elements (cognitive-behavioural therapy, CBT) if children are sufficiently mature.

Child behaviour therapy, as it is often called, has a very extensive and well-established history (Bloomquist & Schnell 2005; Hersen 1989). Most interventions involve the systematic reinforcement and punishment of responses to produce more desirable behaviours. It is assumed that inappropriate behaviours can be modified through rewards and punishments and that children are capable of learning the relationship (or contingency) between their behaviours and consequences (Fahlberg 1991). Ultimately, the aim is to teach children to form new habits and to make more socially appropriate and adaptive behavioural choices. The usual process is for the therapist or caregiver (parent, foster parent or residential staff) to apply positive reinforcement or rewards for positive behaviours and punish or ignore (fail to reward) undesirable behaviours. In this way, the incidence of bad behaviour should decrease while desirable behaviour increases (Meadowcraft 1989). Only very simple rewards (e.g., praise or privileges) and punishments (e.g., loss of privileges or withdrawal of attention) are used during the modification process. In general, few of these programs are punitive in nature or involve any sort of physical punishment or harsh disciplinary techniques (Bloomquist & Schnell 2005).

Many of these programs will employ a form of behaviour modification based upon the principle of conditioned reinforcement. The central idea here is that people can often be encouraged to perform behaviours to achieve specific outcomes (secondary reinforcers) which can then be used to obtain highly desirable outcomes (primary reinforcers). Primary reinforcers usually include such things as money, privileges and luxuries, whereas secondary reinforcers usually take the form of points, tickets or tokens. Often such programs use what is termed a 'token economy' procedure (Bloomquist & Schnell 2005; Chamberlain 1990). A token economy is a system whereby tokens are used as reinforcers to increase desirable behaviour in individuals. Programs for older children that employ this form of behavioural modification usually supplement the process of conditioned reinforcement with the use of behavioural contracts. Behavioural contracts are, in most cases, mutually negotiated obligations established between the young person and their caregiver (parent, foster parent, residential youth worker, therapist etc.) (Patterson 1974).

Multidimensional treatment foster care

Internationally, one of the most well-known programs that utilises token economies as part of its intervention with children is multidimensional treatment foster care (MTFC) (Rhoades et al. 2013). MTFC is used predominantly as a service for adolescents and particularly those with offending histories or complex externalising behaviours. It has been used widely in the US, but has also been trialled elsewhere, including in the UK, Australia and New Zealand. The program goals are to decrease problem behaviour and increase developmentally appropriate normative and prosocial behaviour. These treatment goals are accomplished by providing: close supervision, fair and consistent limits, predictable consequences for rule breaking, a supportive relationship with at least one mentoring adult, and reduced exposure to peers with similar problems. Often these are achieved by using a stepped process of rewards or privileges. For example, when young people enter the program they may be given very few possessions and privileges. As their behaviour then improves over time, they accumulate points which can then be exchanged for things that they desire (i.e. more furniture, a radio). In another approach, young people might not be deprived initially but have the option to accumulate more points to obtain additional luxuries, greater responsibilities or variations in the level of freedom in the program. Such accumulation of points is often referred to in terms of 'levels' or 'stages', so that as the young person accumulates the points they are then able to graduate to a higher level or stage in the program. Eventually, once the young person graduates from each of the levels, they are then able to be discharged from the program, in most cases to a less restrictive setting.

MTFC has generally proven to be quite effective and the youth have shown significant reductions in antisocial behaviour (Chamberlain & Reid 1991; Rhoades et al. 2013), and significant decreases in criminal referrals and days spent in detention facilities (Chamberlain 1990); thus, it appears to be a cost-effective alternative to residential treatment, leading to better outcomes for children and families. The only downside to this type of program, however, is that it can be very labour intensive and time consuming (due to the high amount of monitoring and documentation of behaviours that is required). The technique also does not address the underlying emotions and attitudes that may be driving the behaviour. Some researchers (e.g., Levy & Orlans 1998) have also suggested that such transactional styles of interaction may inhibit young people's capacity to form more emotionally fulfilling relationships with adults, in that it may reinforce the young people's view of adults as rigid and authoritarian. Another potential point of caution is that relatively few evaluations have been conducted independently on the principal designers of the program. Despite this, it provides a useful model that could potentially be applied in family preservation programs or in some forms of residential care where there may be a case–plan to transition young people back home.

Cognitive-behavioural therapy (CBT)

Many of the behaviourally focused programs often try to incorporate additional cognitive elements that recognise children and young people as 'thinking beings' who have their own ability to shape and plan their own behaviour (Ollendick & King 1998). CBT involves, in addition to the behavioural therapy techniques, the use of cognitive therapy to teach the child or young person the link between how certain thinking patterns can cause certain symptoms. For example, the therapist might teach the child how to change their thought patterns from ones that lead to maladaptive behaviour to ones that produce adaptive behaviour and positive feelings (Hinswaw, Henker & Whalen 1984; Hodges 2004).

CBT-based techniques may also be a useful strategy to consider for serious problems such as sexualised behaviours (Saunders, Berliner & Hanson 2004). For example, studies have shown that CBT in combination with Dynamic Play Therapy can be used to assist younger children (6–12 years) who exhibit inappropriate and/or aggressive sexual behaviour. The children attend 12 weekly sessions that involve both cognitive-behavioural therapy and dynamic therapy components including: impulse control; learning and applying sexual behaviour rules for children; cognitive reframing to prevent re-abuse of or by the child; weekly assessment of acquisition of information; positive re-informing of appropriate behaviour; reflection to increase child's self understanding; acceptance to convey positive regard for child and improve child's self-esteem; and, facilitating group interaction to improve peer relationships (Bonner, Walker & Berliner 2000).

II. Building resilience

PRACTICE ISSUE: Children from vulnerable families where abuse is present often have poorer social skills which often leads to problems at school, difficulties in forming relationships and a danger of being further mistreated as teenagers and young adults.

Social skills training

A lot of social work practice and philosophy is based on the assumption that children have strengths and abilities that need to be harnessed so that they can cope with future challenges. Accordingly, there are a number of programs that practitioners can draw upon to encourage the development of positive and adaptive social behaviours (Evans, Axelrod & Sapia 2000). Common program elements include anger management, social skills training, personal skill development and assertiveness training. Many of these interventions use behavioural principles, but there is a much greater focus on the development of skills as opposed to just controlling or removing problematic behaviours. Furthermore, these interventions generally do not ascribe to just one theoretical model but often incorporate a broader range of theoretical approaches including cognitive therapy, social learning theory and general counselling techniques.

Conflict resolution and anger management skills are likely to be beneficial for both younger and older children. Although they take several different formats, programs generally involve a counsellor or therapist helping the young person to recognise the nature, the causes and the consequences of their anger and what situations appear to act as triggers. There may, for example, be a focus on simple relaxation, behavioural, or social methods for dealing with the situation and their anger and how the young person can learn to avoid the escalation of their anger by relaxing, taking deep breaths or simply by counting to ten before making a response. Other important elements may include the inclusion of role-playing, modelling and rehearsal to teach the client effective and appropriate ways to respond in anger-inducing situations. The client may practice such strategies with the therapist or may practice in a group therapy context with others who share similar problems. Such approaches may be combined with cognitive elements such as being able to avoid interpretation of situations in a way that induces anger or which leads it to escalate.

As might be expected, these broader social skills programs tend to vary depending upon a child's age, mental ability and the nature of the areas for development. In very young children, training may focus on simple things such as: eye contact, taking turns in conversation and in tasks or sharing toys with other children. By contrast, programs for older children, will commonly focus on improving communication skills (e.g., how to talk respectfully to adults, how to make requests or express certain ideas, initiate conversations and keep them going). There may also be a greater emphasis on limit setting or 'boundaries' of behaviours, including: the appropriate standards of personal attire or personal hygiene for different situations; appropriate emotional or physical boundaries (who can be approached, touched or contacted), or social rules and obligations (e.g., what is impolite, inappropriate or selfish). Some of the programs may include elements of:

- *Social learning or role-modelling*: Opportunities are given to demonstrate and practise the social skills observed in others. Subtle reinforcements (praise, positive affective responses) can encourage repetition of behaviours which are more adaptive and increase confidence in social interactions (Bandura 1977).
- *Self-assertiveness training*: Young people can learn to protect their interests, deal with bullying and interact with others in appropriate and non-aggressive ways (Thompson 2000; Wise et al. 1991).
- *Self-discipline and obligations:* Young are taught life skills, independent living skills, about how to organise their lives and daily routines and the obligations that exist between people. Some programs and, particularly some good residential care programs, may encourage such skill development by giving young people tasks, responsibilities and routines.

Dealing with early developmental harm

CP practitioners will often be aware from case notes and their own observations that many children have been significantly harmed by abuse. This means that once they have moved beyond any immediate focus on very visible behavioural problems, there is need to seek specialist help to deal with the deeper underlying problems caused by early traumatic experiences. Such problems may commonly manifest themselves in the form of unusual attachment behaviours or PTSD-like symptomology. But it is important that any such diagnosis is not rushed or made without appropriate assessment or evaluation. As McLean et al. (2013) points out: not all social-behavioural problems necessarily reflect disrupted attachments, and attachment- and trauma-related behaviours can often be confused. Each must be assessed by a trained clinical psychologist or psychiatrist to understand the specific causes of the symptomology observed. Thereafter, however, children may benefit from multidisciplinary approaches deriving from a number of disciplines including social work, occupational therapy as well as psychology.

Trauma-informed counselling

One option that could be considered is trauma counselling or some form of trauma-informed therapy (Allen & Hoskowitz 2017; Kolko, Iselin & Gully 2011). Such approaches are predicated on the assumption that young people need to come to terms with their experiences by discussing them. In a non-judgmental way, the therapist helps them understand why and what happened to them and how this can affect the way that they function today. One of the best empirically supported approaches is Trauma Focused CBT (Cohen, Mannarino & Deblinger 2016). This technique, based on learning and cognitive theories is designed to reduce children's negative emotional and behavioural responses. Common treatment components include: psychoeducation about child abuse; gradual exposure techniques of abusive events (i.e. utilising dolls, puppets etc.); cognitive reframing, consisting of exploration and correction of inaccurate attributions about the abuse; stress management techniques; parental participation in parallel or conjoint treatment; parental instruction in child behaviour management strategies; family work to enhance communication and create opportunities for therapeutic discussion regarding the abuse (Carr, Duff & Craddock 2018; Saunders Berliner & Hanson 2004).

Activity scheduling and play therapies

Children may also benefit from some form of Activity Scheduling involving play therapy, art therapy and music therapy. Although the evidence base for these techniques is less developed than for programs such as MTFC, such methods may service a variety of useful functions. Therapeutically, the aim is to take advantage of children's natural means of expression as embodied in their play behaviour to assist them in coping with emotional stress or trauma. Play therapy can be implemented in a variety of formats including sensorimotor, art, fantasy, and game play (Hall, Kaduson & Schaefer 2002). Play therapy has also been applied to initiate change and help children in transition, especially those children experiencing multiple moves in the care system. Play therapists use the therapeutic powers of play (e.g. relationship enhancement, role-playing, catharsis, attachment formation, etc.) to help clients prevent or resolve psychological difficulties.

The therapists believe that this method allows the child to manipulate their world on a small scale. Therefore, by playing with specially selected materials (i.e. crayons, painting supplies, dolls and figures of various sizes and ages, toy cars, toy guns, stuffed animals) and with the guidance of the therapist, the child can play out their feelings, bringing them to the surface where they can face them and cope with them. The therapist also works from a non-judgemental, non-punitive position and creates an environment whereby children feel safe to express themselves in any manner they wish (Ray et al. 2001).

Attachment therapy/Attachment-focused approaches

Attachment refers to the enduring ties that children form with their primary caregivers during early development (Ainsworth 1979). The quality of these earliest relationships lays the foundation for later psychosocial and cognitive development (Fahlberg 1991). Effective attachments enhance conscience development, the ability to empathise with others, the ability to trust others, inner feelings of security, the ability to express a range of emotions and the internal regulation of emotions and impulses (Delaney 1998; Levy & Orlans 1998). Disruption to these attachments can lead to attachment disorder. Such children may feel rejected and worthless, be unable to control and regulate their emotions or have the have the ability to form productive relationships with others. Children may present as either very withdrawn or mistrustful, or conversely, overly controlling and demanding due to their inability to negotiate with others, or understand what should be expected of others. Others may be lacking in empathy or indiscriminately affectionate (absence of stranger anxiety) (Delaney 1998).

Attachment therapy has been a controversial topic because it has been associated with questionable practices involving the physical restraint or 'holding-therapy'. However, in more acceptable practices, the approach focuses on the regulation of emotions and behaviours to help develop more productive and fulfilling relationships with other people (Becker-Weidman 2006; Hughes 2004; Newman & Mares 2007). Attachment therapy does not specify that any single style of intervention is best (Moretti et al. 1997). Rather the purpose is to emphasise the importance of parent–child relationships and how the low quality of such relationships can impact greatly on the development of a wide range of social, cognitive and emotional impairments. Theoretically grounded approaches to attachment disorder recognise that the disorder is complex and multifaceted with behavioural, emotional, social and cognitive components. Moretti et al. (1997) argue that interventions need to be diverse and individually tailored to meet each child's particular needs. Therefore, the therapist and caregiver need to create an environment in which the young person feels protected, cared for to reduce their anxiety and uncertainty and so that they know what is expected of them. Attachment therapy focuses on providing the young person with opportunities and choices as attachment-disordered children do not generally respond to the same rewards as other children.

A fundamental element of attachment therapy is to teach the child empathy and emotional regulation; two parts of social development that the child with attachment disorder often fails to acquire. During therapy it is imperative that the child goes through a process of self-reflection whereby they are better able to understand their own actions and also understand how certain behaviours influence the emotional states for others. Children will be taught self regulation of their own emotional expression and to recognise what are appropriate or inappropriate behaviours with certain people and in certain environments. Such approaches can often be combined with some of the play and social skills methods described above. As Fahlberg (1991) points out, a child's sense of self-worth and the predictability and safety of the environment will be enhanced by making things seem positive and worthwhile. By engaging in activities that the young person is interested in, the expectation is that their confidence in their own abilities will increase in conjunction with their level of trust in other people. The hope is that their ability to interact with others without the need to manipulate or control their behaviour is also likely to improve.

III. Parental skill training and enhancing family functioning

PRACTICE ISSUE: Parents of children who are abused often face parenting challenging, including how to deal with complex behaviour and how to make the right choices in parental behaviours.

Effective family preservation and reunification also requires that birth parents are able to cope effectively with their children's behaviour. To this end, many interventions have been developed to enhance the skills and well-being of parents and to improve family functioning. Some of the best documented programs are summarised in this section.

Parent–Child Interaction therapy (PCIT)

Parent–Child Interaction therapy (PCIT) is an empirically supported therapy that has been used for parents of children aged 2–8 years, including in cases involving abuse (Thomas et al. 2017; Urquiza et al. 2011). CP practitioners may be able to locate psychologists who are trained in this method by contacting peak bodies or seeking specialist referrals. PCIT attempts to improve parent–child interactions with a focus on nurturance and boundary-setting, both of which are the hallmarks of Baumrind's authoritative parenting style (Baumrind 1966). PCIT usually commences with a component termed Child-Directed Interaction (CDI) which aims to restructure the parent–child relationship and provide the child with a secure attachment to his or her parent. The CDI phase is similar to play therapy in that parents engage with their children in play to help strengthen their relationship with the child. The second phase of PCIT is based on social learning theory and emphasises the contingencies that shape interactions of conduct-disordered children and their parents; referred to as the Parent-Directed Interaction (PDI). The PDI phase often uses a step-by-step, live-coached (e.g., from behind one-way glass) behavioural parent training model. It provides the parents with immediate prompts, from the therapist in an observation room, to a parent while they are interacting with their child through an ear-mounted receiver worn by the parent to develop new more effective interaction strategies.

A number of studies have shown that this can lead to significant improvements in the conduct-disordered behaviour of preschool children (Bell & Eyberg 2002), in reducing parental distress (Schuhmann et al. 1998) and maladaptive interactions that might lead to abuse (Ware, Forston & McNeil 2003). Although some studies have not supported sustained improvements in behaviours beyond 18 months (Funderburk et al. 1998), it is generally accepted this is a promising approach for assisting parents at risk of being physically abused (Chadwick 2004).

Parent Management Training (PMT)

If children are older and particularly if there is a history of offending, CP practitioners may find that parents may need to be trained to deal with more complex and serious behaviours. One good example of this type of program is Parent Management Training or PMT. PMT usually involves older children and often those with more serious behaviours or offending histories. Most of these programs are usually behavioural or cognitive-behavioural in nature and focus on teaching parents the skills that will enable them to create a home environment that is less likely to trigger and reinforce problematic behaviour in children. Interventions can be individually administered or also involve both parents and children (Pearl 2009). One well-known PMT program was developed at the Oregon Social Learning Centre (Patterson, Chamberlain & Reid 1982; Reid, Patterson & Snyder 2002) and focuses on breaking down maladaptive and ultimately destructive behavioural cycles between parents and their children. Attempts are made to recognise and modify the patterns of control, coercion and factors that lead to the mutual escalation of behaviour, often by using the behavioural techniques described above. Studies conducted by Patterson Chamberlain and Reid (1982) as well as Bank et al. (1991) have indicated positive results in the form of reductions in offending and other anti-social behaviours.

The Incredible Years

The Incredible Years programs were developed by Carolyn Webster-Stratton for children (aged 2 to 10 years) who are highly aggressive, disobedient, hyperactive and inattentive. The program has also been used with parents at risk for abusing or neglecting their children. Influenced by the work of Patterson, Chamberlain and Reid (1982), the program includes a parent, teacher and child training series that is designed to promote social competence and prevent, reduce and treat aggression and related conduct problems in young children. The program uses group discussion, videotape modelling, and rehearsal intervention techniques to help adults living and working with children.

The interventions that make up this series (parent training, teacher training, and child training programs) are guided by developmental theory concerning the role of multiple interacting risk and protective factors (child, family and school) in the development of conduct problems. The parent training intervention is focused on strengthening parenting competencies (monitoring, positive discipline, confidence) and developing parents' involvement in children's school experiences in order to promote children's academic and social competencies and reduce conduct problems. The child social skills and problem-solving training programs involve strengthening children's social and emotional competencies (i.e. effective problem-solving strategies, managing anger, practising friendship and conversational skills), as well as appropriate classroom behaviours. The teacher training programs are focused on strengthening teacher classroom management strategies, promoting children's prosocial behaviour and school readiness (reading skills), and reducing classroom aggression and non-cooperation with peers and teachers. Additionally the intervention focuses on ways teachers can effectively collaborate with parents to support their school involvement and promote consistency from home to school.

Multisystemic therapy (MST)

Multisystemic therapy (MST) (Henggeler et al. 1993) was developed in the late 1970s and also focuses parent management and skills training. MST is an intensive family- and community-based treatment that views individuals as being nested within a complex network of interconnected systems that include individual, family and extra-familial (i.e. peer, school and neighbourhood) factors. The MST approach believes that interventions must deal with each of these systems. Originally designed to treat chronic, violent or substance abusing offenders at high risk of out-of-home placement, MST is now being tested and used with a variety of populations including children and young people with emotional and behavioural disturbance (Huey et al. 2000), abused and neglected youth (Brunk, Henggeler & Whelan 1987) substance abusing or dependent adolescent offenders (Henggeler et al. 1997; Schoenwald et al. 2000). MST is based on two behavioural theories; namely systems theory and social ecology, and on causal modelling studies of serious anti-social youth (Burns et al. 2000). The program seeks to intervene in a way that alters both the surrounding environment and the individual's behaviour. Accordingly, MST is a strengths-focused approach in that it endeavours to promote behaviour change in the youth's natural environment through using existing strengths within each system (e.g., family, peers, school, neighbourhood, informal support networks). The ultimate goal of MST is to empower parents with the skills and resources needed to address the difficulties that may arise in the home with the youth and also enable the youth to cope with the family, peer, school, and neighbourhood problems.

MST helps the family to function more successfully in their immediate environment (Burns et al. 2000). Interventions are integrated into a social–ecological context and include a variety of approaches such as strategic family therapy, structural family therapy, behavioural parent training and cognitive behaviour therapies. MST is provided to families using a home-based model of services delivery. The reason for this type of service delivery model is to help overcome barriers to service access, increase family retention in treatment, allow for the provision of intensive services and enhance the maintenance of treatment gains. Core treatment principles focus on the use of child strengths as the level for change and developmental appropriateness, target specific behaviours and try to address the causes across the different levels or domains of the child's life (e.g., both in the home and at school). Evidence generally supports the view that MST can be an effective family preservation approach (Schoenwald et al. 2000), but some authors (e.g., Littell, Popa & Forsythe 2006) have pointed to some inconsistencies in results, and whether this, being a very intensive and, by implication, expensive program, is necessarily better than other parenting skills programs.

Positive Parenting Program (PPP)

Many stand-alone parenting programs exist around the world and CP practitioners would be encouraged to consider a range of options. However, one useful starting point would be the Australian program, Triple P, developed by Professor Matthew Sanders and his colleagues from the Parenting and Family Support Centre in the School of Psychology at the University of Queensland, which uses a multi-level framework to tailor information, advice and professional support to the needs of individual families. Triple P offers five levels of intervention of increasing strength, ranging from basic tip sheets and videos, to brief targeted interventions to more intensive parent training in positive parenting that targets broader family issues such as parental depression, anger and stress, and aims to prevent severe emotional, behavioural and developmental problems in children (Sanders, Markie-Dadds & Turner 2003). PPP is designed to promote family independence by enhancing parents' knowledge, skills and confidence to create safe and nurturing environments that foster healthy child development.

The program aims to use the minimally sufficient intervention a parent requires, working from level 1 up to level 5 to avert the child from developing more serious problems. The program targets five different developmental periods: infants, toddlers, preschoolers, primary schoolers and teenagers and within each developmental period the intervention is very flexible and therefore tailored to the specific needs of the individual. The program also uses a variety of flexible delivery modalities including individual, face-to-face, group, telephone-assisted and self-directed programs. Triple P has a 25- year history of implementation and research evidence and is considered to be evidenced-based family intervention. Many of the studies conducted by Sanders and his colleagues (see Sanders et al. 2003) reported very positive changes in child behaviour problems, reductions in aversive parenting practices and parenting conflict, and improvements in relationship satisfaction and communication.

Summary

CP practitioners will often encounter children and families who face multiple, complex and often overlapping problems. Effective therapeutic approaches for these families involve multiple elements. While much of the early stages of engagement with children and families is likely to have a stronger social work focus (e.g., building trust) and dealing with practical problems such as housing, contact and support services, therapeutic needs will eventually need to be considered. Such services are likely to have a dual focus. One will be to recognise and identify the deeper underlying causes and effects of any ongoing trauma (e.g., trauma focused and attachment therapies); the other will be to deal with the immediate behaviours and symptomology (e.g., CBT or social skills training). Such approaches are not in competition, but are likely to be complementary. A best practice approach would, therefore, involve recognition of the importance of the early identification and standardised clinical assessment of child problems followed by tailored interventions. Effective interventions should also involve the development of a strengths-based approach that recognises the importance of developing skills and capacity in both children and their families so as to gradually encourage greater self-determination and resilience to face future challenges.

Discussion questions

- Complex behaviours often reflect deeper underlying psychological problems arising from earlier abuse and trauma. How do practitioners balance the needs to deal with the practical challenge of outward behaviours while also dealing therapeutically with the underlying causes?
- How should multidisciplinary expertise be best utilised in situations involving abused children with complex psychological and social needs?
- What are the most promising strategies which might be used to enhance the skills of parents to look after children with complex needs?

References

Ainsworth, M., 1979, 'Infant–mother attachment', *American Psychologist*, vol. 34, pp. 932–937.

Allen, B. & Hoskowitz, N.A., 2017, 'Structured trauma-focused CBT and unstructured play / experiential techniques in the treatment of sexually abused children: A field study with practising clinicians', *Child Maltreatment*, vol. 22, pp. 112–120.

Applegate, J.S. & Shapiro, J.R., 2005, *Neurobiology for clinical social work theory and practice*, New York: WW Norton.

Bandura, A., 1977, *Deviant behaviour: A social learning approach*, Belmont, MA: Wadsworth.

Bank, L., Marlowe, J.H., Reid, J.B., Patterson, G.R. & Weinrott, M.R., 1991, 'A comparative evaluation of parent-training interventions for families of chronic delinquents', *Journal of Abnormal Child Psychology*, vol. 19, pp. 15–33.

Baumrind, D., 1966, 'Effects of authoritative parental control on child behaviour', *Child Development*, vol. 37, 887–907.

Becker-Weidman, A., 2006, 'The report of the APSAC Taskforce in Attachment Therapy: Reactive attachment disorder and attachment problems', *Child Maltreatment*, vol. 11, pp. 379–380.

Bell, S. & Eyberg, S.M., 2002, 'Parent–child interaction therapy', in L. VandeCreek, S. Knapp & T. L. Jackson (eds), *Innovations in clinical practice: A source book*, Sarasota, FL: Professional Resource Press, pp. 57–74.

Bloomquist, M.L. & Schnell, S., 2005, *Helping children with aggression and conduct problems*, London: The Guilford Press.

Bonner, B., Walker, C.E. & Berliner, L., 2000, *Children with sexualised behaviour problems: Assessment and treatment*, Washington DC: National Clearinghouse on Child Abuse and Neglect.

Bruce, M., Young, D., Turnbull, S., Rooksby, M., Chadwick, G., Oates, C., Nelson, R., Young-Southward, G., Haig, C., & Minnis, H., 2018, 'Reactive attachment disorder in maltreated young children in foster care', *Attachment and Human Development*, vol. 21, no. 2, pp. 152–169.

Brunk, M., Henggeler, S. W. & Whelan, J.P., 1987, 'Comparison of multisystemic therapy and parent training in the brief treatment of child abuse and neglect', *Journal of Consulting and Clinical Psychology*, vol. 55, pp. 171–178.

Burns, B.J., Schoenwald, S.K., Burchard, J.D., Faw, L. & Santos, A.B., 2000, 'Comprehensive community-based interventions for youth with severe emotional disorders: Multisystemic therapy and the wraparound process', *Journal of Child and Family Studies*, vol. 9, pp. 283–314.

Carr, A. Duff, H. & Craddock, F., 2020, 'A systematic review of the outcome of child abuse in long-term care', *Trauma, Violence and Abuse*, vol. 21, pp. 660–677.

Chadwick Center on Children and Families, 2004March, *Closing the quality chasm in child abuse treatment: Identifying and disseminating best practices*, San Diego, CA: Kauffman Foundation.

Chamberlain, P., 1990, 'Comparative evaluation of specialized foster care for seriously delinquent youths', *Community Alternatives: International Journal of Family Care*, vol. 2, pp. 21–36.

Chamberlain, P. & Reid, J.B., 1991, 'Using a specialized foster care community treatment model for children and adolescents leaving the state mental hospital', *Journal of Community Psychology*, vol. 19, 266–276.

Cohen, J.A., Mannarino, A.P. & Deblinger, E., 2016, *Trauma focused CBT for children and adolescents: Treatment applications*, London: Guilford Press.

Delaney, R., 1998, *Fostering changes: Treating attachment disordered foster children*, Oklahoma City, OK: Wood 'N' Barnes.

Delfabbro, P.H., 2018, *Aboriginal children in out-of-home care in NSW: Developmental outcomes and cultural and family connections in the Pathways Longitudinal Study*, Sydney, NSW: FACS.

Dorsey, S., Burns, B.J., Southerland, D.G., Revillion-Cox, H., Wagner, R. & Farmer, E., 2013, 'Prior trauma exposure for youth in treatment foster care', *Journal of Child and Family Studies*, vol. 21, pp. 816–824.

Dubner, A.E. & Motta, R.W., 1999, 'Sexually and physically abused foster care children and posttraumatic stress disorder', *Journal of Consulting and Clinical Psychology*, vol. 67, pp. 367–373.

Evans, S.W., Axelrod, J.L. & Sapia, J.L., 2000, 'Effective school-based mental health interventions: Advancing the social skills training paradigm', *The Journal of School Health*, vol. 70, pp. 191–194.

Fahlberg, V., 1991, *A child's journey through placement*, Indianapolis, IN: Perspective Press.

Funderburk, B.W., Eyberg, S.M., Newcomb, K., McNeil, C., Hembree-Kigin, T. & Capage, L., 1998, 'Parent–child interaction therapy with behaviour problem children: Maintenance of treatment effects in the school setting', *Child & Family Behavior Therapy*, vol. 20, pp. 17–38.

Hall, T.M., Kaduson, H.G. & Schaefer, C.E., 2002, 'Fifteen effective play therapy techniques', *Professional psychology: Research & Practice*, vol. 33, pp. 512–522.

Henggeler, S.W., Melton, G.B., Brondino, M.J., Scherer, D.G. & Hanley, J.H., 1997, 'Multisystemic therapy with violent and chronic juvenile offenders and their families: The role of treatment fidelity in successful dissemination', *Journal of Consulting and Clinical Psychology*, vol. 65, pp. 821–833.

Henggeler, S.W., Melton, G.B., Smith, L.A., Schoenwald, S.K. & Hanley, J.H., 1993, 'Family preservation using multisystemic treatment: Long-term follow-up to a clinical trial with serious juvenile offenders', *Journal of Child and Family Studies*, vol. 2, 283–293.

Hersen, M., 1989, *Innovations in child behaviour therapy*, New York: Springer.

Hinswaw, S.P., Henker, B. & Whalen, C.K., 1984, 'Self-control in hyperactive boys in anger-inducing situations: Effects of cognitive-behavioral training and methylphenidate', *Journal of Abnormal Child Psychology*, vol. 12, pp. 55–77.

Hodges, K., 2004, *Evidence-based treatments for children and adolescents: A compilation of resources and guide for matching CAFAS profiles to evidence-based treatments*, Ann Arbor, MI: Functional Assessment Systems.

Hughes, D., 2004, 'An attachment-based treatment of maltreated children and young people', *Attachment and Human Development*, vol. 6, pp. 263–278.

Huey, S.J., Henggeler, S.W., Brondino, M.J. & Pickrel, S.G., 2000, 'Mechanisms of change in multisystemic therapy: Reducing delinquent behaviour through therapist adherence and improved family and peer functioning', *Journal of Consulting and Clinical Psychology*, vol. 68, pp. 451–467.

Kolko, D.J., Iselin, A.M.R. & Gully, K.J., 2011, 'Evaluation of the sustainability and clinical outcome of alternatives for families: A cognitive-behavioral therapy (AF-CBT) in a child protection center', *Child Abuse & Neglect*, vol. 35, pp. 105–116.

Levy, T.M. & Orlans, M., 1998, *Attachment, trauma and healing: Understanding and treating attachment disorder in children and families*, Washington DC: Child Welfare League of America.

Littell, J.H., Popa, M. & Forsythe, B., 2006, 'Multisystemic Therapy for social, emotional, and behavioural problems in youth aged 10–17', *The Cochrane Database of Systematic Reviews*, New York: John Wiley.

Mclean, S., Riggs, D., Kettler, L. & Delfabbro, P., 2013, 'Challenging behavior in out-of-home care: mis-application of attachment ideas in practice', *Child and Family Social Work*, vol. 18, pp. 243–252.

Meadowcraft, P., 1989, 'Treating emotionally disturbed children and adolescents in foster homes', *Children and Youth Services*, vol. 12, pp. 23–43.

Moretti, M.M., Emmrys, C., Grizenko, N., Holland, R., Moore, K., Shamsie, J. & Hamilton, H., 1997, 'The treatment of conduct disorder: Perspectives from across Canada', *The Canadian Journal of Psychiatry*, vol. 42, 637–648.

Newman, L. & Mares, S., 2007, 'Recent advances in the theories of and interventions with attachment disorders', *Current Opinion in Psychiatry*, vol. 20, pp. 343–348.

Ollendick, T.H. & King, N.J., 1998, 'Empirically supported treatments for children with phobic and anxiety disorders: Current status', *Journal of Clinical Psychology*, vol. 27, pp. 156–167.

Patterson, G.R. 1974, 'Interventions for boys with conduct problems: Multiple settings, treatments and criteria', *Journal of Consulting and Clinical Psychology*, vol. 42, pp. 471–481.

Patterson, G.R., Chamberlain, P. & Reid, J.B., 1982, 'A comparative evaluation of a parent-training program', *Behavior Therapy*, vol. 13, pp. 638–650.

Pearl, E.S., 2009, 'Parent management training for reducing oppositional and aggressive behaviour in preschoolers', Aggression and Violent Behavior, vol. 14, pp. 295–305.

Perry, B., 2002, 'Childhood experience and the expression of genetic potential: What childhood neglect tells us about nature and nurture', *Brain and Mind*, vol. 3, pp. 79–100.

Perry, B., 2009, 'Exploring maltreatment through a neurodevelopmental lens: Child applications of the neurosequential model of therapeutics', *Journal of Loss and Trauma*, vol. 14, pp. 240–255.

Ray, D., Bratton, S., Rhine, T. & Jones, L., 2001, 'The effectiveness of play therapy: Responding to the critics', *International Journal of Play Therapy*, vol. 10, pp. 85–108.

Reid, J.B., Patterson, G.R. & Snyder, J., 2002, *Antisocial behavior in children and adolescents: A developmental analysis and model for intervention*, Washington, DC: American Psychological Association.

Rhoades, K.P., Chamberlain, P., Roberts, P. & Leve, L.D., 2013, 'MTFC for high-risk adolescent girls: A comparison of outcomes in England and the United States', *Journal of Child and Adolescent Substance Abuse*, vol. 22, pp. 435–449.

Sanders, M.R., Markie-Dadds, C. & Turner, K.M.T., 2003, 'Theoretical, scientific and clinical foundations of the Triple-P- Positive Parenting Program: A population approach to the promotion of parenting competence', *Parenting Research and Practice Monograph*, no. 1, pp. 1–24.

Saunders, B.E., Berliner, L. & Hanson, R.F., 2004, *Child physical and sexual abuse: Guidelines for treatment*, Seattle, WA: Office for Victims of Crime.

Sawyer, M., Carbone, J., Searle, A. & Robinson, P., 2007, 'The mental health and wellbeing of children and adolescents in home-based foster care', *Medical Journal of Australia*, vol. 186, pp. 181–184.

Schoenwald, S.K., Ward, D.M., Henggeler, S.W. & Rowland, M.D., 2000, 'Multisystemic therapy versus hospitalization for crisis stabilization of youth: Placement outcomes 4 months post-referral', *Mental Health Services Research*, vol. 2, pp. 3–12.

Schuhmann, E.M., Foote, R., Eyberg, S.M., Boggs, S. & Algina, J., 1998, 'Parent–child interaction therapy: Interim report of a randomised trial with short-term maintenance', *Journal of Clinical Child Psychology*, vol. 27, pp. 34–45.

Tarren-Sweeney, M., 2008, 'The mental health of children in out-of-home care', *Current Opinion in Psychiatry*, vol. 21, pp. 345–349.

Tarren-Sweeney, M., 2013, 'An investigation of complex attachment and trauma-related symptomology among children in foster and kinship care', *Child Psychiatry and Human Development*, vol. 44, pp. 727–741.

Thomas, R., Abell, B., Haley, J.W., Avdagic, E. & Zimmer-Gembeck, M., 2017, 'Parent–child interaction therapy: A meta-analysis', *Pediatrics*, vol. 140

Thompson, R., 2000, 'The legacy of early attachments', *Child Development*, vol. 71, pp. 145–152.

Urquiza, A., Zebell, N., Timmer, S., McGrath, J. & Whitten, L., 2011, Course of Treatment Manual for PCIT-TC, http://pcit.ucdavis.edu/wp-content/uploads/2013/01/Section-1_General-Information2.pdf, accessed 25 September 2019.

Ware, L.M., Forsten, B.L. & McNeil, C.B., 2003, 'Parent–child interaction therapy: A promising intervention for abusive families', *The Behavior Analyst Today*, vol. 3, pp. 375–378.

Wise, K.L., Bundy, K.A., Bundy, E.A. & Wise, L.A., 1991, 'Social skills training for young adolescents', *Adolescence*, vol. 26, pp. 233–241.

Part 3

The protective care continuum

Chapter 9

Prevention and early intervention with children, young people, and families

Carmel Devaney

Introduction

Children's future is the present (Cosaro 1997). Notwithstanding the fact that children are active agents in their own right they remain a vulnerable group dependent on adults to protect, support, nourish and educate them. Supports therefore need to be available to children and young people as early as possible and usually require the involvement of family members who, as Devaney (2008) emphasised, can be either the subject of the intervention or a partner for change. As will be shown in this chapter, any supports that are provided need to be underpinned by the principles of accessibility, responsiveness and inclusivity in their how they are planned and delivered. To illustrate the application of these principles, this chapter will examine models and approaches applied in children and families services in Ireland. The Republic of Ireland is geographically a relatively small country of just over 70,000 square kilometres, with a population of 4,761,865, of which 1,251,796 are children. The average number of children in each family is 1.38, with 18 per cent of families having one parent, the vast majority of whom (86.4%) are one-parent mothers (CSO 2016). The chapter firstly debates the conceptual issues involved in taking a preventative stance in service provision and in day-to-day child welfare practice. The chapter will use this context to highlight the implementation of, and evidence base supporting a programme for prevention and early intervention in the child protection and welfare system.

Prevention and early intervention in supporting children and young people

Supportive welfare services play a central role in preventing issues escalating to the point that they cause significant harm to children's welfare and a delays to their development. This includes an emphasis, not only on preventing difficulties arising in the first instance, but also on intervening early where difficulties have occurred. In line with this view, Barlow and Schrader McMillan (2010) draw a conceptual distinction between preventive interventions, designed to reduce the likelihood of maltreatment, and more specialist or therapeutic interventions, designed to prevent its recurrence and/or address the psycho-social consequences. Although such interventions may differ in content and focus, they are all nonetheless preventative in nature. It is widely accepted that prevention and early intervention approaches can reduce risk factors, enhance protective factors as well as help achieve better outcomes than interventions that are implemented later (Harvey 2014).

Other authors such as Frost and Parton (2009) further argue that the role of prevention is not only to combat risk (the negatives) for children and families, but also to enhance the positives which may include opportunities to strengthen child development by maximising protective factors and processes (p. 20).

It is also increasingly accepted that best practice in supporting children and young people involves supporting family members and, in particular, parents or carers. MacMillan et al. (2009) found that protective factors for children included access to resources and support for parents (for example, material resources, human capital and social support), nurturing responsive parenting and care, and nurturing supportive family and friendship relationships. Factors such as strong relationships between parents and children, good parental understanding of child development, parental resilience, strong social support and social networks, and child emotional and social competence can serve as protective factors in relation to child maltreatment (Sethi et al. 2013).

In both conceptual and practical terms, the word 'family' can extend beyond immediate biological relatives to include other important people who are both related and unrelated (Morris 2012). The evidence from family decision making in care and protection suggests that the family networks identified by children and those close to them have few boundaries, with factors such as geographical location, blood ties and proximity not necessarily being key determinants of the membership of a child's network (Morris & Barnes 2008). Many families involve complex unconventional networks of relationships. New relationships due to divorce, separation, and changing partners have to be negotiated within families and between families and practitioners (Saltiel 2013). It makes sense to therefore adopt a fluid definition of 'family' that recognises that family structures or networks will vary considerably.

However, although modern families display diversity in their structure, how they are described and how they are viewed by practitioners, the legislation and policies that govern child protection work continue to be situated within a conventional paradigm based on the nuclear family (Morris 2012). In effect, a standard model of family life and operation is presumed by Governments to allow easier legislation, but, in reality, it is very difficult to identify a standard model of what families do or indeed what they ought to do. For this reason, Morgan's (1999) notion of family practices has been particularly helpful in directing attention away from focusing on family structure to the practices that sustain or impede love, connection and support (Featherstone 2004). Understanding family practices allows practitioners to consider how each individual family operates and this extends the debate about who is in the family (what the family composition is) or the role of families (are they good for children) (Morris 2013). Building upon this literature, advocates of prevention, early intervention and Family Support have therefore begun to encourage a change in focus from supporting family structures to family practices (Morris 2012). Such an approach directs attention towards understanding what is happening to individual family members and how the needs of different family members may change over time. It also aligns with international family support literature that provides important insights into what people value, when and how (see Katz & Pinkerton 2003). It opens debate about the type and level of need each individual might have, and what family members and close networks can offer in terms of care and support, and it extends practice and policy considerations away from a narrow focus on time-limited prescriptive interventions as the only possible response.

The importance of timing

Delaying services and support provision to families with complex needs can have a cost, both in terms of individual and family wellbeing and individual and family outcomes (Nupponen 2007). Moreover, risk factors for child maltreatment can be cumulative in nature, meaning that the more a child or family experiences, the more vulnerable they are to child maltreatment. Currently, in many jurisdictions, services for children and families can be driven and shaped by political interests, funding, media focus, individual interests and energy. The actual needs of children and young people are often underplayed or even ignored in this process, resulting in costly interventions later in life (Harvey 2014). However, child maltreatment and the devastating impacts it has on young people throughout their lives can often be prevented through appropriate policies and interventions (Nupponen 2007). However, it is also clear that earlier and timely interventions and those which prevent the occurrence of maltreatment are likely to be more effective than those that address its consequences. Studies show that the outcomes of interventions are influenced by the age of the children or young person entering the services and the length of time he/she is in receipt of a service, with an earlier starting age and a longer time in receipt of services associated with a greater number of positive outcomes (Raspa et al. 2010). As Allen (2011) suggests, one great merit of early intervention is that it can help families under stress to fulfil their mission of giving children a secure and loving environment in which to grow. Early intervention can keep families together and save many from the trauma of break-up and removal (p. ix).

At a broader level, prevention and early intervention can be understood from the perspective of social investment. Early intervention, particularly targeted at early years, can be a more cost-effective investment than those which come later. This is because child maltreatment is associated with numerous longer-term negative outcomes including: increased use of health services, poorer educational outcomes, greater risk of correctional involvement and poorer job and housing outcomes. Indeed, studies focused on return of investment of prevention and early interventions have described a return of between £1.37 and £9.20 per every pound invested (Harvey 2014).

Early intervention approaches place a greater emphasis on people's strengths and potential and can serve to reduce the level of dependency on the state by investing in children, young people and their families as active contributors to society (Gray 2014). Such approaches can be particularly effective when attention is given to children who are predicted to cost the most in terms of service provision and who have a diminished future early capacity and contribution to state taxation revenue (Heckman 2006). This, however, requires government policies to be focused on tackling causes and not symptoms and an overarching shift of investment towards the implementation of prevention and early intervention (or primary) services rather than tertiary interventions once the harm has been caused. It requires the implementation of proactive, empowered and partnership relationships between service providers and children, young people and families that are involved with social services. A public health response recognises that public health issues sit on a continuum of severity and many families with access to universal services may occasionally require secondary services to support their parenting or address other areas of need (Scott, Lonne & Higgins 2016). Furthermore, the long-term impact of childhood abuse on mental and social wellbeing can mean that adults who have suffered abuse as children are at increased risk of maltreating their own children. Daro (2011) outlines strategies and interventions that have been proven to reduce child maltreatment and suggests consideration should be given to:

- Improving the nation's ability to prevent child maltreatment through a public health model of universal program delivery
- Designing programs to support a diverse population
- Employing technology to increase access to programs; and
- Balancing enhancement of formal services and informal supports.

She concludes that preventing child maltreatment is not simply a matter of *parents* 'doing a better job'; it is about creating a *context* in which 'doing a better job' is easier (2011: 11). Heckman's (2006) work shows the value of investing in early childhood as a viable alternative to increased welfare. He notes that, without supportive social services, merely providing increased welfare benefits to families experiencing difficulties merely throws good money after bad.

Importance of social conditions

Social and economic conditions are also key determinants of the health and wellbeing of children and adults. They can be of an economic, social, political and cultural nature. Based on an ecological approach, fundamental aspects of life and living such as occupation, social class, education, gender, ethnicity, income and housing all have a role in the adversities and vulnerabilities that affect individuals and their families (Titterton & Taylor 2018). The difficulties faced by families and their ability to cope with and manage presenting adversities vary from family to family and household to household. Families living in areas of deprivation and with low levels of services available to them experience child maltreatment to a greater extent than those living in less deprived areas and with higher access to supports and resources. Child welfare inequality is defined as occurring 'when children and/or their parents face unequal chances, experiences or outcomes of involvement with child welfare services that are systematically associated with structural social dis/advantage and are unjust and avoidable' (Bywaters et al. 2015: 100). The annual European Union (EU) Survey on Income and Living Conditions (SILC), conducted in Ireland by the Central Statistics Office (CSO) is part of a programme to obtain information on the income and living conditions of different types of households and is used to measure poverty in Ireland. The most recent SILC figures on poverty relate to 2016 and show that, in 2016, 11.1 per cent of children in Ireland lived in consistent poverty, which equates to approximately 138,949 children or one in nine children. The proportion of children living in consistent poverty in Ireland almost doubled during the economic recession from 6.3 per cent in 2008 to 11.1 per cent in 2016. Of all households with children, lone parents had the highest poverty and deprivation rates in 2016, with a deprivation rate of 50.1 per cent (CSO 2016). In the UK, recent research highlights large inequalities in child welfare intervention rates with children living in deprived areas much more likely to be involved in child protection processes or to be taken into state care than children living in more affluent neighbourhoods (Bywaters et al. 2016). A small number of studies in the United States of America have also highlighted a link between family income and involvement in child protection services (Cancian, Yang & Shook Slack 2013). Of note also is that child maltreatment has been shown to be both a cause and a consequence of poverty (Bunting et al. 2018). Most recent Irish policy around tackling poverty for children and families is articulated in Better Outcomes, Brighter Futures (BOBF), the national policy framework for children and young people 2014–2020. This approach includes, among others, a significant focus on prevention and early intervention services for children, young people and their families in disadvantaged communities (Department of Children and Youth Affairs 2014).

Prevention and early intervention in practice in Ireland

Responding to the needs of children and young people from a prevention and early intervention approach and implementing policies such as Better Outcomes, Brighter Futures implies a change in the provision of services for families, which has been described as a paradigm shift. Agencies need to be flexible and adapt to fit with family needs instead of expecting families to adjust to immovable structures and procedures within agencies (Nupponen 2007). This is an ongoing challenge in the design and delivery of child welfare systems worldwide with many commentators debating this issue (Gilbert 2012). In Ireland, the establishment of a new dedicated state agency responsible for improving wellbeing and outcomes for children has afforded an opportunity to reimagine the orientation of the child protection and welfare service. Tusla, the Irish national Child and Family Agency (Tusla) was established in 2014 by the Child and Family Agency Act 2013. The Agency was established as part of a comprehensive reform and consolidation of child protection, early intervention and family support services in Ireland. The Child and Family Agency's services include a range of universal and targeted services, including: Child protection and welfare services, Educational Welfare Services, Psychological Services, Alternative Care (including foster care, residential care and special care), Family and Locally-based Community Supports, Early Years Services and Domestic, Sexual and Gender-based Violence Services. Prior to the Child and Family Agency Act, child protection and welfare services was under the remit of the wider Health Services Executive (HSE) and the Health Boards as was legislated for in the Child Care Act of 1991.

The Agency is committed to the principle that the family affords the best environment for raising children and the objective of external intervention should be to support families within the community. Similar to international developments in child welfare policy and practice, there has been a decisive shift away from institutional, residential type care towards foster care arrangements in Ireland (Devaney & Rooney 2018) and Ireland now has one of highest rates of family-based care placements globally and is similar to countries such as Australia. In May 2018, there were 6,160 children in the care of the Irish state, with approximately 92 per cent of these in either relative or general foster care arrangements; 2,067 young adults (all ages) were in receipt of aftercare services. In Australia, as of 30 June 2018 just over 45,800 children were in out-of-home care. Of these children, 51 per cent were in relative/kinship care, 39 per cent were in foster care, and 6 per cent were in residential care (Australian Institute of Health and Welfare 2019). Overall, at the end of the first quarter of 2018, there were 24,669 open cases in the Irish child protection and welfare system. The average monthly rate of referral to child protection and welfare services was just under 4,000 (61 per cent of which are classified as child welfare concerns) with 'no further action' recorded in just over 50 per cent of these referrals (Tusla Quality Assurance Directorate 2018).

Within its child welfare remit there is a new programme of action being undertaken by Tusla as part of its Service Delivery Framework. The programme, known as Prevention, Partnership and Family Support (PPFS) seeks to transform child and family services in Ireland by providing services which are provided when and where families need them, are responsive to the difficulties families are having and include the views of family members. The programme has five distinct but complementary and interwoven components: Parenting Support and Parental Participation (i.e. in the services they are involved in); Public Awareness (i.e. increasing awareness of where and how to access help among the general public); Children's Participation (i.e. enhancing child and youth participation at all levels of their involvement with Tusla); Commissioning, which focuses on the funding of services; and the development of the 'Meitheal' model. The latter is a distinct stream but it also acts as a fulcrum for much of the development of the other aspects of the programme. Meitheal is defined as

> a national practice model to ensure that the needs and strengths of children and their families are effectively identified, understood, and responded to in a timely way so that children and families get the help and support needed to improve children's outcomes and to realise their rights.
>
> (Gillen et al. 2013: 1)

The model is a process-based system, which is not linked to a physical infrastructure or network but rather revolves around the development of an approach that can be applied by organisations in the community and voluntary sector, by Tusla and other statutory services. This is grounded in a set of principles and structures that help to ensure a consistent application of this model regardless of where a family lives or which practitioner is working with them. These principles include:

- involvement in the process is voluntary and all aspects of the process are led by the parent and child or young person. This includes the decision to enter the process, the nature of information to be shared, the outcomes desired, the support delivered, and the agencies involved. Review Meetings cannot take place without the involvement of at least one parent.
- The process privileges the voices of the parent and child, recognising them as experts in their own situations and assisting them to identify their own needs and ways of meeting them.
- The model looks at the whole child in a holistic manner, in the context of their family and environment. It considers strengths and resilience, as well as challenges and needs.
- The overall focus is on outcomes and implemented through an agreed key worker known as the 'Lead Practitioner' who has an existing relationship with the family.

(Tusla 2015: 15–16)

Additionally, the model operates outside of the child protection system in that, for instance, families cannot be involved with Meitheal and the child protection system at the same time. Should child protection concerns be raised during the process, a referral will be made to the child protection system and the process will be closed. However, support can continue to be provided by individual agencies and practitioners.

While Meitheal activity is relatively low compared with the general family support service, it is rising. For example, at the end of 2017, there were 21,526 children in receipt of family support services with a total of 39,065 children referred to family support services throughout the year. During the same period there were 1,409 Meitheal processes requested. Of these, 52 per cent (736) were direct requests (i.e. without going through the child protection system), 39 per cent (554) were diverted from the child protection team and 8 per cent (119) were requested after the involvement of the child protection workers. In 2018, by the end of the first quarter, 802 Meitheals had been requested and processed (Tusla Quality Assurance Directorate 2018).

A number of Meitheal case studies are published by Cassidy, Devaney and McGregor, 2016. (See the following extracts from 'Early Implementation of Meitheal and the Child and Family Support Networks: Lessons from the field', pp. 65–66).

Family A

An Educational Welfare Officer described a family they were involved with where there was a young child with serious behavioural issues in school. The school was struggling to support the child, it did not have supportive resources to draw on. It was also challenging to engage the child's parents, who rarely attended meetings and were reluctant to get involved with statutory services. They eventually agreed to a Meitheal and the situation improved considerably for the child, who now attended school almost full time whereas previously they only attended a couple of hours a day. The parents were supported not only during the Meitheal Review Meetings but also afterwards by the services involved in the case. The parents' engagement in the process increased because they were active participants who felt listened to.

Family B

A number of different services had been working separately in one family with the children and the parent. In the case of the teenage son, a Meitheal process was initiated and at a meeting that he, his mother and a number of agencies attended it was decided that he would enrol in an alternative education programme. Meitheal had enabled a more coordinated approach to be taken to the case, which also made it easier for the parent, as the agencies were brought together simultaneously at a meeting where a joint decision could be taken.

Discussion points

1. Can you identify Meitheal principles and structures that made a difference to the outcomes of these families?
2. Would you consider this a preventative early intervention?
3. What would a likely outcome be if the families did not engage in the Meitheal process?
4. What are the strengths of this model as exemplified in these case vignettes?

The evidence base

Recent research with families who participated in the Meitheal process showed significantly improved outcomes for mothers and that mothers reported improved outcomes for children, young people and families as a whole. Father's wellbeing improved significantly (Rodriguez, Cassidy & Devaney 2018). This is an important finding as poor parental mental health is strongly associated with child maltreatment. Children and young people's self-reports on their wellbeing and family outcomes improved but this was not statistically significant (Rodriguez et al. 2018). The positive impact of Meitheal on most outcomes is a very important finding as currently policy and practice are targeted at outcomes as evidence of best practice, promoting the effectiveness of services, and evidence of accountability for funders and the public (Devaney, Canavan & Landy 2013). Tusla's Child Protection and Welfare Strategy (2017–2022) is informed by the principles that 'early intervention is key to getting better outcomes'. This evidence supports the argument to intervene early to prevent difficulties in families escalating. The introduction of Meitheal in the system has made Tusla's 'continuum of care' a reality by making Tusla's work at a low prevention level accountable in their overall performance reports published quarterly. Tusla (2017) defined low prevention services as those which target children and young people that may have additional needs requiring support without which they may not fully achieve their potential. Meitheal is specifically targeted at this low level of need for families that do not meet the threshold for child protection services although they may have complex and significant needs as well as following involvement with the child protection system.

Families who participated in the research also report positive experience of taking part in the Meitheal process with its capacity to ensure a range of supports are coordinated to meet identified needs. It also appears that Meitheal can lead to improvements in families' experiences of help-seeking by enabling parents to develop better relationships with professionals and take a greater role in decisions about what supports they receive. This empowerment has been identified in the literature as crucial to supporting children and young people's development (Devaney et al. 2013). Furthermore, Dunst and Trivette (2009) identified that having a family focus, and not just viewing the child as the unit of intervention, is one of the principles to enable and empower families, allowing parents to acquire the knowledge and skills to be able to cope with daily living and improve their sense of mastery and control.

The research emphasised the importance of the process characteristics of the model with relationship a key component of its success. The relationship between the family members and practitioners has long been considered the 'bedrock' of good practice, with emphasis placed on its importance (Mason 2012). Nonetheless, despite all the rhetoric on relationship-based practice, it remains a persistent challenge for child welfare practitioners. Along with the ever-decreasing time available to spend with families, a key question for practitioners involves determining what exactly constitutes a positive relationship. What are the skills and qualities that a practitioner needs to possess to develop a warm, helpful yet professional relationship? Mason usefully highlights four elements that enable relationships between practitioners and family members to work successfully:

1 **Respectful communication, this includes trust, honesty and feeling safe.**
When families feel they can trust practitioners, and where there is honesty in the communication exchange there is an increased likelihood of open communication about the difficulties faced and the associated needs. This includes families feeling that practitioners listen to them and take into account what they have to say. It has been suggested that the style adopted by practitioners in how they carry out their work with family members is as important as what they actually do (Devaney & Dolan 2017).

2 **A shared goal**
An agreed goal related to the family's needs has been shown to improve outcomes for family members. An inclusive approach to identifying individual needs, strengths and appropriate helpful responses to them allows for agreed goals which family members are motivated to try and achieve. Opportunities, without blame or judgement, to review and redefine these goals when necessary is also critical.

3 **Practical assistance and understanding parents' own needs**
Being available to support parents and children or young people is a critical factor in building a positive relationship. The importance of providing parents with both practical and emotional support has been highlighted as an important aspect of building relationships as it can convey a sense of understanding and caring.

4 **Reliability – being available**
An emphasis on direct contact with family members is central with a strong degree of flexibility included. Spending time together (the antithesis of busy 'case' driven proceduralised practice) is essential in order to build a trusting relationship.

At a wider level Meitheal also had an unexpected impact on the help-seeking behaviours and awareness of support services for families. Taking part in Meitheal has increased access to formal support networks and families who had had little understanding of how the service provision system worked now had a greater understanding of how to access help. Many of the parents who had a positive experience of Meitheal had begun to recommend the process to their own informal social networks which arguably could have positive consequences for earlier help-seeking in the general community (Rodriguez et al. 2018). It can also be argued that the positive formal support networks families develop with professionals through the Meitheal process could act as a protective factor against future risk, help to ensure that support is sought before issues reach a crisis point or reduce their reliance on continued access to one key service or individual. This could be particularly significant in the long term, as research demonstrates that help-seeking behaviours are strongly influenced by family and community behaviours and attitudes and that in the Irish context most individuals rely on their own informal networks for support (McGregor & NicGabhainn 2018). Given that current public awareness of formal services in Ireland is low (McGregor & NicGabhainn 2018), these parents could be agents of change in the perception of services and help seeking behaviours in their local areas. This has been identified as an especially crucial form of support for families, which is most likely to be utilised in times of need.

At a system-wide level, Meitheal appears to have the potential to affect change in the provision of the child welfare service in Ireland in terms of improving the continuum of support for families who do not meet thresholds for intervention from the child protection workers. It enables issues to be addressed early in a coordinated and prompt fashion based on clear identified needs within a transparent process. It also can lead to the development of stronger inter-agency cross-discipline relationships that are utilised outside of this process.

Conclusion

Maltreatment of children and young people is not inevitable. In many instances it is preventable and undoubtedly intervening early where there are difficulties is more cost-effective than dealing with the consequences of doing nothing. It is early stages in the use of the Meitheal model as an approach to prevention and early intervention but it is expected that this approach to help-seeking and help-provision will continue to evolve and become firmly established in the Irish child welfare system. Time is needed to further evaluate its impact. Research studies have suggested that it may require up to five years for prevention and early interventions to achieve long-term and permanent benefits (Norman et al. 2017). Ongoing attention to, and most likely balancing of, the prevention and early intervention approach and the requirement to ensure children and young people are safe will be ongoing. The need for integration across this continuum has been highlighted as a way to maximise potential of all services and to achieve better outcomes for children and families (Devaney & McGregor 2017; McGregor & Devaney 2019). Continued efforts will be required to reach the most vulnerable families who will not necessarily present themselves or make their way to services.

Responding to the needs of children, young people and their families and improving their outcomes is the ultimate goal of support services. This paper has presented the issues involved in prevention and early intervention using recent developments and research in the Irish context as a case study. Contexts differ and, as this chapter has emphasised, families differ; however, the values and principles that underpin this approach have transferability and applicability across jurisdictions and within diverse settings. This approach has delivered a service that is welcomed by families (and practitioners) that makes a positive difference to their outcomes and wellbeing.

References

Allen, G., 2011, *Early intervention: The next steps. An independent report to HM Government*, London: Cabinet Office.

Australian Institute of Health and Welfare, 2019, Child protection Australia: 2017–18. Child welfare series no. 70. Cat. no. CWS 65. Canberra: AIHW.

Barlow, J. & Schrader McMillan, A., 2010, *Safeguarding children from emotional maltreatment: What works*, London: Jessica Kingsley.

Bunting, L., Davidson, G., McCartan, C., Hanratty, J., Bywaters, P., Mason, W. & Steils, N., 2018, 'The association between child maltreatment and adult poverty: A systematic review of longitudinal research', *Child Abuse & Neglect*, vol. 77, pp. 121–133.

Bywaters, P., Brady, G., Sparks, T. & Bos, E., 2016, 'Inequalities in child welfare intervention rates: the intersection of deprivation and identity', *Child & Family Social Work*, vol. 21, pp. 452–463.

Bywaters, P., Brady, G., Sparks, T., Bos, E., Bunting, L., Daniel, B., Featherstone, B., Morris, K. & Scourfield, J., 2015, 'Exploring inequities in child welfare and child protection services: Explaining the "inverse intervention law"', *Children and Youth Services Review*, vol. 57, pp. 98–105.

Cancian, M., Yang, Mi-Y. & Shook Slack, K., 2013, 'The effect of additional child support income on the risk of child maltreatment', *Social Service Review*, vol. 87, pp. 417–437.

Cassidy, A., Devaney, C. & McGregor, C., 2016, *Early implementation of Meitheal and the child and family support networks: Lessons from the field.* Galway: The UNESCO Child and Family Research Centre, the National University of Ireland.

CSO, 2016, Households and families, www.cso.ie/en/media/csoie/releasespublications/documents/population/2017/Chapter_4_Households_and_families.pdf, accessed 30 September 2018.

Cosaro, W., 1997, *The sociology of childhood*, London: Pine Forge Press.

Daro, D., 2011, *Child maltreatment prevention: Past, present, and future.* Chicago, IL: Chapin Hall at the University of Chicago.

Department of Children and Youth Affairs, 2014, Better outcomes, brighter futures: the national policy framework for children and young people 2014–2020. www.dcya.gov.ie/viewdoc.asp?fn=/documents/cypp_framework/BetterOutcomesBetterFutureReport.pdf, accessed 31 August 2018.

Devaney, J., 2008, 'Chronic child abuse and domestic violence: Children and families with long-term and complex needs', *Child & Family Social Work*, vol. 13, pp. 443–453.

Devaney, C., Canavan, J. & Landy, F., 2013, *What works in family support? National guidance & local implementation*, Dublin: Tusla Child and Family Agency.

Devaney, C. & Dolan, P., 2017, 'Voice and meaning: The wisdom of Family Support veterans', *Child & Family Social Work*, vol. 22, pp. 10–20.

Devaney, C. & McGregor, C., 2017, 'Child protection and Family Support practice in Ireland: A contribution to present debates from a historical perspective', *Child and Family Social Work*, vol. 22, no. 3, pp. 1–9.

Devaney, C. & Rooney, C., 2018, *The feasibility of conducting a longitudinal study on children in care in Ireland*, Galway: UNESCO Child and Family Research Centre, National University of Ireland.

Dunst, C. & Trivette, C., 2009, 'Capacity-building family-systems intervention practices', *Journal of Family Social Work*, vol. 12, no. 2, pp. 119–143.

Featherstone, B., 2004, *Family life and family support*, Basingstoke, UK: Palgrave Macmillan.

Frost, N. & Parton, N., 2009, *Understanding children's social care politics, policy and practice.* London: Sage.

Gray, M., 2014, 'The swing to early intervention and prevention and its implications for social work', *The British Journal of Social Work*, vol. 44, pp. 1750–1769.

Gilbert, N., 2012, 'A comparative study of child welfare systems: Abstract orientations and concrete results', *Children and Youth Services Review*, vol. 34, pp. 532–536.

Gillen, A., Landy, F., Devaney, C. & Canavan, J., 2013, *Guidance for the implementation of an area-based approach to prevention, partnership and family support*, Dublin: HSE.

Harvey B., 2014, *The case for prevention and early intervention. Promoting positive outcomes for children, families and communities*, Dublin: Prevention and Early Intervention Network.

Heckman, J.J., 2006, 'Skill formation and the economics of investing in disadvantaged children', *Science*, vol. 312, pp. 1900–1902.

Katz, I. & Pinkerton, J. (eds), 2003, *Evaluating family support: Thinking internationally, thinking critically*, Chichester, UK: John Wiley.

McGregor, C. & Devaney, C., 2019, 'Protective support and supportive protection for families "in the middle": Learning from the Irish context', *Child & Family Social Work*, vol. 25, no. 2, pp. 277–285.

McGregor, C. & NicGabhainn, S., 2018, *Public awareness*, Galway: UNESCO Child and Family Research Centre, National University of Ireland.

MacMillan, H.L., Wathen, N.C., Barlow, J., Fergusson, D.M., Leventhal, J. & Taussig, N., 2009, 'Interventions to prevent child maltreatment and associated impairment', *The Lancet*, vol. 373, pp. 250–266.

Mason, C., 2012, 'Social work the "art of relationship": parents' perspectives on an intensive family support project', *Child & Family Social Work*, vol. 17, pp. 368–377.

Morgan, D.H.J., 1999, *Risk and family practices: Accounting for change and fluidity in family life – The new family*, London: Sage.

Morris, K., 2012, 'Thinking family? The complexities of family engagement in care and protection', *British Journal of Social Work*, vol. 42, pp. 906–920.

Morris, K., 2013, 'Trouble families: Vulnerable families' experiences of multiple service use', *Child & Family Social Work*, vol. 18, pp. 198–206.

Morris, K. & Barnes, M., 2008, 'Prevention and Social Exclusion: New Understandings for Policy and Practice', *British Journal of Social Work*, vol. 38, pp. 1194–1211.

Norman, R., Anderson, K., MacDougall, A., Machanda, R., Harricharan, R., Subramanian, P., Richard, J. & Northcott, S., 2017, 'Stability of outcomes after 5 years of treatment in an early intervention programme', *Early Intervention and Psychiatry*, vol. 12, pp. 720–725.

Nupponen, H., 2007, 'Prevention and early intervention: Innovative practice model "down under" in South-east Queensland, Australia', *Child Care in Practice*, vol. 13, pp. 367–386.

Raspa, M., Bailey, D.B., Olmsted, M.G., Nelson, R., Robinson, N., Simpson, M., Guillen, C. & Houts, R., 2010, 'Measuring family outcomes in early intervention: Findings from a large-scale assessment', *Exceptional Children*, vol. 76, pp. 496–510.

Rodriguez, L., Cassidy, A., & Devaney, C., 2018, *Meitheal process and outcomes study*, Galway: UNESCO Child and Family Research Centre, National University of Ireland.

Saltiel, D., 2013, 'Understanding complexity in families' lives: the usefulness of "family practices" as an aid to decision-making', *Child and Family Social Work*, vol. 18, pp. 15–24.

Scott, D., Lonne, B. & Higgins, D., 2016, 'Public health models for preventing child maltreatment: Applications from the field of injury prevention', *Trauma, Violence, & Abuse*, vol. 17, no. 4, pp. 408–419.

Sethi, D., Bellis, M., Hughes, K., Gilbert, R., Mitis, F. & Galea, G. (eds), 2013, *European report on preventing child maltreatment*, Copenhagen: WHO.

Titterton, M., & Taylor, J., 2018, 'Rethinking risk and resilience in childhood and child maltreatment', *The British Journal of Social Work*, vol. 48, pp. 1541–1558.

Tusla, 2015, *Meitheal toolkit*, Dublin: Tusla Child and Family Agency.

Tusla, 2017, The Prevention, Partnership and Family Support Programme. Collaborative leadership for better outcomes, www.tusla.ie/uploads/content/PPFS_Low_Prevention_Services_Brochure.pdf , accessed 12 April 2018.

Tusla Quality Assurance Directorate, 2018, Integrated performance and activity report. Quarter 1 2018, Dublin: Tusla.

Chapter 10

Foster family care as a response to child maltreatment

June Thoburn

Introduction

Across the world, a version of foster family care forms part of the response to the abuse and neglect of children. Informal foster care, especially with relatives and friends, is a part of every society, although the proportion of children who are in foster care varies over time and across jurisdictions. This chapter focuses on foster care in 'global north' nations, and on the formally provided services, while recognising its presence in a less regulated form in poorer countries. In some countries, including the USA and Australian states, out-of-home care in general, and foster family care in particular, is mainly court-mandated and triggered by concerns about abuse or neglect. In other countries such as the UK and much of Europe, state-provided foster family care is part of a service to a wider range of children and families 'in need of additional services' including disabled children needing a 'shared care' family support service (Thoburn 2010b). But even when they enter care on a voluntary basis (53% of care entrants in England in 2017–18), there are in most cases some concerns about actual or likely harm if the service is not provided. So foster family care as part of the response to maltreatment has much in common across jurisdictions.

In this chapter foster care services and foster carer 'careers' are considered in terms of whether they are in the main providing a short-term, birth family-focused service or a longer-term substitute family service. Information is provided on the extent to which foster family care is used in different jurisdictions. This is then followed by a summary of what is known about the outcomes of foster family care.

Which children and families need a family foster care service?

Children in different jurisdictions enter care for similar reasons and therefore often have similar needs. A large proportion will have experienced trauma, often because of parental mental ill-health, addictions or inter-partner violence which is frequently exacerbated by material deprivation. Except for infants removed at birth and placed directly with long-term foster families, or those placed with kinship foster parents they have known since birth, children placed with foster carers will have experienced the traumas of separation and loss, usually more than once and sometimes on multiple occasions. But there are also notable differences, especially with respect to the numbers and proportions entering care in the different age groups. Table 10.1 shows that, in Anglophone countries, a larger proportion of care entrants is in the younger age groups, whereas in most Western

Table 10.1 0–1 Percentages of those entering care by age group. Data for Australia, England and USA from 2016 to 2017 and for other countries from 2010 to 2013

Country	*0–4 (<12 months)*	*5–9*	*10+*
Australia	47% (20%)	26%	27%
England	35% (17%)	18%	47%
Denmark	12% (5%)	12%	76%
Germany	(0–5 yrs) 15% (4%)	28% (6–11 yrs)	56% (aged 12+)
Sweden	(0–3 yrs) 12%	15% (4–9 yrs)	79%
USA	44% (19%)	23%	33%

Sources: AFCARS 2019; Australian Institute of Health and Welfare 2018; Department for Education 2018; Thoburn 2010a.

European and Nordic countries a higher proportion enter care when of school age or even in late adolescence. The reasons for this are complex, but in part are related to the availability of family support services within the community (Thoburn 2010a).

All jurisdictions seek to provide appropriate placements for children in all age groups, but the table indicates several differences. For example, care services in Germany and Denmark and other similar countries have to be ready to care appropriately for smaller numbers of infants and larger numbers of teenagers entering care than is the case for Australia, the USA and English service agencies. In both the UK and US, and increasingly is some Australian states though not in others, there is a strong emphasis on young children leaving care quickly via adoption. Foster care for the youngest children in these countries tends to be very short term to facilitate a rapid return home or transition to adoptive families. By contrast, in European countries, when infants do come into foster care, they are more likely to stay with those foster families on a long-term basis. With older children, most jurisdictions place greater emphasis on continuing family links and the role of foster carers in helping children maintain birth family links and be comfortable, if the placement is long term, with their membership of two families (Schofield & Beek 2009; Schofield et al. 2013). Such age differences will influence the needs that the care system has to meet.

Although in theory, one might anticipate that countries which emphasise the importance of birth family links might recruit, train and support foster carers who can empathise with and have particular skills in working with birth families, it is not at all clear from research that this happens (an exception is reported in Fernandez 2012; Fernandez & Lee 2011: see Thoburn 2018 for a review of research on birth family contact with children in temporary and long-term care.)

The proportion of children entering care in the different age groups will clearly have an impact on the proportion placed in foster family as opposed to group care (see Table 10.2), and also on the ways in which foster families meet their needs. Unsurprisingly, there is a greater use of residential care and a consequently lower use of foster care in those countries where a larger proportion of care entrants are already teenagers (see Thoburn 2013 and Ainsworth & Thoburn 2014). Children who enter care later and have spent longer with their families (even if there are difficulties in the family) often prefer a group care placement or need foster families who are comfortable with and skilled at facilitating birth family links as well as providing a secure base (Schofield & Beek 2014). At the other end of the age continuum, it

Table 10.2 0–2 Percentages of children in care in different placement types. Data for Australia, England and USA from 2016 to 2017 and for other countries from 2010 to 2013

	Australia	*England*	*Norway*	*Denmark*	*Sweden*	*USA*
Non-kin foster care	32%	61%	55%	60%	65%	45%
Kinship foster care	37%	12%	17%	Included in above	12%	32%
Adoption **		5%				4%
Group care	5%	11%	28%	39%	21%	13%
Other (including with parents)	26%	11%			3%	7%

Sources: AFCARS 2019; Australian Institute of Health and Welfare 2018; Department for Education 2018; Thoburn 2010a.

** although some children in care in all countries will be with adoptive families waiting the adoption order, numbers are too small to show in the statistics.

can be hypothesised that when pre-school or school-age children do come into care, in some Western European and Nordic countries with higher investment on generally available child and family welfare services, more has been tried before the move into care so that it is less possible to get children safely home than in countries with less well developed family support services and higher thresholds for receipt of in-home targeted services (Skivenes & Thoburn 2016; Ubbesen, Gilbert & Thoburn 2015; Vinnerljung & Sallnas 2008). A consequence of these differences is that, although proportions and absolute numbers of pre-school children entering care are lower in most European countries than in Australia, North America and UK nations, these younger entrants are more likely to stay for longer periods in their foster families. If we look at a population of children in care on a given date, more will have joined their foster families at a young age and be still there after several years than is the case in the UK and USA where young entrants to care are likely to leave quickly via adoption or kinship guardianship orders. When adoptions from care do happen in Europe, this is most likely to be by their existing foster carers with whom they have lived for some years (Skivenes & Thoburn 2016).

Foster carer careers

In 1989 Jane Rowe, an influential UK foster care researcher, drew from a large-scale mixed methods study the following list of foster care roles and tasks (subsequently used with respect to more recent studies of foster care by Sinclair et al. 2007 and Thoburn 2010b).

- Emergency care
- Planned temporary care/strengthening families/preparation for reunification
- Regular series of placements with the same family ('respite' or 'support' foster care, often for disabled children)
- Assessment (of child, of parents, of whole family)
- Therapy (of child, of parents, of whole family)

- Preparation for long-term placement, usually of young children and usually with an adoptive family not previously known to the child
- Care and upbringing ('long-term' 'permanent' foster family care, often including members of the child's kin or friendship network)
- A bridge to independence for teenagers entering care following family breakdown or following an adoptive or long-term foster family breakdown.

At one end of the continuum, a foster care career might involve the upbringing of a single foster child or sibling group as 'part of their family' for 16 plus years and on into adult life. Included amongst these are members of the kinship network of a child who cannot safely remain with the birth parents. With respect to kinship foster care, it is important to note that most children living with family members do not enter care, or leave care quickly, sometimes through legal guardianship arrangements and sometimes (as happens most often in the USA) by legal adoption by their kinship foster carers. However, there are sound reasons why some children, especially those who have been maltreated, remain within the formal care system. The wishes of the kinship carers and the child are important in this respect. Other reasons are the need for continuing financial support (more relevant in some countries than others depending on the adequacy of the social security systems).

Some long-term kin and non-kin carers opt for the child to remain in care rather than taking on legal guardianship because of the continuing importance of a social work service. This may be because of the very special needs of the child; to assist with continuing birth family links if a birth parent's behaviour can be unpredictable or threatening; or because relationships amongst different members of the extended kinship network are so strained that ongoing professional support is needed for an extended period.

In contrast, a different foster care career might involve 30 or more children staying for different lengths of time, some becoming long-term members of the family, others being helped to go safely home; and another might involve 30 or more infants and young children being cared for for a few weeks or months and moving to an adoptive family.

Between the two ends of the continuum, some foster carers provide a medium or longer-term 'shared care', 'family support' or 'short break' service to children with special needs or parents experiencing a period of stress or with a long-term mental or physical health condition. Carers are matched with a particular family and child/sibling group and provide care in their own homes at agreed periods over a few months but sometimes for years. In some countries this service is provided outside the formal out-of-home care system and in others, as in England, the children are formally in the care system.

The foster care service

In many countries the foster care service is an integral part of the statutory child welfare or child protection service, with foster carers recruited, 'licensed' and monitored by public employees, most often social workers. Mostly, foster carers are private contractors but in some countries (France for example) some foster carers are directly employed by the statutory child welfare agency. In some countries the service is fully contracted out to a third sector agency, either a charitable agency/NGO or a private for-profit agency, whilst in others (England for example), there is a 'mixed economy' of provision, with some 'in-house' foster carers and other children placed with foster carers recruited and remunerated by NGOs or private for-profit companies (Narey & Owers 2017). Once the children are placed, the arrangements for supervision, monitoring, support and remuneration of the foster family also vary. Most often a single worker (usually the child's allocated social worker) is required to visit and support the foster family as a whole, but in some countries (including England) a separate 'supervising' social worker is allocated to the foster family and the child retains their own allocated social worker. In many countries foster carers, nationally or in a particular state or area, are members of a support body which lobbies policymakers on their behalf and provides training materials and other services (as an example see for England, The Fostering Network 2019).

Countries differ in how they conceptualise the role of 'foster carer' and the services required to support a thriving foster care service. In some countries a clear distinction is made between the services needed by carers taking on the different roles. Although research from across jurisdictions points to there being many similarities in the way in which care services recruit, assess, train and support foster carers and match children with foster carers (Fernandez & Barth 2010), there are differences in how service systems in different countries adapt the service to the intended role of the foster carers. In general, therapeutic foster care appears to be conceived in similar ways across national boundaries. Such care, usually designed for older children with challenging behaviour, was first introduced in Sweden as 'professional foster care' in the 1980s and most recently provided as a manualised programme (Multidimensional Treatment Foster Care (MTFC) see Biehal, Ellison & Sinclair 2011; Chamberlain 2003; Hansson & Olsson 2012 for evaluations of its use in different countries).

In some countries, there appears to be an uneasy tension between the legislation requiring carers to facilitate reunification with birth families, and the reality that many foster *carers* have become, in effect, foster *parents*, with whom the child may wish to remain as 'part of the family' (Schofield 2003; Schofield et al. 2013). Given these findings, the emphasis on children's need for a sense of permanence in England has resulted in a recognition of the differences between 'task-focused' foster *carers* and 'family for life' foster *parents*. Statutory Guidance (DfE 2015) recognises long-term foster family care as a permanence option and provides for changes in social work practice that give foster carers an enhanced 'sense of permanence' and children a more secure sense of being part of the family.

The knowledge base on motivations, values, qualities skills and support needs of successful foster carers (referred to in the next section) has increased greatly in recent years, a development enhanced by researchers in different countries working together or building on each other's work. Many of the attributes and skills needed by successful foster carers are shared across all the different roles and foster care careers. For example, the ability to empathise with the child and also with the birth family is as essential for long-term foster carers who go on to adopt (even those who have little or no contact with birth parents) as it is for treatment foster carers (Schofield & Beek 2014). Enjoying being with children and also being able to rise to (and even enjoying) a challenge is an attribute that all those caring for children placed from care are likely to need to draw on at some point. Neil, Beek and Ward (2014) found that, even amongst children mostly under two when placed for adoption, only around half were 'thriving' between 16 and 18 years after placement and that many were demonstrating seriously challenging behaviour. Schofield and Beek (2014) found that long-term foster families met similar challenges and needed similar skills.

Scoping the research on family foster care

The knowledge base on family foster care is growing rapidly. Some studies are descriptive, usually including the views of foster carers, young people in or who have left foster care, service providers and, less frequently, the voices of birth parents. Soundly conducted randomised control trials of specific interventions with children in foster care, or the training of foster carers are also a valuable source of information for those planning a foster care service (see for example Chamberlain 2003 and Macdonald & Turner 2008). However, such research needs to be based on a clearly identified group of children with similar needs and a specific intervention, with valid outputs and outcomes that can be identified and measured within a reasonably short time frame. Mixed methods and longitudinal studies are needed to provide valid and reliable information on long-term processes and outcomes (Fernandez 2008). To this end, recent advances in statistical techniques have also been important for the more rigorous analysis of routinely collected administrative data as evidenced by the Sebba et al. (2015) study which compared educational outcomes for children in care with similar children not in care.[1]

Such quantitative evidence can be combined with other more qualitative evidence obtained by practitioner and action research methods such as through the involvement of peer researchers, the use of texts and photos to obtain information concerning the satisfaction of children and young adults with their experience of foster care, as well as their detailed views on what they found more and less helpful. When such evidence is combined with robustly conducted prospective longitudinal studies (using mixed quantitative and some increasingly imaginative qualitative methodologies), the combined analysis can be particularly valuable. But for some of the questions for which we need answers, a range of qualitative methodologies is often necessary to explore the value of new techniques to assist and support children, carers and birth parents.

From the available research using a range of methodologies it is possible to identify variables that have been associated with good or less good outcomes. Information is needed about:

- the child;
- the child's family and biography;
- the profession and training and characteristics of those providing services to the children, their parents and carers;
- the approaches and methods used by social work and other services for
  - decision making,
  - placement practice/therapy;
- law, systems and procedures for care planning, review and service delivery.

There are helpful overviews to be found in the edited volumes of Schofield and Simmonds (2009) (mainly UK); and Fernandez and Barth (2010) (covering several countries).

Although there is a growing literature on outcomes of foster family placement, across and within countries, comparisons are often complicated because researchers make different decisions about when and how to measure outcomes. These differences are related to differences in historical and cultural context, and political as well as professional choices (Gilbert, Parton & Skivenes 2011; Thoburn 2013). As an example, different choices are made about whose outcome is to be measured. Policymakers and researchers agree that it is the outcome for the child/ren that is to be prioritised and that children's views should be heard and taken seriously, but recognise a 'duty of care' and a 'right to a fair hearing' of the adults who are likely to be affected by the service provided to a child.

Rich and poor countries alike share a commitment to meeting the needs of children as set out in the UN Convention on the Rights of the Child (United Nations 1989). Birth and/or alternative parents and carers must meet the basic human needs as summarised by Maslow (1954) for:

- Adequate nutrition and shelter
- Protection from danger, including all types of abuse and neglect
- Health care
- Opportunities and encouragement to learn.

But for children who need more than a short stay in care, all countries recognise the additional needs for a 'sense of permanence' and a 'sense of identity' (Figure 10.1, Thoburn 1994).

To summarise, although there are differences in emphasis and prioritisation depending on country, context and research design, the wellbeing outcomes that policymakers seek to achieve, and researchers seek to evaluate are:

- Physical, emotional, 'educational' wellbeing into adulthood;
- Stability – keep any moves to a minimum;
- The child having a sense of permanence;
- Family membership (foster family and birth family);
- Continuity – links with relatives, friends and community;

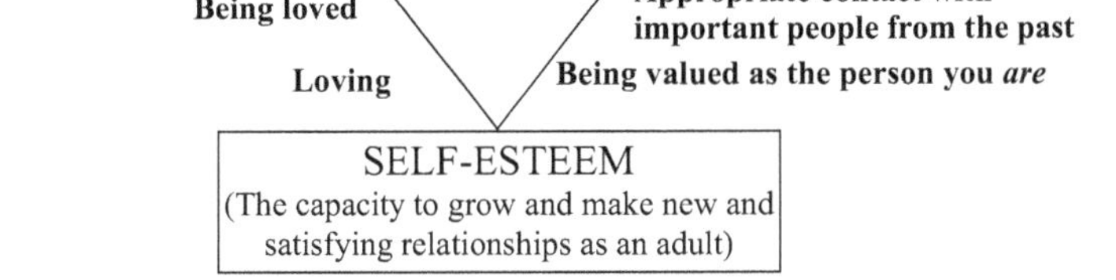

Figure 10.1 The special needs of children who are looked after by the local authority

- Minimum length of stay in out-of-home care – a key aim in USA and UK policy but less apparent in other countries (Skivenes & Thoburn 2016);
- Normality – but different family forms including being part of a foster family should not be seen as conveying the stigma associated with the 'abnormal', as recounted by many care leavers (Stein & Munro 2008).

Some of the listed measures are 'outputs' (was a particular service received? was the child adopted? did the child leave care to a recognised legally permanent family arrangement or did he or she 'age out' of care?). As a sub-text to much of the discourse on children in care is the aim of keeping costs and therefore numbers as low as possible. This is often justified by a commonly held view especially among politicians and service planners, that outcomes for care entrants are generally poor. This prevailing view is not supported by research going back over the years (the latest being Sebba et al., 2015) and summarised by Biehal et al. (2010), Boddy (2013), Bullock et al. (2006) and Thoburn and Courtney (2011). Whilst qualitative studies provide evidence that the care system badly fails a minority of those who experience it, the majority (including in the eyes of the young people themselves (Children's Commissioner for England 2015)) do as well or better than if they had remained at home or returned quickly home. Those who go home too quickly, have inadequate support, and return to care on more than one occasion do least well (Farmer et al. 2011; Wade et al. 2011).

Studies that measure child and young adult wellbeing, including changes in wellbeing over time, are needed to assist service providers in securing the best interest of each child, but these usually require longitudinal studies which are costly to undertake. Because most children entering care will have additional obstacles and challenges to overcome, it is generally agreed that wellbeing outcomes cannot be assessed until young people are well into their twenties. For example, a young person entering care at 15 in part because of school problems is unlikely to be having good exam results 18 months later, though he or she may well pick up their education at 18 and go through college and gain qualifications in their twenties.

Data on outputs can serve as useful proxy interim outcome measures if longer-term outcome information is not yet available. Multiple changes of placement (placement instability) comes through in qualitative studies as a proxy for a poor outcome, at least in terms of what young people have to say about their experience. But young people contributing to research report that one or even two moves as teenagers from placements that were not working for them could be followed by more successful foster family placements (Schofield 2003).

A growing number of longitudinal studies in different jurisdictions (some large-scale cohort studies, some small-sample and more detailed), have enabled researchers to follow foster children into adult life. As well as providing information on housing, education, criminality, health and employment status, some of these report on 'self-esteem' as an adult and the ability to make satisfying relationships in adult life as indicators of a successful outcome (Anderson 2009; Biehal 2014; Courtney & Dworsky 2006; Fernandez 2012; Schofield et al. 2013; Stein & Munro 2008; Thoburn, Norford & Rashid 2000).

Some of these studies also report on the characteristics of foster families that appear to be associated with higher wellbeing or positive change over time. Some attributes are more important to some foster care roles than others. The ability to be part of the therapeutic team, and to value this part of their role, is essential for treatment foster carers.

'Family for life' foster carers need to be able to work with professionals, but there are examples in the qualitative research literature of foster parents standing up for and advocating for their child, and coming into conflict with the foster care agency. Schofield and colleagues (2013) explore this question of different role identities. Some identify primarily as foster carers, but also embrace the role of parent; others primarily identity as parents, but also embrace the professional elements of their foster carer role. These researchers conclude that successful long-term foster parents can have different role identities, but there must be an element of each of these role identifications.

Countries which recognise the differences between different foster care careers tend to be more relaxed about the discourse of the service – is 'foster carer' the required term to be used by social workers and in official reports, and 'foster parent' frowned on? Does the recognition of the importance of children's and family rights allow for the recognition that some foster children will want to call their foster parents 'mum and dad'?

Contexts and policies have an impact on cost-effectiveness as an outcome measure. If the care system is mainly providing for teenagers with challenging behaviour, the cost per child is likely to be higher and the proportion of 'good' outcomes is likely to be lower than in some countries (mainly in Eastern or Southern Europe), in which fairly young children come into care largely because of absolute poverty, family tragedy, are placed in a stable kin or non-kin foster family and remain there until they are ready to make the transition to adulthood. In England and the USA, where all the youngest entrants leave care quickly through reunification or adoption, those who 'age out' of care at 16 or 18 are likely to be the 'unadoptable' ones with more complex histories who are more likely to have less-good outcomes.

Conclusions

This chapter has provided an overview of the cross-national knowledge base on family foster care. But an important warning is needed for those developing foster care services in their own countries or states that what seems to work in one country will not necessarily work in another. As well as more 'technical' questions needing further exploration, some 'public attitude' questions have been highlighted by the existing body of research. To plan for the development or improvement of a foster care service in a particular state or cultural context, information is needed on the prevailing societal opinion of foster carers and foster children. For example, do children growing up in foster care feel 'different' or even stigmatised? do members of the public look on foster families as 'normal' families; special people putting in something extra to meet the needs of special children, or just 'doing it for the money'?

In brief, child welfare systems serving children and families with different characteristics will have different patterns of foster family care and different 'success' rates. There is no 'right' or 'wrong' rate of children in care, or percentage of children in care placed with foster families. But those children who need and can benefit from foster family placement, especially those who have been maltreated, have a right to the highest quality service and most will benefit from and value the experience of being welcomed into foster families for as short or long a period as their individual and family circumstances require.

Questions for discussion

In your country/state/culture do you think most/few/none of the children in foster family care feel stigmatised?

In your country/state/culture what do you think is the general view about why people become foster carers?

In your country/state/culture what is the balance between foster carers who provide short-term respite or therapeutic care and long-term 'part of their family' care?

Think yourself into the position of foster carers who initially cared for three foster children in succession on a short-term basis and helped them to go back successfully to their parents. What were the components of the social work service you found helpful and unhelpful? You have now been looking after Jamie and Billy (brothers now aged 8 and 6) for two years, originally on a short-term basis whilst their single mother had treatment for a mental health difficulty. It becomes clear to the authority that they cannot successfully go back to their mother and it is agreed (including by their mother) that you will become their long-term foster carers. What are the key components of the social work service you will find helpful for the future and how does this differ from the social work service provided when you were short-term foster carers?

Note

1 An important note when reading research reports is that some USA studies use the term 'foster care' to include children in residential placements as well as children in family foster care.

References

Adoption and Foster Care Reporting System (AFCARS), 2019, The AFCARS Report 25, Washington DC: US Department of Health and Human Services.

Ainsworth, F. & Thoburn, J., 2014, 'An exploration of the differential use of residential child care across national boundaries', *International Journal of Social Welfare*, vol. 23, no. 1, pp. 16–24.

Anderson, G., 2009, 'Foster children: A longitudinal study of placements and family relationships', *International Journal of Social Welfare*, vol. 18, pp. 13–26.

Australian Institute of Health and Welfare, 2018, Child Protection Australia 2016–17. Canberra: AIHW.

Biehal, N., 2014, 'A sense of belonging: meanings of family and home in long-term foster care', *British Journal of Social Work*, vol. 44, no. 4, pp. 955–971.

Biehal, N., Ellison, S., Baker, C. & Sinclair, I., 2010, *Belonging and permanence: Outcomes in long-term foster care and adoption*, London: BAAF.

Biehal, N., Ellison, S. & Sinclair, I., 2011, 'Intensive fostering: An independent evaluation of MTFC in an English setting', *Children and Youth Services Review*, vol. 33, pp. 2043–2049.

Boddy, J., 2013, *Understanding permanence for looked after children: A review of research for the Care Inquiry*, London: The Fostering Network, www.fostering.net/sites/www.fostering.net/files/resources/england/understanding-permanence-for-lac-janet-boddy.pdf, accessed 1 November 2018.

Bullock, R., Courtney, M., Parker, R., Sinclair, I. & Thoburn, J., 2006, 'Can the corporate state parent?', *Children and Youth Services Review*, vol. 28, no. 11, pp. 1344–1358.

Chamberlain, P., 2003, 'The Oregon multidimensional treatment foster care model: Features. Outcomes and progress in dissemination', *Cognitive and Behavioural Practice*, vol. 10, no. 4, pp. 303–312.

Children's Commissioner for England, 2015, Children in care and care leavers survey 2015, London: Office of the Children's Commissioner.

Courtney, M.E. & Dworsky, A., 2006, 'Early outcomes for young adults transitioning from out-of-home care in the USA', *Child & Family Social Work*, vol. 11, pp. 209–219.

Department for Education, 2015, *Permanence, long-term foster placements, and ceasing to look after a child: Statutory Guidance for Local Authorities*, London: DFE.

Department for Education, 2018, Children looked after by local authorities in England, London: National Statistics.

Farmer, E., Sturgess, W., O'Neill, T. & Wijedasa, D., 2011, *Achieving successful returns from care: What makes reunification work?*, London: BAAF.

Fernandez, E.A., 2008, 'Unravelling emotional, behavioural and educational outcomes in a longitudinal study', *British Journal of Social Work*, vol. 38, no. 7, pp. 1283–1301.

Fernandez, E.A., 2012, *Accomplishing permanency: Reunification pathways and outcomes for foster children*, New York: Springer.

Fernandez, E. & Barth, R.P. (eds), 2010, *How does foster care work?*, London: Jessica Kingsley.

Fernandez, E. & Lee, J.S., 2011, 'Returning children in care to their families: factors associated with the speed of reunification', *Child Indicators Research*, vol. 4, no. 4, pp. 749–765.

Gilbert, N., Parton, N. & Skivenes, M., 2011, *Child protection systems: International trends and orientations*, Oxford, UK: Oxford University Press.

Hansson, K. & Olsson, M., 2012, 'Effects of multidimensional treatment foster care (MTFC). Results from a RCT Study in Sweden', *Children and Youth Services Review*, vol. 34, no. 9, pp. 1929–1936.

Maslow, A., 1954, *Motivation and personality*, New York: Harper.

Macdonald, G.M. & Turner, W., 2008, 'Treatment foster care for improving outcomes in children and young people', *Cochrane Database of Systematic Reviews*, doi:10.1002/14651858.CD005649.pub2.

Narey, M. & Owers, M., 2017, *Foster care in England*. London: DfE.

Neil, E., Beek, M. & Ward, E., 2014, *Contact after adoption: A longitudinal study of adopted young people and their adoptive parents and birth relatives*, London: BAAF.

Rowe, J., Hundleby, M. & Garnett, L., 1989, *Child care now: A survey of placement patterns*, London: BAAF.

Schofield, G., 2003, *Part of the family: Pathways through foster care*, London: BAAF.

Schofield, G. & Beek, M., 2009, 'Growing up in foster care: providing a secure base through adolescence', *Child & Family Social Work*, vol. 14, pp. 255–266.

Schofield, G. & Beek, M., 2014, *The secure base model: Promoting attachment and resilience in foster care and adoption*, London: BAAF.

Schofield, G. & Simmonds, J. (eds), 2009, *The child placement handbook: Research, policy and practice*, London: BAAF.

Schofield, G., Beek, M., Ward, E. & Biggart, L., 2013, 'Professional foster carer and committed parent: Role conflict and role enrichment at the interface between work and family in long-term foster care', *Child and Family Social Work*, vol. 18, pp. 46–56.

Sebba, J., Berridge, D., Luke, N., Fletcher, J., Bell, K., Strand, S., Thomas, S., Sinclair, I. & O'Higgins, A., 2015, *The educational progress of looked after children in England*, Oxford: Rees Centre.

Sinclair, I., Baker, C., Lee, J. & Gibb, I., 2007, *The pursuit of permanence: A study of the English child care system*, London: Jessica Kingsley.

Skivenes, M. & Thoburn, J., 2016, 'Pathways to permanence in England and Norway: A critical analysis of documents and data', *Children and Youth Services Review*, vol. 67, pp. 152–160.

Stein, M. and Munro, E.R., 2008, *Young people's transitions from care to adulthood*, London: Jessica Kingsley.

The Fostering Network, www.thefosteringnetwork.org.uk/ accessed February 2019.

Thoburn, J., 1994, *Child placement: Principles and practice*, 2nd edn, Aldershot, UK: Ashgate.

Thoburn, J., Norford, L. & Rashid, S., 2000, *Permanent Family Placement for Children of Minority Ethnic Origin*, London: Jessica Kingsley.

Thoburn, J., 2010a, 'Achieving safety, stability and belonging for children in out-of-home care. The search for "what works" across national boundaries', *International Journal of Child and Family Welfare*, vol. 12, no. 1–2, pp. 34–48.

Thoburn, J., 2010b, 'International perspectives on foster care', in E. Fernandez & R.P. Barth. (eds), *How does foster care work?*, London: Jessica Kingston, pp. 29–43.

Thoburn, J., 2013, 'Services for vulnerable and maltreated children', in I. Wolfe & M. McKee (eds), *European child health services and systems: Lessons without borders*, Maidenhead, UK: Open University Press/McGraw Hill.

Thoburn, J., 2018, 'Research on birth family contact for children who need out-of-home care', *Seen and Heard*, vol. 28, no. 3, pp. 28–43.

Thoburn, J. & Courtney, M., 2011, 'A Guide through the knowledge base on children in out-of-home care', *Journal of Children's Services*, vol. 6, no. 4, pp. 210–227.

Ubbesen, M-B., Gilbert, R. & Thoburn, J., 2015, 'Cumulative incidence of entry into out-of-home care: Changes over time in Denmark and England', *Child Abuse and Neglect*, vol. 42, pp. 63–71.

United Nations, 1989, *Convention on the Rights of the Child*, New York: UN.

Vinnerljung, B. & Sallnas, M., 2008, 'Into adulthood: A follow-up study of 718 young people who were placed in out-of-home care during their teens', *Child and Family Social Work*, vol. 13, pp. 144–155.

Wade, J., Biehal, N., Farrelly, N. & Sinclair, I., 2011, *Caring for abused and neglected children: Making the right decisions for reunification or long-term care*, London: Jessica Kingsley.

Chapter 11

Kinship care in Australia and the United Kingdom

Meredith Kiraly and Elaine Farmer

Introduction

The United Nations (UN) defines kinship care as *family-based care within the child's extended family or with close friends of the family known to the child, whether formal or informal in nature* (United Nations 2010). Kinship care is thus very diverse in nature. In this chapter we discuss its role in providing care for children informally and its increasing use as a formal part of child protection systems. We outline the benefits for children, early policy developments, the challenges for carers and the lack of recognition and help provided to children and carers. We also consider drivers of the growth of statutory kinship care, the nexus with permanency planning and issues for practice. We will contend that, as kinship care has grown, traditionally held beliefs about kinship care have been replaced by new myths – or partial truths. These will be considered as they impact on current practice.

Research into kinship care is better developed in the United Kingdom (UK) than in Australia. Significant research studies in the twenty-first century include work by Hunt, Waterhouse and Lutman (2008) and Farmer and Moyers (2008) in the UK, and Brennan et al. (2013) and Kiraly and Humphreys (2016) in Australia. Literature reviews on kinship care include Boetto (2010) in Australia, Nixon (2008) in the UK, and in the USA, Cuddeback (2004) and a systematic review by Winokur, Holtan, and Batchelder (2018). An edited book (Pitcher 2014) provides an overview of key issues in contemporary kinship care, and two journal special issues on kinship care have been published in Australia (Doyle & Kiraly 2018, 2019).

Both authors of this chapter have for a long time been involved in major kinship care research studies. This chapter will therefore mainly address research and practice in Australia and the UK, with a predominant focus on Australia.

Terminology in this area varies. Generic terms include *kinship care* in Australia, and *family and friends care* or *kinship care* in the UK. *Formal kinship care* in Australia is defined as a form of out-of-home care where the caregiver is provided with a reimbursement for the care of the child (AIHW 2020: 102). For Aboriginal and Torres Strait Islander children the definition is extended to include care by other Indigenous people in the child's community, a compatible community, or from the same language group (AIHW 2020: 102). In the UK and the USA, formal kinship care is often referred to as *kinship foster care* (as opposed to *non-kin foster care*). Although these terms are little used in Australia, in some areas kinship care is viewed as a form of foster care, while in others it is regarded as a separate entity. In this chapter we use the terms *kinship care* (or *kin care*) and *foster care* as denoting two discrete forms of care, and the terms *informal kinship care* and *formal kinship care* to identify whether or not the care arrangement has been formalised by a statutory order. Non-family kinship carers are known as *family friends* in the UK and by a range of terms in Australia; here we use the term *non-familial kinship carers*. *Parent* is used for the mother or father of a child in care; *child* is used for people under the age of 18.

Support and services for kinship families are provided differently in Australia and the UK due to the different national and subnational government structures. In the UK services to families are mostly delivered via local authorities. In Australia, statutory child protection and therefore formal kinship care is the remit of the States and Territories. The Commonwealth of Australia provides some limited financial support and services to families, mostly on a means-tested basis to which some informal and formal kinship families may be entitled.

The great majority of children in kinship care in both Australia and the UK are in informal care arrangements (Selwyn & Nandy 2014; Smyth & Eardley 2007). We therefore begin by considering issues that relate to both informal and formal kinship care, before examining formal kinship care in some detail.

Background: informal and formal kinship care

The use of the term 'kinship care' to describe care of children within a child's family and community network is relatively recent (Stack, 1974). As a paradigm, it is still evolving and as such can be subject to varying conceptualisations.

> As a new paradigm arises, and before an older one is discarded, a professional community finds itself in a period of paradigm conflict, which can last for an extended period of time.
>
> (Hegar 1999: 225)

> I get a bit confused about kinship care because I just thought that was normal, but if you're talking about other kinship … Tara didn't know she was in kinship support. She said 'What's that?' I said, 'Apparently it's something that we don't know about'.
>
> (Mother quoted in Kiraly & Humphreys 2015: 109)

The number of Australian children living in kinship care is unknown, as census data do not provide sufficient identification of children's living circumstances (Kiraly 2018). In the UK, however, research using census data has identified the number of children living with relatives and their associated demographic details (Selwyn & Nandy 2014; Wijedasa 2015). However, non-familial kinship care arrangements ('family friends') cannot be identified from the census, nor can the reasons for relative care arrangements. The census analyses showed that 95 per cent of all relative kinship care in the UK is informal.[1,2] Half (51%) of the children were growing up in households headed by grandparents, nearly one-quarter (23%) (surprisingly) in families headed by a sibling, and another quarter (26%) in households headed by another relative, such as an aunt, uncle or cousin. Significantly, around three quarters (76%) of the kinship children were living in a deprived[3] household (Wijedasa, 2015). Compared with children growing up with at least one parent, the kinship children were almost twice as likely to have a long-term health problem or disability that limited their day-to-day activities. These census data analyses also showed that in England the number of children growing up in the care of relatives increased by 7 per cent between 2001 and 2011, which was over three times the rate of population growth of all children in England (2%).

In the UK, families are required to notify the local authority about informal care arrangements with unrelated people or more distant relatives (known as 'private fostering') to ensure a minimum of oversight, but this requirement does not apply to informal care with closer relatives. There is no requirement in Australia to register informal care arrangements of any sort.

Research has tended to focus on the much smaller group of children in formal kinship care, in part due to interest in comparing children's outcomes in this newer form of OOHC with foster care and because their visibility also makes this group much easier to recruit. In addition, much kinship care literature has focused on grandparent carers as the largest group of kinship carers (Cuddeback 2004). One myth that has thus emerged is that kinship care and grandparent care are more or less synonymous; as a result, the diversity of kinship care arrangements is frequently overlooked.

Benefits of kinship care for children

Research has consistently identified significant benefits of kinship care for children as compared with foster care. The systematic review by Winokur, Holtan and Batchelder (2018) found that children have better wellbeing, better reported behaviour and mental health outcomes than those in foster care, and that kinship care ensures greater placement stability (see also Farmer 2010; O'Brien 2013; Webster, Barth & Needell 2000). Children have also been found to have more frequent contact with parents, siblings and their wider family and thus maintain a range of supportive family relationships (which are absent in foster care) and appreciate the relative normality of their family situation (Nixon 2008). Many studies show that children usually make close relationships with their kin carers who show high commitment and rarely give up on them, even when their behaviour is very challenging (see for example Farmer & Moyers 2008; Selwyn et al. 2013). Critically, the Nixon review (2008) also found that kinship care was at least as safe as foster care (although see later discussion of this issue). In addition, Wellard and colleagues (2017) found that young people usually stayed with their carers into adulthood as long as they wished, rather than moving to 'independent living' at the cessation of state support, as frequently occurs in foster care. This more normalised entry into adulthood (Hartley 1993) has obvious benefits for young people's transition from school to further education and employment.

The burden of care

Paradoxically, the many benefits for children in kinship care frequently accrue to children despite huge challenges for their carers (Farmer 2009a). As in foster care, children often arrive with histories of maltreatment, which manifest in emotional and behavioural difficulties and educational deficits. Unlike in foster care however, relationships between the carers and children's parents are intimate and complex and frequently involve tension and conflict relating to parents' issues with substance dependency, mental ill-health and family violence. Contact with parents is often difficult for both children and carers. Whether or not care has been formalised by a court order, families are usually left to manage parental contact issues themselves, frequently in their own homes (see the section on parental contact).

An overwhelming theme in almost all the kinship literature is the difficult financial circumstances of kinship families, and many publications conclude with a call for a greater response by governments to this unmet need (see for example, Boetto 2010; Brennan et al. 2013; Cuddeback 2004; Farmer 2009b; Nixon 2008; Palacios & Jimenez 2009).

The preponderance of grandparent carers means that, as a cohort, carers are older and in poorer heath than foster carers; they also typically have lower educational attainment (Boetto 2010). In addition, carers frequently take on larger groups of children than foster carers in order to keep siblings together, exacerbating financial and housing stress as well as the emotional burden of care (McHugh 2013). In a systematic review of 13 surveys in the UK, Australia and New Zealand, over one-third of respondents in each survey were sole carers, usually female, and financial hardship was reported by one-third or more in each survey. Myriad stressors were identified including health issues, severely challenging behaviour from some children, and isolation. Remarkably, despite the burdens of care, these carers expressed much joy and satisfaction in caring for the children (Kiraly 2015).

Indigenous kinship carers in Australia experience even greater poverty, poorer health and more crowded housing than others. The legacy of the Stolen Generations[4] includes an imperative amongst Indigenous people to care for children in order to prevent their further alienation from family, community and culture. Indigenous carers assume the care of even larger numbers of children than non-Indigenous carers (Kiraly, James & Humphreys 2015). Nevertheless, despite a call from the Indigenous child care peak body (SNAICC 2004), there is as yet little published research on Indigenous kinship care in Australia.

Informal kinship care

Informal kinship care arrangements attract little or no financial or social support in Australia and the UK. Such carers frequently experience particularly acute financial difficulties, and also a lack of help to address children's trauma histories, emotional and behavioural difficulties, and the challenges of parental contact. In a study of informal kinship care in the UK, two-thirds of the carers were found to be clinically depressed, although only just over one-quarter had actually been diagnosed as such (Selwyn et al. 2013).

Informal kinship carers in the UK can receive a very small *Guardian's Allowance* if one parent has died and the other is unable to look after the children, but many carers are unaware of its existence (Selwyn et al. 2013). It is also technically possible for local authorities to provide a small amount of time-limited financial support to informal kinship carers for designated 'children in need'.

In Australia the Commonwealth Government agency Centrelink provides financial support to families, mostly on a means-tested basis. The *Grandparent Advisor program* and *Additional Child Care Subsidy for Grandparents* provide limited assistance for children in both informal and formal grandparent care, occasionally including a child care subsidy, and some of these benefits are now being extended to other kinship families. The small *Double Orphan's Allowance* is available for those children in circumstances similar to those for the UK *Guardian's Allowance*.

Much concern has been raised about the lack of government recognition and support for children in kinship care in Australia, especially where care is informal. The 2014 Senate Inquiry into grandparents who take primary responsibility for raising their grandchildren (the 'Grandparent Inquiry') (Senate Community Affairs References Committee 2014) recommended the development of policy and practice to support Australian children in grandparent care (both informal and formal), including greater financial, housing, legal and practical assistance, respite care and training programs, and better information about community services. Regrettably given its remit, this Inquiry was unable to promote better recognition of the existence and unmet needs of the many *other* groups of kinship carers. Following this Inquiry, some steps were taken, including staving off threatened cuts to Commonwealth benefits. Overall, however, less has been achieved to date as a result of this Inquiry than might have been hoped.

A study exploring informal kinship care in the UK (Selwyn et al. 2013) and another examining the differences in support, need and legal status between different kinds of kinship care placements (Hunt and Waterhouse 2013) both identified significant deprivation and unmet need among children in informal kin care and made recommendations that financial support should be based on need rather than legal status, a principle which is actually set out in government guidance there (Department for Education UK 2011).

Poverty affects life chances independently of other circumstances (Tucker 2016). Children in informal kinship care are thus clearly the most disadvantaged children in alternative care. The challenge of protecting these children from the risks associated with poverty, intrafamilial conflict and the untreated impacts of trauma is one with which both Australia and the UK have yet to come to grips. With limited budgets for child welfare services, governments fear that widening eligibility for help would 'open the floodgates' to demand.

We now turn to consider formal kinship care.

Formal kinship care

Kinship care for statutory child protection is a relatively new phenomenon, having developed in a number of Western countries in the late twentieth century. Recognition of the advantages of placing children within their family network initially sprang from the family preservation movement of the 1990s which included the development of intensive family support programs (Gilligan 2006; McFadden 1998; Pine, Warsh & Maluccio 1993). Family Group Conferencing (FGC) also emerged in New Zealand around this time as an approach consistent with the values of the Indigenous Māori community (Maxwell & Morris 1992). Family Group Conferences bring together a wide range of extended family members to address the care of a child at risk, prior to (or later, alongside) any statutory child protection intervention. This process led to hitherto undiscovered options for children's care within their kinship networks, and was quickly adopted in many other countries.

Concomitant with the family preservation movement, increasing difficulty in recruiting sufficient foster carers – particularly in Australia following the progressive closure of children's residential facilities (Ainsworth & Maluccio 1998) – led to more pragmatic reasons for exploring this new care option. The old adage, 'The apple doesn't fall far from the tree' that had previously deterred exploration of extended family care options was gradually replaced by a new dominant idea, 'If they're with family, they're safe'.

> The juxtaposition of the philosophical shift to the family continuity paradigm of maintaining significant family and kinship ties, and a desperate need for more placement resources created the phenomenon of a sudden pendulum swing towards kinship care. The placement of last resort had become the placement of choice.
>
> (McFadden 1998: 8)

Kinship care is a radical departure from earlier forms of out-of-home care that to a greater or lesser extent separated vulnerable children from their family and community according to a 'child rescue' ideology (Farmer & Owen 1995). Debate continues about whether kinship care is in fact best viewed as a form of out-of-home care, or as a family preservation intervention (Scannapieco & Hegar 1999) that might warrant a 'lighter touch' to regulation and casework.

The use of formal kinship care varies from country to country, possibly in part due to variations in foster care capacity and different governance arrangements placing existing kinship care arrangements inside or outside the formally designated out-of-home care system. Australia has one of the highest rates of usage, along with New Zealand (Connolly, de Haan & Crawford 2013), Spain (del Valle et al. 2009), to a lesser extent Ireland (Munro & Gilligan 2013), and some areas of the Netherlands, Canada and the US (Connolly 2003; Gough 2006; Strijker, Zandberg & van der Meulen 2003).[5] Kinship care now appears in legislation as the preferred formal placement option in the UK and in all Australian jurisdictions.

Data on the number of Australian children in out-of-home care is collected annually by the Australian Institute of Health and Welfare (AIHW) and shows a progressive increase of children in kinship care year on year. On 30 June 2019, 23,351 Australian children were in formal kinship care, which was 52 per cent of all children in out-of-home care (AIHW 2020).

Aboriginal and Torres Strait Islander children

Aboriginal and Torres Strait Islander (Indigenous) children are greatly over-represented in out-of-home care, and thus also in formal kinship care; the rate of Indigenous children in out-of-home care is nearly 11 times the rate for non-Indigenous children. In 2019, 40 per cent of Australian children in formal kinship care were Indigenous (AIHW 2020). Kinship care provides the opportunity for Indigenous children to maintain strong connections to family, culture and community (SNAICC 2005). The Aboriginal Child Placement Principle now in legislation in all Australian jurisdictions prioritises the care of Indigenous children with carers in their family and kin networks, followed by Indigenous non-related carers in the child's community, and then carers in a compatible Indigenous community. If no other suitable placement with Indigenous carers can be found, this Principle provides for children to be placed with non-Indigenous carers who are able to maintain the child's connections to their family, community and culture (see for example, State of Victoria 2005a).

The relationship between child and carer

Central to the notion of kinship care is the assumption of a meaningful pre-existing relationship between child and carer that is seen to be inherently protective and nurturing. The UN definition of kinship care nevertheless provides for family care arrangements regardless of whether the child and carer are known to each other, presumably on the assumption that the family tie will invoke a commitment to care. However, a distant family connection may not always be a sound basis for loving care. UK research on children in kinship care under Special Guardianship Orders (SGOs) (a permanency order) has found that the strength of the pre-existing bond between child and carer is predictive both of greater well-being for the child and a reduced risk of placement breakdown (Wade et al. 2004). Other research in Canada and Sweden has shown that non-familial kinship care arrangements are more prone to break down than familial care (Perry, Daly & Kotler 2012; Sallnäs, Vinnerljung & Westermark 2004). It is therefore of concern that although figures from the Australian Institute of Health and Welfare suggest that around 44 per cent of Australian formal kinship carers are grandparents, an accurate picture cannot be established and the proportion of non-familial kinship carers cannot yet be determined due to a very large component of missing data (AIHW 2020). More information about the prevalence of such care is thus needed, especially as non-familial arrangements may require different supports. Better identification of the percentage of Indigenous children in the care of non-Indigenous, *non-familial* kinship carers is also important in order to ensure that the Aboriginal Child Placement Principle is implemented as intended.

In cases where the pre-existing relationship between child and carer is limited, practice varies in relation to whether placements are regarded as kinship care or foster care. Kinship care practice often includes placement prior to a full assessment being completed (see section, Assessment of care arrangements), an advantage for pressed workers facing a child protection emergency. The temptation towards a loose interpretation of a pre-existing child–carer relationship is naturally greater where care options are in short supply. In Australia there appears to be little in policy to clarify whether such placements should be regarded as kinship care or foster care arrangements.

Regulation and support

Ambiguity and paradox confound kinship care policy and program development, not least because kinship care is actually care in the home, not 'out of home'. This has led to the anomaly frequently heard from kinship families, policymakers and field workers in Australia, that even formal kinship care 'keeps children out of care'. Tensions about regulation and support versus autonomy and expectations of self-sufficiency therefore abound.

In Australia, placement-making always remains with the statutory child protection agency; practice regarding outsourcing of support programs varies across the country. Where kinship programs are outsourced, service may be provided by specialist kinship teams or alternatively by combined kinship and foster care programs. Separation of kinship care and foster care may be advantageous in recognising the unique features of kinship care, but it also has potential to threaten equity regarding assessment, case management, financial and casework support. An observation in both Australia and the

UK is that kinship care support is more effective when separated from the intense and often fraught purview of statutory child protection work.

Casework services for children in kinship care generally fall well below those provided in foster care in both countries (see for example Boetto 2010; Farmer & Moyers 2008). Prominent myths here include the view that as 'normal families', kin families will require little particular assistance, and that in any case, 'Families should look after their own'. There is also a belief that carers will be helped by their extended family, even though research has shown that some kinship carers have little or no such support, and that other family members are in fact sometimes hostile to the arrangement (Selwyn et al. 2013). These myths have thus helped to sustain the paradox that whilst kinship families are known to face greater challenges than foster families in a range of areas, they attract less support.

Other areas of support – provided on a very variable basis to kinship carers – include support groups (much valued by carers), information booklets, and training programs addressing topics such as trauma, attachment disorders, parental contact, statutory processes and schooling issues. Widespread concern has been expressed by both practitioners and researchers about the lack of appropriate services for children in formal kinship care in both countries (Boetto 2010; Farmer 2010; Hunt, Waterhouse & Lutman 2008) and the resulting burden of care on kinship carers (Connolly 2003; Cuddeback 2004).

In recent years, the Senate Inquiry into Out of Home Care (Senate Community Affairs References Committee 2015), and the Royal Commission into Institutional Responses to Child Sexual Abuse (2017) have both addressed the regulation and support of formal kinship carers within their broader remits and made recommendations to improve its governance and support.

Assessment of care arrangements

The practice of placement prior to full assessment depends on a partial truth that a protective family bond may ensure the child's safety in the interim – clearly in some cases a debatable issue. While at least minimal safety screening must occur at the time of placement, children's safety and wellbeing can only be ensured if thorough assessment follows quickly afterwards. Slippage may however occur when workers are pressed for time, and timeliness has been a significant issue in kinship care assessment in Australia (Kiraly 2018). There has been concern by social workers and researchers about the risk of superficial assessments (Kiraly 2018; McHugh 2014a; Nixon 2008; Palacios & Jimenez 2009) particularly when the child is already living with the kin carers or the prospective carers have little or no prior relationship with the child. Kinship care assessments may appropriately prioritise a strong and protective child-carer bond over factors such as a materially less advantaged home than might pertain in foster care, and also a carer possibly being older and in less robust health (Child Welfare League of America 2000, cited in Cuddeback 2004). Nevertheless, assessments should always consider the quality of the carer–child relationship and the carers' parenting skills; the carers' capacity to manage intra-familial dynamics that may affect the child's safety and wellbeing, and carers' willingness to comply with regulatory standards such as the prohibition of corporal punishment. An important consideration is also the extent of social support available to carer and child, and any additional support that may be required. Both Wade et al. (2014) and

Kiraly (2018) argue that if a child does not have a strong pre-existing relationship with the prospective kin carer, a foster care assessment is more appropriate.

To date, no universally accepted kinship care assessment tool has been introduced in either. Australia or the UK. Based upon British research and practice, Hunt (2019) produced a useful overview of the issues involved in good kinship assessment, and some issues for assessment have also been reviewed by Australians McHugh and Hayden (2014). The assessment tool Step by Step (Relative and Kinship Carers) (Mulroney & Roach 2016) has been adapted from foster care in New South Wales, and is being taken up in other jurisdictions. Recognising the unique aspects of Indigenous kinship care, in 2011 Winangay (http://winangay.com/resources/) produced a dedicated Aboriginal Kinship Carer Assessment tool, and subsequently an adapted version for generic use.

Financial support for formal kinship carers

Whilst the lack of financial support is of greatest concern for informal kinship carers, there are also problems for formal kinship carers. A myth suggesting that kinship care is cheaper than foster care appears to have developed in Australia from the establishment of kinship care programs with limited funding and a rudimentary theoretical base from which to identify the actual needs of kinship families. Levels of financial support for formal kinship care vary considerably between the Australian States and Territories, being generally highest in the Australian Capital Territory and lowest in South Australia and Victoria (McHugh 2014b). While allowances are purportedly equal to those in foster care, kinship carers have frequently observed that in practice their allowances and/or additional reimbursements are set at lower levels. This situation came to a head in Victoria with an Inquiry by the Ombudsman whose report included some critical conclusions and recommendations for improved practice (Victorian Ombudsman 2017). In the UK a number of court judgements have affirmed that local authorities must pay kinship carers at the same rate as 'non-kin' foster carers, although it appears that there may still be variations in actual practice there too (Selwyn et al. 2013).

Contact between children and their families

Children's contact with their parents may be complicated because of the previous history between the parents and kinship carers, parents' substance misuse, their problematic behaviour during contact (often in the carers' home) and the fact that parents may live close by. There has been one dedicated research study on family contact in the UK (Roth et al. 2011) and another in Australia (Kiraly & Humphreys 2016). However a considerable body of kinship care research has included some findings about children's parental contact (Kiraly & Humphreys 2013a). Studies generally find that while children in kinship care see more of their parents than children in foster care, their experiences are much more mixed (see for example, Cuddeback 2004; Delfabbro 2017). Studies in both Australia and the UK have found that *half* or more of the children in kinship care experience significant difficulties with parental contact, such as high levels of intrafamilial conflict, parents who were unreliable or exposed them to risk, including a minority of children whose wellbeing or safety may be compromised by parental actions (Farmer & Moyers 2008; Hunt, Waterhouse & Lutman 2008; Selwyn et al. 2013; Kiraly & Humphreys 2016; Wellard et al. 2017). Farmer and Moyers (2008) found that concerns about safety were noted for one-third of children in contact with their mother, and over a quarter during contact with their father; figures in Australia were slightly higher (39% for mothers and 31% for fathers) (Kiraly & Humphreys 2016).

Managing safe contact between children and their parents can be a major challenge for carers. Children and their carers tend to receive far less support for parental contact visits than is the case in foster care and are generally expected to supervise contact themselves (Farmer, 2010). The need for advice and/or individualised support for kinship carers where parental contact is problematic has been widely identified (Farmer & Moyers 2008; Hunt, Waterhouse & Lutman 2010; Kiraly & Humphreys 2013c).

By contrast, numerous studies have reported extensive and positive contact for children with their separated sisters and brothers. The maintenance of relationships with siblings and the wider family has overwhelmingly been viewed by children and their carers as positive and beneficial (see for example, Downie et al. 2010; Kiraly & Humphreys 2013a; Kiraly & Humphreys 2016; Messing 2006).

In a study of Indigenous children in kinship care, carers and support workers stressed the imperative of family contact and cultural connection and described creative approaches to maintaining children's safety. However a lack of cultural support planning[6] for children was frequently noted. The non-Indigenous carers of Indigenous children were particularly concerned about children's loss of contact with family and culture (Kiraly, James & Humphreys 2015).

Stability and quality of care

While research has shown kinship care to be more stable than foster care, stability is particularly associated with grandparent care, followed by care by aunts and uncles (Farmer & Moyers 2008; Zinn 2012) and then 'family friends' (Perry, Daly & Kotler 2012; Sallnäs, Vinnerljung & Westermark 2004). Stability however does not always imply quality, especially as monitoring of kinship care is frequently less rigorous than for foster care. In a study comparing kinship care and foster care, Farmer (2009b) reported that while most carers provided excellent care, a small proportion of both kin and foster care placements were of a very poor standard, and that the unsatisfactory kin placements lasted significantly longer than such placements in foster care. Some continued either because there was little monitoring or because reports about difficulties (often from family members) were disregarded (see also Connolly 2003). In other cases, authorities had allowed standards to fall considerably below those that would have been accepted in foster care. In an Australian study of non-familial kinship care, quality of care was also highlighted as an issue in some cases (Kiraly 2018).

Children's restoration to parents from kinship care

Some studies have found that children are less likely to be restored to parental care than children in foster care (Delfabbro et al. 2013; Scannapieco & Hegar 1999), although the systematic review by Winokur, Holtan and Batchelder (2018) reported that reunification rates were similar for each type of care. A factor that may be influencing the chance of restoration may also be the limited casework with parents associated with kinship care programs.

Permanency planning and the pressure to keep children out of statutory care

As a result of concern about the rising numbers of children in out-of-home care in recent years, efforts in Australia have been directed towards keeping children out of the formal care system by encouraging informal kinship care arrangements without legal protection or by referring families to the Federal Family Court to pursue custody orders (with associated legal costs for carers). However, these dispositions stand to leave kinship carers with insufficient means to bring up the children, given that care allowances are not payable in these circumstances.

Further along the placement pathway, permanency planning legislation may transfer guardianship to the carer, ending requirements for state oversight and support. Removal of children from the formal care system via permanency planning broadly follows an adoption-type discourse that views the reconstituted family as autonomous and capable of managing its own affairs 'as a normal family would' – once again a partial truth. Practice regarding continuing financial support to children on permanent care orders varies across Australia, likewise whether or not permanent care arrangements are counted in the out-of-home care statistics (for example, they are counted in Victoria but not in New South Wales). Similarly in the UK, there has been an increasing push towards permanent care for children in kinship care through the use of SGOs, thus limiting the numbers of children registered as being in out-of-home care (Selwyn et al. 2013; Wade et al. 2014). If the SGO is made at the outset of care (as frequently happens), the child is then ineligible for some significant forms of assistance such as education support funds and (as also in Australia) for Leaving Care services. While some carers indicate that they prefer the autonomy accorded by such permanence orders, others caring for children with additional needs feel abandoned to the challenging task of raising other people's children with limited or no state assistance (Selwyn et al. 2013; Wellard et al. 2017).

Perspectives of children and parents

Much kinship care literature has included the views of kinship carers. We now turn to studies that have reported the views of the children themselves which generally confirm findings from carers, and the views of their parents.

Children often report feeling settled in the kinship care arrangement, having close relationships with their carers and being able to confide in them (for example, Selwyn et al. 2013; Wellard et al. 2017). However, in these studies a minority wished they could return to their parents, and/or felt responsible for them – conflicted feelings that could affect their ability to settle and form strong attachments with their kin carers. Children quite often did not understand why they were living with their carers or what the plans for their future were, and some reported being bullied at school because they did not live with their parents:

> [Other children said] 'You're not normal because you don't live with your parents'.
> (12-year-old girl quoted in Farmer, Selwyn & Meakings 2013: 28)

In a study by Messing (2006), some young people reported feeling angry at being in a different situation from their peers, and others have been observed to turn their anger on their carers (Gleeson 2014; Wellard et al. 2017). In contrast, some children emphasise the relative normality of life with close relatives:

> It's pretty much the same life that everyone else has really. Just different circumstances ... Really I don't think I'm disadvantaged compared to other kids ... We're just normal kids.
>
> (14-year-old boy quoted in Kiraly & Humphreys 2013b: 320)

When carers are in poor health some children give them considerable help. Many children live with the knowledge that their parents' and/or carers' health is fragile and worry that their carer may become ill or die, leaving them without a home (Gleeson 2014; Selwyn et al. 2013). An under-reported finding is that a few 'only' children living with elderly grandparents in poor health and at a distance from friends may feel quite isolated from their peers (Farmer & Moyers 2008). Some children want to see more of their separated siblings (Farmer & Moyers 2008; Kiraly & Humphreys 2013b; Wellard et al. 2017). Kiraly and Humphreys (2016) found that children generally wanted to see their parents unless there were major difficulties; however, multiple disappointments meant they sometimes wanted to stop visits. They felt strongly that their wishes should receive greater consideration and that they should not be forced to see their parents against their wishes.

There are relatively few studies of the views of parents of children in kinship care (Kiraly & Humphreys 2015). Nevertheless, repeated themes appear in these studies. Parents frequently articulate their grief at losing their children; feelings of powerlessness in the face of the child welfare system; the importance of contact with their children but the many difficulties they experience with visits; a lack of social or professional support and feelings of resentment or ambivalence towards the caregivers (Kiraly & Humphreys 2015):

> So I think some focus needs to be on how the parent feels when the child is taken away. Do you still feel like you can be a parent? ... your say in their upbringing gets removed.
>
> (Mother quoted in Kiraly & Humphreys 2015)

The small number of parents interviewed in Farmer and Moyers (2008) showed attitudes to the children's care ranging from positive endorsement to active hostility, but all acknowledged the good care their children were receiving. Gleeson (2014) similarly noted that parents who were positive about their relatives' care could also feel jealous and critical of the carers. This could be exacerbated if the parents felt that their children were receiving the kind of good care from their grandparents that they themselves had lacked from them (Farmer & Moyers 2008).

Conclusions

Kinship care is on the rise in Western societies, yet attention has not yet been accorded to addressing the particular disadvantages experienced by such families. At present the benefits of kinship care for children are often achieved at the expense of their carers, who may be under severe stress because of their financial difficulties and the demands of traumatised children with challenging behaviour. There is a particular gap in financial support and access to direct work for the majority of children in informal kinship care. For children in formal kinship care, the battle continues to ensure that children are supported equitably on the basis of need as compared with children in foster care. In times of financial stringency there is a tendency to consider that kinship care can be a cheaper option than foster care or even, where jurisdictions allow, not to fund placements at all (see for example, Selwyn et al. 2013).

Given the findings of Wijedasa (2015) that the majority of UK children being brought up by relatives are living in deprived households and are disproportionately affected by long-term health problems or disability, it would be useful to ascertain whether the same is true in Australia. However, there is already plenty of evidence that kinship carers in both countries face very considerable challenges often without sufficient support, and that the issues for Australian Indigenous carers are particularly acute. These matters have been raised by researchers now for several decades, but there is a continuing gap between the needs of children and their carers and the services they receive, the greatest need being for informal kinship families. The myth that kinship families can (and indeed should) manage on their own without outside assistance appears to be a powerful one, and the continued silo between foster care and kinship care often allows governments to consider the needs of the first group without regard to the latter. A kinship carer expressed her view of the state of support in a carer survey thus:

> We love caring for all the children and seeing them develop and gain confidence. It is not an easy path at times. Kinship care seems to be the 'Cinderella' of the care system, so I hope your research project might help these people.
>
> (Carer quoted in Kiraly, James & Humphreys 2015)

There is also a need to disaggregate the kinship carer population. Research has shown the severe pressures under which siblings and young aunts and uncles bring up children (see for example, Selwyn et al. 2013) and likewise non-familial kinship carers (Kiraly 2018). Both groups need more help. Other high need groups are carers whose health problems over time leave them dependent on the kinship children, and carers who also support children's parents or other sick relatives (Selwyn et al. 2013). When the outcomes in young adulthood of children brought up in kinship care are considered, the findings are both encouraging and worrying. On the one hand, these young adults do considerably better than those in foster care in most areas but not all. On the other hand, their outcomes still lag considerably behind those of their peers in the general population (Wellard et al. 2017). Without sufficient help, young people growing up in kinship care are at risk of having poor psychological and economic outcomes in adulthood. Governments in both Australia and the UK now need to abandon policy based on myths and partial truths and step up to the real task of supporting all vulnerable children in alternative care equitably and sufficiently.

Discussion questions

1 Do you agree that some policy and practice about kinship care over time has been affected by the dominant ideas or myths that have developed about it? If so, which

myths do you think have been the most influential? What might be done to address these issues?

2 Why do you think governments have not responded more actively to the evidence of financial difficulties and stress among kinship carers even when the outcomes of these care arrangements for children are often so good?

3 Why do you think parental contact is more often fraught for children in kinship care as compared with those in (non-kinship) foster care? What could be done to make direct and indirect assistance more widely available to kinship carers?

Notes

1 In this study, formal relative care was defined by the British term 'kinship foster care'. Included in this informal group therefore is the relatively small number of children in the UK under private law orders such as Special Guardianship Orders (SGO) for which child welfare services have the discretion to pay an allowance and provide some support. An accurate estimate of their numbers is currently difficult to achieve due to data limitations, as reported in Wade et al. (2014).

2 A similar figure has also been established in the USA, see Gleeson (2014).

3 A deprived household was defined as one including a person with one or more of the following conditions: lack of employment, low education, poor health or disability, and substandard housing.

4 The name given to the large number of Aboriginal people who were forcibly removed from their families for several decades up to the 1960s.

5 Whilst rates of formal kinship care (kinship foster care) have remained steady in the UK (Department for Education 2017), the rates of private law orders like Special Guardianship Orders (SGOs) have continued to rise, but as there is no single source of published statistics on SGOs, exact numbers cannot readily be established (Wade et al. 2014).

6 A cultural support plan is an individually tailored plan for Aboriginal children in care that contains information about their traditional links and family connections in order to maintain a strong sense of identity and belonging. In some jurisdictions this is enshrined in legislation as a requirement for all Aboriginal children, for example, see State of Victoria, 2005a, State of Victoria, 2005b.

References

AIHW, 2020, Child Protection Australia 2018–19, Canberra: Australian Institute of Health and Welfare.

Ainsworth, F. & Maluccio, A.N., 1998, 'Kinship care: False dawn or new hope?', *Australian Social Work*, vol. 51, no. 4, pp. 3–8.

Boetto, H., 2010, 'Kinship care: A review of issues', *Family Matters*, vol. 85, pp. 60–67.

Brennan, D., Cass, B., Flaxman, S., Hill, T., Jenkins, B., McHugh, M., *et al.*, 2013, *Grandparents raising grandchildren: Towards recognition, respect and reward*, Sydney: Social Policy Research Centre, University of New South Wales.

Connolly, M., 2003, *Kinship care: A selected literature review*, Wellington: submitted to the Department of Child, Youth and Family, May 2003.

Connolly, M., de Haan, I. & Crawford, J., 2013, 'The safety of young children in care: a New Zealand study', *Adoption & Fostering*, vol. 37, no. 3, pp. 284–296.

Cuddeback, G.S., 2004, 'Kinship family foster care: A methodological and substantive synthesis of research', *Children and Youth Services Review*, vol. 26, pp. 623–639.

del Valle, J.F., López, M., Montserrat, C. & Bravo, A., 2009, 'Twenty years of foster care in Spain: Profiles, patterns and outcomes', *Children and Youth Services Review*, vol. 31, pp. 847–853.

Delfabbro, P., 2017, *Relative/kinship and foster care: A comparison of carer and child characteristics. Pathways of care longitudinal study: Outcomes of children and young people in out-of-home care*, Sydney: NSW Department of Family and Community Services.

Delfabbro, P., Fernandez, E., McCormick, J. & Kettler, L., 2013, 'Reunification in a complete entry cohort: A longitudinal study of children entering out-of-home care in Tasmania, Australia', *Children and Youth Services Review*, vol. 35, pp. 1592–1600.

Department for Education UK, 2011, Family and friends care: Statutory guidance for local authorities, London: Department for Education.

Downie, J., Hay, D., Horner, B., Wichmann, H. & Hislop, A., 2010, 'Children living with their grandparents: resilience and wellbeing', *International Journal of Social Welfare*, vol. 19, pp. 8–22.

Doyle, J. & Kiraly, M. (eds), 2018, Developing practice (Special kinship care issue no.1), vol. 51, Sydney: Association of Children's Welfare Agencies.

Doyle, J. & Kiraly, M. (eds.), 2019, Developing Practice (Special Kinship Care Issue No.2), vol. 52, Sydney: Association of Children's Welfare Agencies.

Farmer, E., 2009a, 'How do placements in kinship care compare with those in non-kin foster care: placement patterns, progress and outcomes?', *Child and Family Social Work*, vol. 14, pp. 331–342.

Farmer, E., 2009b, 'Placement stability in kinship care', *Vulnerable Children and Youth Studies*, vol. 4, no. 2, pp. 154–160.

Farmer, E., 2010, 'What factors relate to good placement outcomes in kinship care?', *British Journal of Social Work*, vol. 40, pp. 426–444.

Farmer, E. & Moyers, S., 2008, *Kinship care: Fostering effective family and friends placements*, London: Jessica Kingsley Publishers.

Farmer, E. & Owen, M., 1995, *Child protection practice: Private risks and public remedies*, London: HMSO.

Farmer, E., Selwyn, J. & Meakings, S., 2013, 'Other children say you're not normal because you don't live with your parents. Children's views of living with informal kinship carers: social networks, stigma and attachment to carers', *Child and Family Social Work*, vol. 18, no. 1, pp. 25–34.

Gilligan, R., 2006, 'Creating a warm place where children can blossom', *Social Policy Journal of New Zealand*, vol. 28, pp. 36–45.

Gleeson, J.P., 2014, 'The views of children in kinship care, their caregivers and their birth parents', in D. Pitcher (ed.), *Inside kinship care*, London: Jessica Kingsley.

Gough, P., 2006, 'Kinship care', in Centre of Excellence for Child Welfare Canada, Toronto: Faculty of Social Work, University of Toronto, pp. 1–4.

Hartley, R., 1993, 'Young adults living at home', *Family Matters (AIFS)*, vol. 36.

Hegar, R.L., 1999, 'Kinship foster care: The new child placement paradigm', in R.L. Hegar & M. Scannapieco (eds), *Kinship foster care: Policy, practice and research*, New York: Oxford University Press.

Hunt, J., 2019, 'Kinship carer assessments: An Anglo-Welsh perspective', *Developing Practice*, vol. 52, pp. 40–57.

Hunt, J. & Waterhouse, S., 2013, *It's just not fair! Support, need and legal status in family and friends care*, London: Family Rights Group.

Hunt, J., Waterhouse, S. & Lutman, E., 2008, *Keeping them in the family: Outcomes for children placed in kinship care through care proceedings*, London: British Agencies for Adoption and Fostering.

Hunt, J., Waterhouse, S. & Lutman, E., 2010, 'Parental contact for children placed in kinship care through care proceedings', *Child and Family Law Quarterly*, vol. 22, no. 1, pp. 71–92.

Kiraly, M., 2015, A review of kinship carer surveys: The "Cinderella" of the care system?, Melbourne: Child Family Community Australia (CFCA) information exchange, Australian Institute of Family Studies, https://aifs.gov.au/cfca/sites/default/files/publication-documents/cfca-paper31.pdf, accessed 25 September 2019.

Kiraly, M. (2019). Non-familial kinship carers – who are they and what support do they need to nurture children? *Child & Family Social Work*, vol. 24, no. 4, pp. 449–457.

Kiraly, M. & Humphreys, C., 2013a, 'Family contact for children in kinship care: A literature review', *Australian Social Work*, vol. 66, no. 3, pp. 358–374.

Kiraly, M. & Humphreys, C., 2013b, 'Perspectives from young people about family contact in kinship care: "Don't push us—listen more"', *Australian Social Work*, vol. 66, no. 3, pp. 314–327.

Kiraly, M. & Humphreys, C., 2013c, 'Policy briefing paper: Kinship care and family contact', *Developing Practice*, vol. 35, Winter, pp. 68–74.

Kiraly, M. & Humphreys, C., 2015, 'A tangled web: Parental contact with children in kinship care', *Child and Family Social Work*, vol. 20, pp. 106–115.

Kiraly, M. & Humphreys, C., 2016, '"It's about the whole family": Family contact for children in kinship care', *Child & Family Social Work*, vol. 21, no. 2, pp. 228–239.

Kiraly, M., James, J. & Humphreys, C., 2015, '"It's a family responsibility": Family and cultural connection for Aboriginal children in kinship care', *Children Australia*, vol. 40, no. 1, pp. 23–32.

McFadden, E.J., 1998, 'Kinship care in the United States', *Adoption and Fostering*, vol. 22, no. 3, pp. 7–15.

McHugh, M., 2013, *An exploratory study of risks to stability in foster and kinship care in NSW: final report*, Sydney: Social Policy Research Centre, University of New South Wales.

McHugh, M., 2014a, 'Australia and New Zealand: Assessing parenting capacity in kinship care', in D. Pitcher (ed.), *Inside kinship care: Understanding family dynamics and providing effective support*, London: Jessica Kingsley, pp. 206–220.

McHugh, M., 2014b, *Victoria's declining foster care allowances: A comparative analysis*, Sydney: Social Policy Research Centre, UNSW.

McHugh, M. & Hayden, P., 2014, 'Australia and New Zealand: Assessing parenting capacity in kinship care', in D. Pitcher (ed.), *Inside kinship care: Understanding family dynamics and providing effective support*, London: Jessica Kingsley, pp. 206–220.

Maxwell, G. & Morris, A., 1992, 'The family group conference: A new paradigm for making decisions about children and young people', *Children Australia*, vol. 17, no. 4, pp. 11–15.

Messing, J.T., 2006, 'From the child's perspective: A qualitative analysis of kinship care placements', *Children and Youth Services Review*, vol. 28, pp. 1415–1434.

Mulroney, L. & Roach, J., 2016, *Step by step relative kinship assessment tool*, Sydney: Association of Children's Welfare Agencies.

Munro, E.R. & Gilligan, R., 2013, 'The "dance" of kinship care in England and Ireland: Navigating a course between regulation and relationships', *Psychosocial Intervention*, vol. 22, pp. 185–192.

Nixon, P., 2008, *Relatively speaking: Developments in research and practice in kinship care*, Dartington, UK: Blacklers.

O'Brien, V., 2013, *Kinship care: Stability, disruption and the place of support services*, Dublin: University College Dublin, School of Applied Social Science.

Palacios, J. & Jimenez, J., 2009, 'Kinship care: Protection or risk?', *Adoption and Fostering*, vol. 33, no. 3, pp. 64–75.

Perry, G., Daly, M. & Kotler, J., 2012, 'Placement stability in kinship and non-kin foster care: A Canadian study', *Children and Youth Services Review*, vol. 34, pp. 460–465.

Pine, B.A., Warsh, R. & Maluccio, A.N. (eds), 1993, *Together again: Family reunification in foster care*, Washington DC: Child Welfare League of America.

Pitcher, D. (ed.), 2014, *Inside kinship care: Understanding family dynamics and providing effective support*, London: Jessica Kingsley.

Roth, D., Tunnard, J., Lindley, B., De Gaye, A. & Ashley, C., 2011, *Managing contact: Research findings on managing contact with parents and relatives for children living in family and friends arrangements*, London: Family Rights Group.

Royal Commission into Institutional Responses to Child Sexual Abuse, 2017, Final Report: Our inquiry, Canberra: Royal Commission.
Sallnäs, M., Vinnerljung, B. & Westermark, P.K., 2004, 'Breakdown of teenage placements in Swedish foster and residential care', *Child and Family Social Work*, vol. 9, no. 141–152.
Scannapieco, M. & Hegar, R.L., 1999, 'Kinship Foster Care in Context', in R.L. Hegar & M. Scannapieco (eds), *Kinship foster care: Policy, practice and research*, New York: Oxford University Press.
Selwyn, J., Farmer, E., Meakings, S. & Vaisey, P., 2013, *The poor relations? Children and informal kinship carers speak out*, Bristol, UK: University of Bristol.
Selwyn, J. & Nandy, S., 2014, 'Kinship care in the UK: using census data to estimate the extent of formal and informal care by relatives', *Child and Family Social Work*, vol. 19, no. 1, pp. 44–54.
Senate Community Affairs References Committee, 2014, Grandparents who take primary responsibility for raising their grandchildren, Canberra: Commonwealth of Australia.
Senate Community Affairs References Committee, 2015, Out of home care, Canberra: Commonwealth of Australia.
Smyth, C. & Eardley, T., 2007, *Out of home care for children in Australia: A review of literature and policy*, Sydney: Social Policy Research Centre, University of New South Wales.
SNAICC, 2004, Research priorities for indigenous children and youth, Melbourne: Secretariat of National Aboriginal and Islander Child Care.
SNAICC, 2005, Policy paper: Achieving stable and culturally strong out of home care for Aboriginal and Torres Strait Islander Children, Melbourne: Secretariat of National Aboriginal and Islander Child Care.
Stack, C., 1974, *All our kin: Strategies for survival in a black community*, New York: Harper & Row.
State of Victoria, 2005a, Children, Youth and Families Act, No. 96 of 2005.
State of Victoria, 2005b, *Aboriginal and Torres Strait Islander cultural support plan: Guide*. Melbourne: Department of Human Services.
Strijker, J., Zandberg, T. & van der Meulen, B.F., 2003, 'Kinship care and foster care in the Netherlands', *Children and Youth Services Review*, vol. 25, no. 11, pp. 843–862.
Tucker, J. (ed.), 2016, *Improving children's life chances*, London: Child Poverty Action Group.
United Nations, 2010, Guidelines for the alternative care of children, New York: United Nations General Assembly.
Victorian Ombudsman, 2017, Investigation into the financial support provided to kinship carers, Melbourne: Victorian Ombudsman.
Wade, J., Sinclair, I., Stuttard, L. & Simmonds, J., 2014, Investigating Special Guardianship: experiences, challenges and outcomes – Research report, London: Department for Education.
Webster, D., Barth, R.P. & Needell, B., 2000, 'Placement stability for children in out-of-home care: A longitudinal analysis', *Child Welfare*, vol. 79, no. 5, pp. 614–632.
Wellard, S., Meakings, S., Farmer, E. & Hunt, J., 2017, *Growing up in kinship care: Experiences as adolescents and outcomes in young adulthood*, London: Grandparents Plus.
Wijedasa, D., 2015, *The prevalence and characteristics of children growing up with relatives in the UK: Characteristics of children living with relatives in England: Part I*, Bristol, UK: Hadley Centre for Adoption & Foster Care Studies, University of Bristol.
Winokur, M., Holtan, A., & Batchelder, K. E., 2018, 'Systematic review of kinship care effects on safety, permanency, and well-being outcomes', *Research on Social Work Practice*, vol. 28, no. 1, pp. 19–32.
Zinn, A., 2012, 'Kinship foster family type and placement discharge outcomes', *Children and Youth Services Review*, vol. 34, no. 4, pp. 602–614.

Chapter 12

Therapeutic residential care

Kenny Kor and Patricia McNamara

Introduction

Deinstitutionalisation spread rapidly across most developed Anglophone countries from the late 1960s, sharply reducing the number of children and young people placed in residential care (Thoburn & Ainsworth 2015; Whittaker 2000). Accordingly, residential programs in the out-of-home care (OOHC) context have gradually moved away from large dormitory settings to smaller group homes. Several drivers have contributed to this shift, not least of which is the continuing evidence of child maltreatment in institutional settings (Fernandez et al. 2017; The Royal Commission into Institutional Responses to Child Sexual Abuse [The Royal Commission] 2017; Uliando & Mellor 2012). Coupled with its high cost and a perceived restrictive environment that may constrain healthy child development, residential care is often utilised as a 'last resort' OOHC option for containment of 'hard cases' (Colton 2002; McLean 2018; McLean, Price-Robertson & Robinson 2011). This approach contributes to a paradox: although residential care is judged to be unconducive to optimal child development, it is continually used for children and young people with the most complex and challenging needs.

In Australia, the vast majority of children (93%) in OOHC were in kinship or foster care, with only about 6% in residential care in 2018 (Australian Institute of Health and Welfare [AIHW] 2019). Deinstitutionalisation has not only reduced the accessibility of various forms of residential care, but also transferred the burden of care to the rest of the OOHC system. Consequently, modern care systems face two principal challenges: an insufficient supply of foster and kinship care placements, and inadequate resources within these placements to support children and young people who often have entrenched behavioural and emotional difficulties (Vicary 2015). For children and young people living with such difficulties, the intimacy and reciprocity demanded of them within family placements frequently proves unsustainable (Ainsworth & Hansen 2005; Bath 2008). Because of these challenges, residential care has remained an integral part of the OOHC service continuum. It has been argued that dismissing this acknowledged reality perpetuates inattention to residential care service development (Ainsworth & Hansen 2005).

Within this context, much international effort has been made in recent years to further develop residential care as a therapeutic OOHC option (Whittaker, del Valle & Holmes 2015). In contrast to general residential care, therapeutic residential care is underpinned by trauma-informed care principles aiming to cultivate an environment conducive to recovery and attainment of developmental competency (McNamara 2015). This represents a significant shift from general provision of accommodation and support to specialised models of care that aim to holistically address educational, emotional and psychosocial needs of children and young people (McLean, Price-Robertson & Robinson 2011). Various definitions and principles of therapeutic residential care have shaped current development (McLean, Price-Robertson & Robinson 2011; Whittaker, del Valle & Holmes 2015). A group of international scholars representing 11 countries, for example, has developed a cross-national definition of therapeutic residential care:

> The planful use of a purposefully constructed, multi-dimensional living environment designed to enhance or provide treatment, education, socialization, support, and protection to children and youth with identified mental health or behavioural needs in partnership with their families and in collaboration with a full spectrum of community-based formal and informal helping resources
>
> (Whittaker, del Valle & Holmes 2015: 24).

This definition is not intended to represent a single model of care (Whittaker, del Valle & Holmes 2015). It is vigorously argued that it should be considered in tandem with the following principles when designing and implementing therapeutic residential care:

1 Safety first: protect children from harm through implementing staff screening, monitoring, reporting and respecting children's right to be heard.
2 Family partnerships: preserve and strengthen family and kinship connections.
3 Community-based service delivery: collaborate with the broader child welfare system to provide holistic services.
4 Relationship driven practice: cultivate positive learning environments through stable relationships with staff.
5 Effective, replicable and scalable services: continue to develop evidence-based service models in light of the needs of children and young people (Whittaker, del Valle & Holmes 2015).

An alternative Australian definition has recently been developed to reflect an important international difference, from the US especially; Australian residential care is primarily used for young people in statutory OOHC care systems as a result of parental abuse and neglect, and multiple unsuccessful home-based placements:

> Therapeutic residential care is an intensive intervention and purposefully constructed living environment which creates a therapeutic milieu that is the basis of positive, safe, healing relationships and experiences designed to address complex needs arising from the impacts of abuse, neglect, adversity and separation from family, community and culture. It is informed by current understandings of trauma, attachment, socialisation and child development theories; which are translated into practice and embedded in the therapeutic care program (National Therapeutic Residential Care Alliance 2016, cited in McLean 2018: 5).

Arguably, both Australian and international definitions are steps in the right direction for advancing therapeutic residential care. However, implementation of these definitions is yet to be fully explored and studied. Research into therapeutic residential care has only recently begun in earnest, yet important findings are emerging. Evidence has been brought together in a number of publications which have focused on a range of different models that appear to accord more strongly with the definitions and principles presented above (Boel-Studt & Tobia 2016; McLean 2016; Pecora & English 2016; Whittaker, del Valle & Holmes 2015). James (2015) suggests that these new models appear to fall into two broad approaches; namely, milieu-based and mental health treatment. To this, we add a third approach, the Australian 'home-grown model' (Lee & McMillen 2017) which is discussed in this chapter. These three approaches have been reviewed and evaluated in Australia, Northern Ireland and the USA respectively. The following sections summarise and appraise key findings and discuss their implications for practice and policy.

When reviewing international evidence, it is important to keep in mind that therapeutic residential care, and more generally residential care, are defined very broadly across different countries. In the USA, for example, residential care encompasses an extensive array of youth services in group settings, from OOHC placements, mental health treatment centres to juvenile detention facilities (Pecora & English 2016). Therapeutic residential care in Australia, as noted previously, typically caters for children and young people aged between 12 and 18 in statutory OOHC (AIHW 2019). These children and young people are placed in houses in the community and looked after by paid staff. These differences need to be taken into consideration when drawing on international research to understand practice and policy implications.

Therapeutic residential care research evidence

The home-grown approach: therapeutic residential care (TRC) pilot program in Australia

The first therapeutic residential care (TRC) pilot program in Australia was launched in 2007 by the Department of Human Services (DHS) in the State of Victoria. It is considered 'home-grown' because the program design has been shaped over time based on local experience specific to a single jurisdiction (James 2017; Lee & McMillen 2017). The pilot program was underpinned by theoretical knowledge of psychological trauma, aiming to provide a therapeutic environment within a trauma-informed framework to address complex and multiple needs of young people (Verso-DHS 2011). The pilot program was conducted at 12 sites operated by nine non-government organisations (NGOs). Each TRC site had specific client foci in relation to gender, age and statutory OOHC orders. Most of the TRC houses accommodated four young people, with others housing up to eight young people, aged between 12 and 18 years (Verso-DHS 2011). The TRC pilot program was designed to improve practice and outcomes. The key features differentiating TRC from general residential care included: consistent rostering of staff, use of therapeutic specialists to provide assessment and care planning, regular interagency meetings, trauma-informed supervision and training (Verso-DHS 2011).

Verso, an independent consultancy, conducted an evaluation of the pilot program between August 2009 and July 2011. Rigorously applying repeated measures, the evaluation tracked progress of young people in the program at seven points in time, from 15 months pre-entry to 27 months post-entry. The project assessed 38 young people from TRC through staff surveys and interviews (Verso-DHS 2011).[1]

Mental health and wellbeing outcomes

Young people's mental health improved, with a general reduction in severity of symptoms: emotional responses to stress, conduct problems, inattention, hyperactivity and impulsivity, and improvement in peer relationships and pro-social behaviours (Verso-DHS 2011). These results were seen only from pre-entry to entry and plateaued thereafter, suggesting that young people had achieved these gains early on and were able to sustain them throughout their stay in the pilot program (Verso-DHS 2011).

TRC staff's perceptions of young people's wellbeing were also measured across different domains: the quality of family contact, relationships with carers, school and community participation, physical health and self-esteem. This part of the evaluation included a comparison group of 16 young people from general residential care to investigate the degree to which their wellbeing outcomes differed from those in the pilot program. Table 12.1 summarises their key differences.

Young people's perspectives

Nine young people were interviewed. They reported two marked differences that separated their experiences in the TRC program from general residential care (Verso-DHS 2011). First, young people reported higher quality family contact and closer relationships with residential care practitioners (Verso-DHS 2011). Second, they felt that residential care practitioners were more readily available to listen to their concerns and provide emotional support (Verso-DHS 2011). This mirrors the key finding that TRC practitioners reported a shift in their attitude towards young people's challenging behaviour, from being 'judgemental' (Verso-DHS 2011: 56) to understanding underlying needs associated with past trauma.

Strengths and limitations

The evaluation provided longitudinal and comparative insights, strengthening the evidence base for therapeutic residential care. It demonstrated that therapeutic residential care, when implemented well, has greater potential than general residential care to improve mental health and wellbeing outcomes. These findings have resulted in the expansion of this TRC approach to 140 additional placements across the state of Victoria (DHHS 2016).

The evaluation, however, identified three concerns that present important challenges and opportunities for future service development and practice. First, upon departure from the pilot program and beyond, young people continued to have more elevated mental health difficulties than their counterparts in the mainstream community (DHS-Verso 2011). This adds to the existing research evidence that there is an urgent need for more responsive post-care support (Cashmore & Paxman 2007; Courtney et al. 2011; Mendes 2009).

Second, whilst the number of young people engaging in risk-taking behaviours declined at the 18-month post-entry point, concern remained that, one year into the pilot program, alcohol was still 'heavily involved' or 'involved' in over 50% of risk-taking behaviours (Verso-DHS 2011). Further, nearly 40% of risk-taking behaviours were associated with sexual behaviour and over 50% of critical incidents were linked with substance abuse

Table 12.1 Key results of the pilot program group vs. the general residential care group in the Victorian Therapeutic Residential Care (TRC) evaluation.

Perceived outcomes by the program's workers	*The TRC group*	*The comparison group*
Quality of family contact	At 27 months post-entry, nearly 60% perceived the quality of family contact as 'high' or 'very high'.	The 'high' and 'very high' ratings remained at 20% at the final data collection point without any marked increase.
Quality of relationship between young people and their program workers	There was a marked increase in the 'high' rating, reaching nearly 60% at the 27 months post-entry point.	The aggregated average ratings for the quality of relationship with residential care workers appeared to be evenly split between 'poor' and 'good' ratings.
Quality of community participation	Over 40% rated 'high' or 'very high' at 27 months post-entry.	Overall, more than 50% were dissatisfied, with fewer than 10% rated 'high' or 'very high'.
School or vocational attendance	School attendance improved slightly over time with the median attendance standing at 4 days per week. Accordingly, a small improvement in language skills and concentration was recorded.	The young people in this group spent less time at school or in vocational training. However, they had more positive experiences at school overall and higher academic functioning.
Quality of peer relationships and social functioning at school	The 'good' or 'high quality' rating went from nought at the entry point to nearly 40% at the 27 months post-entry point.	Nearly 60% of young people were perceived as 'markedly dysfunctional' or 'dysfunctional', with only 5% considered as having good quality peer relationships and social functioning at school.
Frequency of recreation and physical exercise	Over 75% of young people engaged in recreation activities at least twice a week and nearly 60% exercised at least once a day at 27 months post-entry.	20% had recreation activities twice per week and less than 30% exercised more than twice a week.
Self-esteem of the young people	A steady shift towards positive ratings, from less than 10% recorded as having 'very high regard for self' at entry to over 30% at 27 months post-entry. The 'low' sense of self rating also dropped to less than 10%.	Nearly 80% of young people were perceived as having 'low' to 'very low regard for self'.

(Verso-DHS 2011). Previous research indicated that behavioural concerns are not confined to the TRC pilot program but are shared challenges in residential care (Barter et al. 2003; Euser et al. 2013; Huefner et al. 2010; Sinclair & Gibbs 1998). Two perennial questions arise once again from these shared research findings: (1) How are young people in residential care impacted by these risk-taking behaviours? (Dishion, Poulin & Burraston 2001; Whittaker 2017) and (2) for whom might TRC be best suited? (Whittaker 2017).

Finally, the evaluation revealed inconsistent implementation of the pilot program. Staff supervision and training were found to be irregular in both frequency and quality; four of the 12 pilot sites also had a protracted service gap without clinical support from the therapeutic specialist (Verso-DHS 2011). The impact of these implementation issues was also evident in the 2015 inquiry by the Commission for Children and Young People (CCYP) in Victoria. In the six therapeutic residential care sites the Commission visited, only two sites were considered therapeutic, whilst the others were described as 'hostile, bland and institutional' (CCYP 2015: 88). Some of the bedrooms were found to be unhygienic, with food and toys locked away. The Commission was also concerned that some sites had staff offices with a 'viewing window' through which young people were scrutinised (CCYP 2015: 102). Some frontline practitioners told the Commission that they had not received supervision or training on therapeutic care. Deviations from the departmental guidelines on staff recruitment was also reported, revealing that some frontline practitioners had no formal qualifications other than 'life experience' (CCYP 2015: 100). Taking these various aspects of evidence into consideration brings to light the complexities of implementation which is 'neither easy, inexpensive nor straight-forward' (James 2017: 165). Safety, conceptual congruence, professionalisation of staff and enhancement of the physical environment are some learnings from studies of the Australian 'home-grown approach' that clearly need to be consistently applied.

The milieu-based models approach: experience in Northern Ireland

Milieu-based models typically aim to provide safe and nurturing environments for young people who have suffered psychological trauma (James 2015). They emphasise cultural change in the organisation, training practitioners across all service levels to be aware of and sensitive to the impacts of trauma on young people (Bloom 2005). In Northern Ireland, the Institute of Child Care Research at Queen's University Belfast evaluated five milieu-based models commonly deployed in their residential care services. These models were (1) Attachment, Self-regulation and Competency (Blaustein & Kinniburgh 2007); (2) Children and Residential Experiences (CARE) (Holden et al. 2010); (3) Model of Attachment Practice (MAP) (Macdonald & Millen 2012b); (4) Sanctuary model (Bloom 2005) and (5) Social Pedagogy (Bengtsson et al. 2008).

Four of the five models, with the exception of Social Pedagogy, are underpinned by attachment and trauma theories (Macdonald & Millen 2012b). Most of these models aim to broaden practitioners' theoretical knowledge to help them better understand young people's behaviour, and provide descriptive principles for practice, rather than specific therapeutic techniques (Macdonald & Millen 2012b). The five models included in the Northern Ireland study are summarised in Table 12.2.

Key findings

The mixed-method evaluation drew on interviews with 38 practitioners and 29 young people, and questionnaires completed by 116 practitioners from 18 residential care units. Positive attitudinal change was found in the way practitioners approached residential care work, from a disciplinary mindset to a trauma-informed perspective (Macdonald et al. 2012). Irrespective of which milieu-based model was utilised, the evaluation found that training on the model broadened practitioners' understanding of the underlying trauma

Table 12.2 Summary of the milieu-based models evaluated in the Northern Ireland study

Models	*Key Features*
Attachment, Self-Regulation and Competency (ARC)	***Objectives:*** Create a safe environment for children and young people to build and restore developmental competencies (Blaustein & Kinniburgh 2007). ***Core principles:*** (1) Caregiver's self-awareness of emotions; (2) consistent responses to emotional needs; (3) enhance capacity for self-regulation and (4) develop self-care and interpersonal skills (Kinniburgh, Blaustein & Spinazzola 2005).
Children and Residential Experiences (CARE)	***Objectives:*** Build residential care service capacity to serve the best interest of children and young people (Holden et al. 2010) ***Core principles:*** (1) Developmentally focused; (2) family involvement; (3) competency-centred; (4) relationship-based; (5) trauma-informed and (6) ecologically oriented (Holden, Anglin & Nunno 2015).
Model of Attachment Practice (MAP)	***Objectives:*** Enable practitioners to apply attachment and trauma theories to understand children and young people's behaviours (Macdonald & Millen 2012b). ***Core principles:*** (1) Model and practise positive behaviour; (2) developmentally focused; (3) aware of own attachment issues; (3) firm but not confrontational; (4) take control of the environment; (5) self-care and (6) empathy (Macdonald & Millen 2012b)
Sanctuary Model	***Objectives:*** An organisational approach to developing trauma-informed practice to help children and young people change their maladaptive coping responses and develop capacity for emotion regulation and positive interpersonal relationships (Rivard et al. 2004). ***Core principles:*** SELF which stands for (1) Safety; (2) Emotion regulation; (3) Learn to deal with loss and (4) Future-focused (Rivard et al. 2004).
Social Pedagogy	***Objectives:*** Promote young people's social inclusion and competence in the community (Grietens 2015). ***Core principles:*** (1) Holistic child development; (2) relationship-focused; (3) equal power between pedagogues and children; (4) reflect on own practice; (5) use of daily activities to change behaviours; (6) promote peer and family relationships; (7) rights-based approach and (8) teamwork (Petrie 2006, cited in Macdonald & Millen 2012b).

suffered by young people and increased their confidence in managing challenging behaviour (Macdonald et al. 2012). This links with their reports of using fewer punitive measures but more constructive communication with young people. Positive impacts on staff morale and job satisfaction were also noted (Macdonald et al. 2012). Whilst no meaningful differences on service outcomes were found between the five models, practitioners stated that operating within a specified model enabled them to adopt a common language and improve practice consistency (Macdonald et al. 2012).

Young people's experience

Around two-thirds of the 29 young people interviewed were satisfied with their overall care experience. They reported a noticeable improvement in the care environment, commenting that practitioners appeared more relaxed and communicative (Macdonald et al. 2012). More specifically, most young people found practitioners approachable and helpful and valued their positive relationships (Macdonald et al. 2012). However, many young people also reported being bullied and intimidated by other young people in therapeutic residential care. Some young people were also dissatisfied with the institutionalised arrangement in their living environments, such as the locking of certain areas in the house (Macdonald et al. 2012).

Strengths and limitations

This evaluation highlighted that adopting a milieu-based model equips practitioners with a shared language and framework for practice, improving their attitude, confidence and knowledge (Macdonald & Millen 2012a). These changes seem to have benefited young people to the extent that they reported stronger relationships with practitioners (Macdonald et al. 2012). These findings converge with those of previous studies, suggesting that continuous and rigorous staff training on specific practice models such as trauma-informed care can expand their knowledge base and develop new practice perspectives (Conners-Burrow et al. 2013; Redd et al. 2017).

It is, however, noteworthy that enhanced understanding and increased awareness of a particular milieu-based model do not necessarily translate into therapeutic care practice (Holden, Anglin & Nunno 2015). Insufficient staffing and supervision, high numbers of unplanned admissions, and competing priorities between models and organisational needs were identified as key implementation obstacles of these milieu-based models (Macdonald & Millen 2012a). On a policy level, these obstacles must be addressed through stronger investment in building the workforce capacity for therapeutic residential care and a more child-centred approach to admission planning. On a practice level, Anglin (2002) found that service congruency can be enhanced when practitioners are supported by service leaders to uphold a shared set of practice values and principles, highlighting the need for rigorous reflective practice and open communication between management and frontline staff.

When applying milieu-based models in practice, it is also important to recognise that only a small number of evaluations on some of the models were conducted, many of which were undertaken by the model developers (Macdonald & Millen 2012b), which may have affected objectivity. Some milieu-based models such as the CARE model seems more suited for younger children than adolescents with complex behavioural and learning difficulties (Macdonald & Millen 2012a). Other models also seem less applicable to managing aggressive behaviour and crises (Macdonald & Millen 2012a).

The Sanctuary model is widely known in Australia (McLean, Price-Robertson & Robinson 2011; McNamara 2015). The California Evidence-Based Clearinghouse for Child Welfare (CEBC), a children's service assessment platform utilised in the USA and internationally, rated the Sanctuary model as 'promising'[2] (Pecora & English 2016). This reflects longitudinal research evidence that young people in Sanctuary care achieved greater improvement than their peers in general residential care, such as in reduction of verbal aggression and increase in communication and stress management skills (Rivard et al. 2005).

Whilst some promising results of milieu-based models are emerging, more nuanced understandings of their application in therapeutic residential care are needed (Macdonald and Millen 2012b). Other reviews echo this conclusion, indicating that the existing evidence base of the milieu-based models is insufficient to recommend any one model over another (James 2011, 2017). Implications for practice arising from the under-developed evidence base for milieu-based models, which continue to be widely employed internationally, are clearly profound. It has been recognised that implementation of any residential care model lacking rigorous assessment of quality and outcomes against international best practice benchmarks manifests a fundamental failure in duty of care to young people, their families and those who work with them (Whittaker, de Valle &

Holmes 2015). An important mitigating strategy for practice and research is to listen to the voices of young people, ensuring that their lived experiences are taken into account in service model development and implementation (Macdonald & Millen 2012a).

Mental health treatment approaches: experience in the USA

This approach incorporates specific individual-focused mental health treatments within residential care programs. Contrary to milieu-based models, this approach relies heavily on manualised treatment protocols and may not require extensive service reorganisation (James 2011). This may explain why 88% of agencies in the USA used one or multiple mental health treatments in residential care services (James et al. 2015). The three most utilised mental health treatments reported in the USA were Dialectical Behavioural Therapy (DBT), Trauma-Focused Cognitive Behavioural Therapy (TF-CBT) and Cognitive Behavioural Therapy (CBT) (James, Thompson & Ringle 2017). Many of these treatments are typically delivered by clinical specialists, focusing on specific psychiatric diagnoses; for example, DBT is designed for borderline personality disorder, whilst CBT is commonly used to treat anxiety and depression (Pecora & English 2016).

Despite the popularity of the mental health treatment approach in the USA, its applicability in therapeutic residential care settings remains 'a relatively new endeavour that, at the present time, is guided by little theory or data' (James et al. 2017: 14). Research into this therapeutic residential care approach is, in fact, limited. A meta-analysis spanning over 20 years from 1990 to 2012 identified 13 outcome studies with mixed and inconclusive results (James, Alemi & Zepeda 2013). As Chorpita and Daleiden (2009) argue, lumping different mental health treatments together in evaluations generally yields weak evidence for treatment recommendations because they tend to lack descriptions of what each treatment entails and overlook similarities and differences between treatments. Generally, treatments targeted at behavioural modification tended to show positive outcomes (Knorth et al. 2008). However, this may reflect that changes in observable behaviour are more readily detected by research than improvement in cognition and emotion.

Other research evidence found noticeable effects in some specific domains. DBT, for example, was found to have improved young people's emotional regulation (Sunseri 2004; Wasser et al. 2008) whilst Aggression Replacement Training (ART®) appeared to be effective in reducing anti-social behaviour (Coleman, Pfeiffer & Oakley 1992; Nugent, Bruley & Allen, 1999). Further, trauma-focused CBT has consistent evidence in randomised controlled trials for reducing young people's post-traumatic stress and behavioural difficulties (Cohen, Mannarino & Knudsen 2005; Cohen, Mannarino & Deblinger 2017; Jensen et al. 2014). Similarly, providing standard CBT to young people in residential care appeared to be marginally more effective in reducing emotional stress than general residential care without treatment (De Swart et al. 2012). Whilst many of these therapies have long-established research evidence as standalone treatments in individual clinical settings, James (2017) points out that there is little evidence to demonstrate that they can be effectively incorporated into residential care programs.

Strengths and limitations

The high utilisation of an individualised mental health treatment approach is a positive development, signifying a growing emphasis on psychosocial difficulties (James et al.

2015). Residential care practitioners also perceive it to be a clear advantage that many mental health treatments are accompanied by step-by-step implementation guidelines (James et al. 2015). However, research has also revealed that, even for treatments with clear protocols and well-developed training programs, implementation fidelity is poor across residential care services (James 2017; James, Thompson & Ringle 2017). Low staff retention and inadequate supervision are major barriers (James, Thompson & Ringle 2017). Therefore, whilst the mental health treatment approach may seem less resource intensive, its efficiency may be compromised without a sustainable and specialised workforce (James, Thompson & Ringle 2017; Pecora & English 2016).

Further, the individual-focused and therapy-based orientation may not address the therapeutic needs in 'the other 23 hours' (Trieschman, Whittaker & Brendtro 2002), overlooking other therapeutic components such as care stability, education, social activities and positive peer relationships. Research also indicates that direct care practitioners in residential care are mostly excluded from training in and delivery of mental health treatments (James, Thompson & Ringle 2017). As Pecora and English (2016) emphasise, the 'add-on' mental health approach is unlikely to be effective if direct care practitioners are not involved in the treatment process to cultivate safe environments and stable relationships to enable young people to participate in and benefit from treatments.

James (2017) also draws attention to the fact that many mental health treatments are not specifically designed for therapeutic residential care; some are, in fact, intended to prevent residential care admissions. These concerns raise the question of how such individualised and time-limited mental health treatments can be successfully integrated within group care environments to fully address young people's multiple needs (Pecora & English 2016). Accordingly, whilst mental health treatment approaches are often regarded as evidence-based practice (EBP), 'it needs to be stated clearly that, from a scientific standpoint, definitive conclusions about the effectiveness of EBPs in residential care in comparison to "usual care" services cannot be drawn at this point' (James, Thompson & Ringle 2017: 15). This reality too, has important practice implications, especially in relation to matching complex needs of young people to a specific residential care option. Too often, placement matching assessment and decisions are driven by operational and financial imperatives rather than thorough appraisal of specific needs (Whittaker, del Valle & Holmes 2015).

Implications for practice

The three emerging therapeutic residential care approaches discussed in this chapter have demonstrated varying degrees of improvement in mental health, general wellbeing, school attendance, family contact, community participation and social skills. The evaluations in Australia and Northern Ireland manifest positive attitudinal change in practice and improved knowledge. Children and young people confirm this, expressing greater satisfaction in care experience and relationships with residential care practitioners. Whilst these are promising results, concerns about safety, risk-taking behaviour, leaving care vulnerability and inconsistent implementation remain. Taking all aspects of evidence into account, it is premature to draw definitive conclusions about the effectiveness of these therapeutic residential care approaches or make recommendations for one particular approach over another. The overall trend emergent from research findings is that residential care with a therapeutic focus holds greater potential than general residential care to improve practice and outcomes. It is also important to recognise the reality that, for a population whose needs are as diverse and complex as children and young people in therapeutic residential care, it is likely to require not one but multiple approaches across various service systems and disciplines.

The recurrent findings about risk-taking behaviour and inconsistent implementation clearly warrant further attention. The substandard care environment and practice found by the Commission for Children and Young People (CCYP) in Victoria, Australia is evidently antithetical to therapeutic residential care practice principles. Prioritising safety, whilst seemingly obvious, remains a concerning practice gap in therapeutic residential care. Abuse in care remains a significant concern. The Royal Commission and international research have provided clear evidence that children and young people continue to experience various forms of maltreatment in contemporary residential care, including peer-to-peer victimisation (Attar-Schwartz 2011, 2017; Euser et al. 2013, 2014). As Herman (1992) argued several decades ago, a safe, nurturing and stable care environment is the foundation on which children and young people build their capacity to engage in therapeutic work. A commitment to child-safe organisational principles, such as those developed by the Australian Human Rights Commission in 2017, is therefore paramount internationally in ensuring that all aspects of practice in therapeutic residential care are driven by the 'first, do no harm' service goal (Whittaker, del Valle & Holmes 2015: 96).

Mental health support for young people also requires more concerted effort. Although there is evidence of improvement in mental health and general wellbeing, many young people continue to have elevated mental health concerns after leaving care. This adds weight to the concern that the transition to adulthood for young people in care is 'both accelerated and compressed' (Stein 2015: 192), urging the need to re-examine the unrealistic expectation that young people leaving care have the required maturity and resources to establish independent living. Although the importance of leaving care support is increasingly recognised in legislation and policy, in practice, after-care support 'remains discretionary rather than mandatory' (Mendes, Baidawi & Snow 2014: 402). Therefore, there is a clear need to improve practice and adopt a more inclusive and flexible approach to addressing individual disadvantages and reducing structural barriers to accessing leaving care services.

Implications for policy

In making policy recommendations for therapeutic residential care, it is important to carefully weigh and balance the potential benefits and limitations of the range of approaches reviewed in this chapter to understand not only *what* has worked but also *how* it may work in specific local contexts (Harder & Knorth 2015). This task requires policymakers to consult practitioners, implementers, children and young people more widely, whose first-hand experiences are invaluable but not always incorporated into policy development.

It is also crucial for policymakers to take stock of other research evidence that flexible service options, child-centred assessment, family-focused services, extended post-care support and integrated cross-sector collaboration improve engagement and long-term outcomes for children, young people and their families (Geurts et al. 2012; Huefner et al. 2010; Malvaso & Delfabbro 2015; Purtell & Mendes 2016; Schofield, Larsson & Ward 2017; Trout et al. 2012; Whittaker, del Valle & Holmes 2015).

Furthermore, as the Australian and Northern Ireland evaluations have clearly indicated, quality staff development, grounded in trauma-informed frameworks, promote positive attitudes and practice consistency. However, high staff turnover, poor working conditions and inadequate specialised support and training have been repeatedly identified as barriers to achieving professionalisation and sustainability (Ainsworth & Hansen 2008; Bath & Smith 2015; Boel-Studt & Tobia, 2016; James, Thompson & Ringle 2017). Williams and Lalor (2001) argue that failure to address these prevailing workforce issues trivialises the work in residential care and undermines young people's right to be looked after by qualified practitioners. Building and sustaining a robust workforce for therapeutic residential care should be a policy priority.

Conclusions

This chapter has reviewed three emerging therapeutic residential care approaches, showcasing the breadth of development currently under way internationally. Evidence on these three approaches points to the benefits of therapeutic residential care over general residential care in terms of mental health, general wellbeing, school attendance, family contact, community participation and social skills. These encouraging results are a testament to the concerted effort researchers and practitioners have made in recent years, providing an important lead for continued improvement.

This chapter has also examined the limitations associated with each therapeutic residential care approach. The key challenges and opportunities ahead are clear. In order to fully actualise the potential of therapeutic residential care and achieve meaningful changes in the lives of children and young people, we must first prioritise the 'do no harm' principle; continually develop our understandings of what therapeutic residential care entails and for whom it may be appropriate; collect evidence to demonstrate how various practice and systemic components associate with outcomes; and improve implementation both within residential care services and across the wider OOHC service system.

Case study

Jacob (13) lives in therapeutic residential care with three other young people, Brian (15), Lucas (16) and Victor (16). Not only is Jacob the youngest in the placement, he is also the newest, having moved in only a month ago. The other three young people have been living there for over 2 years. Jacob has been in OOHC since he was 5 years old, following substantiated sexual abuse by his father (against Jacob and his siblings).

Jacob has an older sister Lauren (14) and a younger brother, Matthew (12). All three children were initially placed together into foster care. Over the past year, their foster carer became increasingly concerned about Jacob's challenging behaviour including aggression towards his siblings, stealing, property damage and experimenting with drugs. As a result of these concerns, Jacob was removed from foster care and placed in therapeutic residential care.

Jacob has maintained contact (four times a year) with his mother Mandy. However, he has not seen his siblings Lauren and Matthew since being separated from them two months ago, and has no contact with other family members. Jacob's school attendance is sporadic but he is generally liked by his teachers and peers. He enjoys football and fishing but the recent change of placement has meant that he needs to change school and live in a different neighbourhood unfamiliar to him.

Discuss:

1 In applying the five key therapeutic residential care principles (Whittaker, del Valle & Holmes 2015), what would you include in your case planning for Jacob? What other key people and agencies would you consult in formulating your case plan?
2 Examine the research evidence reviewed in this chapter; what have young people told us about their experiences in therapeutic residential care? What have they found helpful and unhelpful? How would you take this knowledge to support Jacob and his residential care organisation?
3 Taking into account the current evidence base on therapeutic residential care and Jacob's circumstances, would you recommend moving Jacob's siblings from foster care and placing them together with Jacob in therapeutic residential care? List the pros and cons of your decision.

Notes

1 The number of young people included in the evaluation varied, from 38 at the entry point to 12 at the 24-month post entry, due to the different lengths of time they spent in the pilot program.
2 The CARE model has also been rated as 'promising' by CEBC. The other three models summarised in this chapter were not able to be rated on the CEBC rating scale because of insufficient research evidence. For the full rating criteria used by CEBC, refer to the website: www.cebc4cw.org/ratings/scientific-rating-scale/

References

Ainsworth, F. & Hansen, P., 2005, 'A dream come true – no more residential care. A corrective note', *International Journal of Social Welfare*, vol. 14, pp. 195–199.
Ainsworth, F. & Hansen, P., 2008, 'Programs for high needs children and young people: Group homes are not enough', *Children Australia*, vol. 33, no. 2, pp. 41–47.
Anglin, J.P., 2002, *Pain, normality and the struggle for congruence: Reinterpreting residential care for children and youth*, Birmingham, NY: Haworth Press.
Attar-Schwartz, S., 2011, 'Maltreatment by staff in residential care facilities: The adolescents' perspectives', *Social Service Review*, vol. 85, no. 4, pp. 635–664.
Attar-Schwartz, S., 2017, 'Experiences of victimization by peers and staff in residential care for children at risk in Israel from an ecological perspective', in A.V. Rus, S.R. Parris, & E. Stative (eds), *Child maltreatment in residential care: History, research, and current practice*, Switzerland: Springer International, pp. 269–299.
Australian Institute of Health and Welfare (AIHW), 2019, *Child protection Australia, 2017–18*, Canberra: Australian Institute of Health and Welfare.
Barter, C., Renold, E., Berridge, D. & Cawson, P., 2003, *Peer violence in children's residential care*, Basingstoke, UK: Palgrave MacMillan.
Bath, H., 2008, 'Residential care in Australia, Part I: Service trends, the young people in care, and needs-based responses', *Children Australia*, vol. 33, no. 2, pp. 6–17.
Bath, H. & Smith, B., 2015, 'Practice challenges in the shift to therapeutic residential care', *Developing Practice*, vol. 41, pp. 62–70.

Bengtsson, E., Chamberlain, C., Crimmens, D. & Stanley, J., 2008, *Introducing social pedagogy into residential child care in England*, London: NCERCC/SET.

Blaustein, M.E. & Kinniburgh, K.M., 2007, 'Intervening beyond the child: The intertwining nature of attachment and trauma', *British Psychological Society Briefing Paper*, vol. 26, pp. 48–53.

Bloom, S., 2005, 'Creating sanctuary for kids: Helping children to heal from violence', *Therapeutic Community: The International Journal for Therapeutic and Supportive Organizations*, vol. 26, no. 1, pp. 57–63.

Boel-Studt, S.M. & Tobia, L., 2016, 'A review of trends, research, and recommendations for strengthening the evidence-base and quality of residential group care', *Residential Treatment for Children & Youth*, vol. 33, no. 1, pp. 13–35.

Cashmore, J. & Paxman, M., 2007, *Wards leaving care: Four or five years on. A longitudinal study*, Sydney: Social Policy Research Centre, University of New South Wales.

Chorpita, B.F. & Daleiden, E.L., 2009, 'Mapping evidence-based treatments for children and adolescents: Application of the distillation and matching model to 615 treatments from 322 randomized trials', *Journal of Consulting and Clinical Psychology*, vol. 77, no. 3, pp. 566–579.

Cohen, J.A., Mannarino, A.P. & Knudsen, K., 2005, 'Treating sexually abused children: 1 year follow-up of a randomized controlled trial', *Child Abuse & Neglect*, vol. 29, no. 2, pp. 135–145.

Cohen, J.A., Mannarino, A.R. & Deblinger, E., 2017, *Treating trauma and traumatic grief in children and adolescents* (2nd edn), New York: Guilford Press.

Coleman, M., Pfeiffer, S. I. & Oakley, T., 1992, 'Aggression replacement training with behaviorally disordered adolescents', *Behavioral Disorders*, vol. 18, no. 1, pp. 54–66.

Colton, M., 2002, 'Factors associated with abuse in residential child care institutions', *Children & Society*, vol. 16, no. 1, pp. 33–44.

Commission for Children and Young People (CCYP), 2015, '... as a good parent would ...' Inquiry into the adequacy of the provision of residential care services to Victorian children and young people who have been subject to sexual abuse or sexual exploitation whilst residing in residential care, Melbourne: Commission for Children and Young People.

Conners-Burrow, N.A., Kramer, T.L., Sigel, B.A., Helpenstill, K., Sievers, C. & McKelvey, L., 2013, 'Trauma-informed care training in a child welfare system: Moving it to the front line', *Children and Youth Services Review*, vol. 35, no. 11, pp. 1830–1835.

Courtney, M.E., Dworsky, A., Brown, A., Cary, C., Love, K. & Vorhies, V., 2011, *Midwest evaluation of the adult functioning of former foster youth: Outcomes at age 26*. Chicago, IL: Chapin Hall Center for Children at the University of Chicago.

De Swart, J.J.W., Van den Broek, H., Stams, G.J.J.M., Asscher, J.J., Van der Laan, P.H., Holsbrink-Engels, G.A. & Van der Helm, G.H.P., 2012, 'The effectiveness of institutional youth care over the past three decades: A meta-analysis', *Children and Youth Services Review*, vol. 34, no. 9, pp. 1818–1824.

Department of Health and Human Services (DHHS), 2016, *Program requirements for the delivery of therapeutic residential care in Victoria*, Melbourne: Department of Health and Human Services.

Dishion, T.J., Poulin, F. & Burraston, B., 2001, 'Peer group dynamics associated with iatrogenic effects in group interventions with high-Risk young adolescents', *New Directions for Child and Adolescent Development*, vol. 91, pp. 79–92.

Euser, S., Alink, L.R.A., Tharner, A., van IJzendoorn, M.H. & Bakermans-Kranenburg, M.J., 2013, 'The prevalence of child sexual abuse in out-of-home care: A comparison between abuse in residential and in foster care', *Child Maltreatment*, vol. 18, no. 4, pp. 221–231.

Euser, S., Alink, L.R.A., Tharner, A., van IJzendoorn, M.H. & Bakermans-Kranenburg, M.J., 2014, 'Out-of-home placement to promote safety? The prevalence of physical abuse in residential and foster care', *Children and Youth Services Review*, vol. 37, pp. 64–70.

Fernandez, E., Lee, J.-S., Foote, W., Blunden, H., McNamara, P., Kovacs, S. & Cornefert, P , 2017, '"There's more to be done; 'Sorry' is just a word": Legacies of out-of-home care in the 20th century', *Children Australia*, vol. 42, no. 3, pp. 176–197.
Geurts, E.M.W., Boddy, J., Noom, M.J. & Knorth, E.J., 2012, 'Family-centred residential care: The new reality?', *Child & Family Social Work*, vol. 17, no. 2, pp. 170–179.
Grietens, H., 2015, 'A European perspective on the context and content for social pedagogy in therapeutic residential care', in J.K. Whittaker, J.F. del Valle, & L. Holmes (eds), *Therapeutic residential care for children and youth: Developing evidence-based international practice*, London: Jessica Kingsley, pp. 288–300.
Harder, A.T. & Knorth, E.J., 2015, 'Uncovering what is inside the "Black Box" of effective therapeutic residential youth care', in J.K. Whittaker, J.F. del Valle & L. Holmes (eds), *Therapeutic residential care for children and youth: Developing evidence-based international practice*, London: Jessica Kingsley, pp. 217–230.
Herman, J., 1992, *Trauma and recovery: The aftermath of violence from domestic abuse to political terror*, London: Pandora.
Holden, M.J., Anglin, J.P. & Nunno, M.A., 2015, 'Engaging the total therapeutic residential care program in a process of quality improvement: Learning from the CARE model', in J.K. Whittaker, J.F. del Valle & L. Holmes (eds), *Therapeutic residential care for children and youth: Developing evidence-based international practice*, London: Jessica Kingsley, pp. 301–315.
Holden, M.J., Izzo, C., Nunno, M., Smith, E.G., Endres, T., Holden, J.C. & Kuhn, F., 2010, 'Children and residential experience: A comprehensive strategy for implementing a research-informed program model for residential care', *Child Welfare*, vol. 89, no. 2, pp. 131–149.
Huefner, J.C., James, S., Ringle, J., Thompson, R.W. & Daly, D.L., 2010, 'Patterns of movement for youth within an integrated continuum of residential services', *Children and Youth Services Review*, vol. 32, no. 6, pp. 857–864.
James, S., 2011, 'What works in group care? – A structured review of treatment models for group homes and residential care', *Children and Youth Services Review*, vol. 33, no. 2, pp. 308–321.
James, S., 2015, 'Evidence-base practices in therapeutic residential care', in J.K. Whittaker, J.F. del Valle, & L. Holmes (eds), *Therapeutic residential care for children and youth: Developing evidence-based international practice*, London: Jessica Kingsley, pp. 142–155.
James, S., 2017, 'Implementing evidence-based practice in residential care: How far have we come?', *Residential Treatment for Children & Youth*, vol. 34, no. 2, pp. 155–175.
James, S., Alemi, Q. & Zepeda, V., 2013, 'Effectiveness and implementation of evidence-based practices in residential care settings', *Children and Youth Services Review*, vol. 35, no. 4, pp. 642–656.
James, S., Thompson, R., Sternberg, N., Schnur, E., Ross, J., Butler, L., Triplett, D., Puett, L. & Muirhead, J., 2015, 'Attitudes, perceptions, and utilization of evidence-based practices in residential care', *Residential Treatment for Children & Youth*, vol. 32, no. 2, pp. 144–166.
James, S., Thompson, R.W. & Ringle, J.L., 2017, 'The implementation of evidence-based practices in residential care: Outcomes, processes and barriers', *Journal of Emotional and Behavioral Disorders*, vol. 25, no. 1, pp. 4–18.
Jensen, T.K., Holt, T., Ormhaug, S.M., Egeland, K., Granly, L., Hoaas, L.C., Hukkelberg, S.S., Indregard, T., Stormyren, S.D. & Wentzel-Larsen, T., 2014, 'A randomized effectiveness study comparing trauma-focused cognitive behavioral therapy with therapy as usual for youth', *Journal of Clinical Child & Adolescent Psychology*, vol. 43, no. 3, pp. 356–369.
Kinniburgh, K.J., Blaustein, M. & Spinazzola, J., 2005, 'Attachment, Self-regulation, and Competency: A comprehensive intervention framework for children with complex trauma', *Psychiatric Annals*, vol. 35, no. 5, pp. 424–430.
Knorth, E.J., Harder, A.T., Zandberg, T. & Kendrick, A.J., 2008, 'Under one roof: A review and selective meta-analysis on the outcomes of residential child and youth care', *Children and Youth Services Review*, vol. 30, pp. 123–140.

Lee, B. & McMillen, J., 2017, 'Pathways forward for embracing evidence-based practice in group care settings', *Journal of Emotional and Behavioral Disorders*, vol. 25, no. 1, pp. 19–27.

Macdonald, G. & Millen, S., 2012a, *Implementing therapeutic approaches to residential child care in Northern Ireland: Report of interviews with trust staff*, Belfast: Social Care Institute for Excellence.

Macdonald, G. & Millen, S., 2012b, *Therapeutic approaches to social work in residential child care settings: Literature review*, Belfast: Social Care Institute for Excellence.

Macdonald, G., Millen, S., McCann, M., Roscoe, H. & Ewart-Boyle, S., 2012, *Therapeutic approaches to social work in residential child care settings*, Belfast: Social Care Institute for Excellence.

McLean, S., 2016, *Report on therapeutic residential care: Report to the South Australian Child Protection Systems Royal Commission*, Adelaide: Australian Centre for Child Protection, University of South Australia.

McLean, S., 2018, *Therapeutic residential care: An update on current issues in Australia*, Melbourne: Australian Institute of Family Studies.

McLean, S., Price-Robertson, R. & Robinson, L., 2011, *Therapeutic residential care in Australia: Taking stock and looking forward*, Melbourne: National Child Protection Clearinghouse, Australian Institute of Family Studies.

McNamara, P., 2015, 'A new era in the development of therapeutic residential care in the State of Victoria', in J.K. Whittaker, J.F. del Valle, & L. Holmes (eds), *Therapeutic residential care for children and youth: Developing evidence-based international practice*, London: Jessica Kingsley, pp. 126–141.

Malvaso, C. & Delfabbro, P., 2015, 'Young people with complex needs leaving out-of-home care: Service issues and the need to enhance practice and policy', *Children Australia*, vol. 41, no. 1, pp. 69–79.

Mendes, P., 2009, 'Young people transitioning from out-of-home care: A critical analysis of Australian and international policy and practice', *Australian Social Work*, vol. 62, no. 3, pp. 388–402.

Mendes, P., Baidawi, S. & Snow, P.C., 2014, 'Young people transitioning from out-of-home care: A critical analysis of leaving care policy, legislation and housing support in the Australian state of Victoria', *Child Abuse Review*, vol. 23, no. 6, pp. 402–414.

Nugent, W.R., Bruley, C. & Allen, P., 1999, 'The effects of Aggression Replacement Training on male and female antisocial behavior in a runaway shelter', *Research on Social Work Practice*, vol. 8, no. 6, pp. 637–656.

Pecora, P.J. & English, D.J., 2016, Elements of effective practice for children and young people served by therapeutic residential care: Research Brief. Casey Family Programs, www.casey.org/media/Group-Care-complete.pdf, accessed 12 August 2019.

Purtell, J. & Mendes, P., 2016, 'Stand By Me – flexible and holistic support for young care leavers: Smoothing transitions from care', *Children Australia*, vol. 41, no. 3, pp. 208–213.

Redd, Z., Malm, K., Moore, K., Murphy, K. & Beltz, M., 2017, 'KVC's bridging the way home: An innovative approach to the application of Trauma Systems Therapy in child welfare', *Children and Youth Services Review*, vol. 76, pp. 170–180.

Rivard, J.C., Bloom, S.L., McCorkle, D. & Abramovitz, R., 2005, 'Preliminary results of a study examining the implementation and effects of a trauma recovery framework for youths in residential treatment', *Therapeutic Community: The International Journal for Therapeutic and Supportive Organizations*, vol. 26, no. 1, pp. 83–96.

Rivard, J.C., McCorkle, D., Duncan, M., Pasquale, L., Bloom, S.L. & Abramovitz, R., 2004, 'Implementing a trauma recovery framework for youths in residential treatment', *Child and Adolescent Social Work Journal*, vol. 21, no. 5, pp. 529–549.

Schofield, G., Larsson, B. & Ward, E., 2017, 'Risk, resilience and identity construction in the life narratives of young people leaving residential care', *Child & Family Social Work*, vol. 22, no. 2, pp. 782–791.
Sinclair, I. & Gibbs, I., 1998, *Children's home: A study in diversity*, Chichester, UK: John Wiley & Sons.
Stein, M., 2015, 'Supportive pathways for young people leaving care', in J.K. Whittaker, J.F. del Valle & L. Holmes (eds), *Therapeutic residential care for children and youth: Developing evidence-based international practice*, London: Jessica Kingsley, pp. 189–202.
Sunseri, P.A., 2004, 'Preliminary outcomes on the use of Dialectical Behavior Therapy to reduce hospitalization among adolescents in residential care', *Residential Treatment for Children & Youth*, vol. 21, no. 4, pp. 59–76.
The Royal Commission into Institutional Responses to Child Sexual Abuse (The Royal Commission), 2017, Final Report: Contemporary out-of-home care, Canberra: Commonwealth of Australia.
Thoburn, J. & Ainsworth, F., 2015, 'Making sense of differential cross-national placement rates for therapeutic residential care', in J.K. Whittaker, J.F. del Valle & L. Holmes (eds), *Therapeutic residential care for children and youth: Developing evidence-based international practice*, London: Jessica Kingsley, pp. 37–48.
Trieschman, A.E., Whittaker, J.K. & Brendtro, L.K., 2002, *The other 23 hours: Child-care work with emotionally disturbed children in a therapeutic milieu*, London: Routledge.
Trout, A.L., Tyler, P.M., Stewart, M.C. & Epstein, M.H., 2012, 'On the way home: Program description and preliminary findings', *Children and Youth Services Review*, vol. 34, no. 6, pp. 1115–1120.
Uliando, A. & Mellor, D., 2012, 'Maltreatment of children in out-of-home care: A review of associated factors and outcomes', *Children and Youth Services Review*, vol. 34, pp. 2280–2286.
Verso Consulting and the Department of Human Services (Verso-DHS), 2011, Evaluation of the therapeutic residential care pilot programs: Final summary and technical report, Victoria: Verso Consulting.
Vicary, D., 2015, 'Children Australia–A 40 year retrospective of Australian out-of-home care: Reflections of the past and future directions', *Children Australia*, vol. 40, no. 4, pp. 274–279.
Wasser, T., Tyler, R., McIlhaney, K., Taplin, R. & Henderson, L., 2008, 'Effectiveness of Dialectical Behavior Therapy (DBT) versus Standard Therapeutic Milieu (STM) in a cohort of adolescents receiving residential treatment', *Best Practice in Mental Health*, vol. 4, no. 2, pp. 114–125.
Whittaker, J.K., 2000, 'The future of residential group care', *Child Welfare*, vol. 79, no. 1, pp. 59–74.
Whittaker, J.K., 2017, 'Pathways to evidence-based practice in therapeutic residential care: A commentary', *Journal of Emotional and Behavioral Disorders*, vol. 25, no. 1, pp. 57–61.
Whittaker, J.K., del Valle, J.F. & Holmes, L. (eds), 2015, *Therapeutic residential care for children and youth: Developing evidence-based international practice*, London: Jessica Kingsley.
Williams, D. & Lalor, K., 2001, 'Obstacles to the professionalisation of residential child care work', *Irish Journal of Applied Social Studies*, vol. 2, no. 3, pp. 73–90.

Chapter 13

Educational interventions that improve the attainment and progress of children in out-of-home care

Judy Sebba

What the chapter will cover

This chapter provides a review of the research evidence on the effectiveness of educational interventions aimed at improving the outcomes of children in out-of-home care (OOHC). The focus is limited to educational interventions during the school years, focused specifically on children in OOHC that have educational outcomes. As the literature reviews in this area have suggested (Evans et al. 2017; Forsman & Vinnerljung 2012; Liabo, Gray & Mulcahy 2013; Mannay et al. 2015; Riitano & Pearson 2014), much of the available evidence is insufficiently theorised and not robust enough to be trusted as a basis for decision making and resource allocation. However, some reviews and studies can help to identify more promising approaches. Previous analysis (Sebba et al. 2015) has shown that children in OOHC do better in those schools that are higher performing for children in general, though some research (e.g. Wiegmann et al. 2014 in California) suggest they are over-represented in under-achieving schools. Reflecting this potential role of schools in outcomes, the chapter looks first at systemic interventions involving whole-school approaches before considering the individual interventions targeting children in OOHC specifically and then those interventions targeting their foster carers. Finally, the implications from the evidence reviewed for policy and practice are drawn out. 'Case study' illustrations are provided and some discussion questions are provided at the end of the chapter.

Background

The educational outcomes of children in OOHC

Children in OOHC are reported to have poorer educational outcomes than their peers in all countries that collect these data. In Australia, those in out-of-home care scored 13–39 percentage points lower across assessment domains and year levels than all school students (Australian Institute of Health and Welfare (AIHW) 2015) and only 45% of those in foster care complete Year 12 schooling compared with 77% of the general population (Harvey et al. 2015). In the US, children living in foster care have a high risk of academic failure, special education placement, and an increased dropout rate (Pears, Kim & Brown 2018).

In England, in 2017 (DfE 2018a) the average attainment at age 16 for children in OOHC[1] across eight school subjects was 19 (out of a possible 64 points that make up the benchmark at that age). For children previously in care (usually adopted[2]), on average it was 30, and for all children, 44. At age 11, the expected level in English, mathematics and science was achieved by 32% of children in care, 39% of children previously in care and 61% of all children. Even considering the very high levels of special educational needs of children in OOHC, significant differences are evident.

Young people in care experience other outcomes that are much poorer than those of their peers including greater year retention in the US (Scherr 2007), fixed-term exclusions from school which are five times higher in England for children in OOHC than for their peers (DfE 2018a).

Access to higher education is at least seven times higher in the general population (more than 50% rather than 7%, DfE 2018b), although data on care leavers in their late twenties in England nearly doubles this figure (Harrison 2017). Rates of offending are much higher and 40% of 19–21-year-old care leavers were not in education, training or employment in 2017, compared with 13% of their peers (DfE 2018b). In the US, former foster youth earn half as much and have an employment rate that is much lower than young adults matched on educational attainment (Okpych & Courtney 2014). However, Okpych and Courtney (2014) reported that former foster youth benefitted significantly more than other young adults from increased levels of education. This highlights the importance of improving the educational attainment of young people in OOHC.

Finally, the type and duration of care received seems to make a difference to educational outcomes. Controlling for differences in disadvantage and severity of behavioural problems, those who are in foster care achieve better outcomes than those in residential care (Scottish Government 2018; Sebba et al. 2015) as do those who spend longer in care (Font et al. 2018; Sebba et al. 2015). Font et al. (2018) in the US reported that youth who aged out of (foster) care had significantly higher odds of graduating high school and enrolling in college than did reunified youth and youth who exited to guardianship. While earnings were similar across these groups, both high school graduation rates and earnings were higher for youth who spent more time in foster care prior to 18 years of age. Courtney and Hook (2017) similarly noted that extending foster care beyond 18 years of age increased educational attainment. This seems to conflict with the US policy which places strong emphasis on establishing permanence for children taken into care through reunification with birth families in contrast with 'ageing out' of foster care.

Possible explanations of why the educational outcomes of children in OOHC are poor

More recently, the previously held assumptions that children in OOHC were either receiving poorer 'parenting' than their peers or that care itself was detrimental to their development, has been challenged (O'Higgins, Sebba & Luke 2015). In a systematic review and meta-analysis of 33 studies, Luke and O'Higgins (2018) concluded that there was very little evidence that being in care is, of itself, detrimental to the educational outcomes of children. Research consistently suggests that pre-care factors make a more important contribution to the poor educational outcomes of young people in care. For example, Brännström et al. (2017) concluded from a prospective longitudinal study that maltreatment, socio-economic deprivation, and ethnic minority status, were associated with both entry into care and later educational disadvantage.

Policy and practice context in the UK, US and Australia

In the US, the care system prioritises permanency through reunification with birth families, guardianship (placing the child permanently with a relative) or adoption. The least acceptable outcome is for a child in the legal custody of the state to reach the age of majority without obtaining a permanent family. In Australia, there were 43,399 children in home-based care on June 2015 which represented 93% of those in care, with 52% of these being Aboriginal and Torres Strait Islander children (AIHW 2016). Of those children in OOHC, 47% were in kinship care and a further 40% in foster care, a much higher proportion in kinship care than in England, where of the 75% of all children in OOHC who are in foster/kinship care, only 18% are in kinship care (with relatives or friends). In Australia, eight different child protection systems operate, since each state or territory has its own system and legislative framework, policies, procedures and practices.

In England, a child is referred to as 'looked-after' if they receive accommodation from a local authority for more than 24 hours, are subject to a placement order (which puts the child up for adoption), or are subject to a care order (which puts the child in the care of a local authority). On 31 March 2018, there were 75,420 looked-after children in England, up 4% on 31 March 2017, with 39% aged 10–15 years, around 6% coming into care due to 'absent parenting' (almost all unaccompanied asylum-seeking children aged 16–17 years). The average duration of the latest period of care was just over two years in 2018.

Local authority care includes residential care (around 9%) or foster/kinship care (73%), where the young person lives in a family environment with foster carers/relatives. Fostering placements are provided directly by local authorities (61%), or contracted out to independent fostering agencies (39%). A small number are in secure facilities for offenders or remain at home with birth parents but under the scrutiny of the local authority. The long-term goal of foster care in England is reunification of the child with their birth parents. However, while 31% were reunified with their birth families in the year ending March 2018 (DfE 2018b), previous research (Farmer & Wijedasa 2012) reported 47% coming back into care during a two-year follow up. In Tasmania, Australia, Delfabbro et al. (2013) found that just under half the children in foster care had reunified with their parents over a two-year period.

Provision for supporting the education of children in OOHC

In response to the poor educational outcomes of children in OOHC, England introduced the 'Virtual School' as a pilot in 2007. Not a physical school as such, the Virtual School in each local authority is a team, mainly of teachers who work with schools and other services to improve educational provision for children in OOHC. In 2014, the appointment of a Virtual School Headteacher in each area was made a legal requirement. Informed by the English model, the Virtual School model was introduced in Victoria, Australia[3] in 2017. There is little research evidence on the impact of the Virtual Schools in England to date (Berridge et al. 2009; Sebba & Berridge 2019) and none on their impact in Victoria.

Statutory Guidance published in England in 2018[4] set out the role of Virtual Schools in promoting the education of children in care or previously in care (e.g. adopted, subject of a Special Guardianship Order[5]). It included creating a culture of high educational aspirations, ensuring access to high quality education placement options and ensuring that each child has an effective Personal Education Plan (PEP – a plan which states the child's needs and how they will be met). The small number or in some cases no children in OOHC that are attending each school makes this a particular challenge for the Virtual School in establishing the commitment and investment of time by the school staff.

Furthermore, every school, whether currently having OOHC on roll or not, must identify a designated teacher (DT) to promote the education of these children. A recent survey of teachers in England (Become 2018), suggests that this provision has yet to impact significantly on teaching staff. It reported that 87% of teachers said they had received no training about children in care before they qualified as a teacher; 31% identified 'not enough support from children's services' as their biggest challenge in working with children in care; and 87% of respondents said they had heard at least one colleague express a negative generalisation about children in care.

A centrally allocated Pupil Premium Plus grant (currently £2,300 per pupil) for every child in care for at least one day during that academic year is provided to meet the needs identified in their PEP. Ofsted, the inspection agency, is required to check that it is spent on implementing the PEP, but other than that, little is known about how it is spent and to what effect. Ofsted's (2012) review of Virtual Schools concluded that there was some evidence of effective support for individual children, enhanced stability and well-being but outcomes were variable. Ofsted also noted that (the c. 40%) children placed outside the local authority were less likely to receive effective educational support than those living within it.

Systemic educational interventions

Providing widescale positive experiences and addressing the negative influences on the educational progress of children in OOHC involves systemic interventions. Accordingly, reducing children's school mobility and grade retention (not used in England), both associated with poorer outcomes for children in OOHC (Pears, Kim & Brown 2018; Scherr 2007 respectively), would be predicted to improve educational outcomes. Similarly, use of alternative education and non-mainstream schools that are statistically associated with poorer outcomes, even when special educational needs and other characteristics are controlled (Sebba et al. 2015), should be minimised for children in OOHC. US legislation[6] and guidance in England[7] emphasise the need to ensure educational stability but the limited availability of placements when disruption occurs can sometimes lead to school moves. When such moves cannot be avoided, Höjer et al. (2018) note the importance of ensuring that accurate records of the child's progress and behaviour are available promptly in the new setting.

School climate has been demonstrated by Dube and McGiboney (2018) to be particularly important for children who have faced adversity. These authors suggest that a growing body of research identifies its importance in social, emotional and intellectual development; sense of safety and well-being; mental health; and healthy relationships. School staff beliefs about behaviour need to be changed from attributing behaviour of students to their characteristics (e.g. as 'naughty'), to the understanding that previous stress and trauma may underlie these behaviours. They note that a 'school climate characterised as unsupportive, unduly critical, overly competitive, and unsafe will compromise, threaten, or weaken the potentially positive impacts of any educational practice, programme, policy, or intervention geared to improve student outcomes' (Dube & McGiboney 2018: 4). They review studies suggesting that a positive school climate gives interventions and prevention programmes a chance to be effective.

The Virtual Schools in England have been the focus of only limited research (e.g. Berridge et al. 2009; Drew & Banerjee 2018; Sebba & Berridge 2019) thus far on contributions that might be linked to educational outcomes. Drew and Bannerjee noted that Virtual School Heads undertook specific transition support when children changed schools such as accompanying a child to school, nurture sessions and providing transition mentors. The heads in their survey offered support for well-being and relationships through attachment training in schools, linkages with other services and well-being interventions such as *Thrive*. [8] A major role in the work of the Virtual School Head was raising awareness through specific training for teachers, examples of which are given below.

In Sebba and Berridge's (2019) interviews with Virtual School Heads, they stated that they would like to be more involved in direct work in schools, but staffing constraints and prioritising statutory work such as PEPs limited this. Their main activities with schools were training staff and trying to circumvent or address the implications of exclusions of children in OOHC from schools (several reported having been successful in reducing exclusions). The quality of the Virtual School Headteachers' relationships with schools, in particular their headteachers, was crucial in this process, helping schools to find other ways of dealing with these children's behaviour. Confirming Dube and McGiboney's findings, they felt that lack of understanding by school staff of behaviours was the greatest challenge. Training whole school staff in the Attachment Aware Schools Programme[9] was mentioned by several heads as providing better understanding of why the children in OOHC behaved as they did and strategies to address this.

Evaluation of attachment and trauma training in schools is reported in detail on the Rees Centre website.[10] Published evaluations by Sebba and colleagues of attachment and trauma training in three areas in which 12, 16 and 24 schools were involved, respectively, are available. Of these 52 schools, 33 were primary (elementary), 12 secondary (high) and seven special schools. The aims of the training were to develop all school staff's (including those who are not teachers) understanding of attachment, the impact of trauma on the developing brain and subsequent behaviours, and to teach staff to use 'Emotion Coaching'[11] to understand the triggers and causes of behaviours and use of language needed to de-escalate the anger and emotions. Evaluation measures included looking at attendance and attainment before, after and at one-year follow-up of all pupils in the school and undertaking surveys of all staff and interviews with staff and pupils in around one-fifth of the schools involved.

Findings on attendance and attainment measures showed huge variation with no consistent patterns, although improvements in attendance were observed in primary schools in one of the three areas and two-thirds of primary schools improved their attainment in all three areas. The secondary schools generally made less progress improving their attendance rates in one area and around half improved their attainment in two areas. However, due to the small numbers, changes in the way benchmark grades were defined and in the absence of a control group, these findings need to be treated with caution.

Findings from the surveys and interviews in these evaluations were more encouraging. Participants reported increased confidence and greater understanding of the reasons behind the behaviour, changes in their own and others' practices, acknowledging children's emotions, changing communication styles and language used with pupils and other staff, and for many, use of emotion coaching.

> Because they [teachers] talk with them, they talk about their feelings and what might happen and things that you might get upset about.
>
> (Young person, post-Programme interview)

The impact on pupils' well-being was reported by both participants and children who suggested that the schools were calmer, more nurturing. Two findings were particularly prevalent: the impact of providing 'safe' areas in which children calmed down and self-regulated, and having a significant adult in school that the pupils trusted.

Case Study 1: Creating safe areas and acknowledging the role of key adults in schools

The importance of having a significant adult in school (not necessarily a teacher) and a 'safe area' to go to in order to calm down emerges strongly from the research. These two examples are quotes from the Rees Centre evaluations of Attachment and Trauma training in schools.

Safe spaces

> Given time and space in which to explain their feelings in a calm safe place.
> (Secondary teacher, survey)

> Miss [name] was basically there for me through everything ... I had to work in her room just to get back into school because I stopped coming into school completely, so for me to come back into school I worked up in Miss [name's] room so I felt more comfortable getting into the routine of school again and just becoming more confident. So, there is still some lessons that I work upstairs just so I can have her support. If I need time out I go up there and I get that time out, like she is literally like my life support in a way because she does everything, she understands me completely.
> (Pupil, post-Programme interview)

Significant adults

> Miss ... is basically like all of us are like planets, right, and she's like the sun because like without her we could not be in this school.
> (Pupil, post-Programme interview)

RESEARCHER: Joe, anything in particular that stops you working?
JOE: I always think of my Mum when she's not there ... I start scribbling on my book ...
RESEARCHER: Right. Is that when you go and see ... Miss?
JOE: Smith [the teaching assistant] .... She takes me out of class for a bit ... She is a nice woman. I stay outside for a bit.

Adapted from evaluation reports on: http://reescentre.education.ox.ac.uk/research/evaluation-of-attachment-aware-schools/

Interventions aiming to increase liaison between social care and education

Zetlin, Weinberg and Shea (2006) report on a US intervention which placed education liaison personnel in child welfare offices to help social workers address the educational issues of the children on their caseloads. Issues they addressed included barriers to obtaining a child's school records, children not being on the roll of a school, lack of recognition of special education eligibility or provision of services, inappropriate school placement, or threatened suspension or expulsion of a child. These are key functions of the Virtual School Head in England and Victoria, Australia although provided through a different model. The evaluation reported by Zetlin et al. suggested positive impact on the social workers and the children in OOHC and improvements in maths and reading scores.

In a more recent study of education liaison personnel for youth in OOHC, Weinberg, Oshiro and Shea (2014) reported increases in Grade Point Averages though these were not high enough to reach statistical significance, and other data in this study suggested that education liaisons reduced risks and developed positive practices by providing support and addressing educational barriers. Liaison personnel worked with the social workers, teachers and caregivers as well as with the young people themselves to ensure that appropriate school placements were secured. They also monitored grades, attendance and behaviour and provided support that avoided or reduced unnecessary school transfers.

Child-focused interventions

The systematic reviews of educational interventions (Evans et al. 2017; Forsman & Vinnerjlung 2012; Liabo, Gray & Mulcahy 2013; Mannay et al. 2015; Riitano & Pearson 2014) while all concluding that study designs are too weak to provide robust evidence of what works, also indicate that tutoring programmes have to date some of the best evidence of efficacy. Promising educational gains were also noted from the provision of tailored individual support (of the type identified in the Personal Education Plan) and the use of an educational liaison person between home and school.

Tutoring programmes

Zinn and Courtney (2014) found no beneficial effects of an individualised in-home tutoring programme for adolescents but noted inconsistencies in the implementation such that 40% of those in the intervention group did not receive tutoring, while others in the control did so. Harper and Schmidt (2016) note that it is important that the evaluations of tutoring interventions, when effectively delivered, are not confounded with the limiting effects of implementation challenges that occur in the field. The balance of evidence overall on tutoring is positive as indicated by the findings from a number of other studies.

Flynn et al. (2012) reported on a randomised trial of an individualised direct instruction tutoring intervention with 6–13-year-old children in OOHC in which the foster carers were the tutors. The intervention group made statistically and practically greater gains than those in the control group on sentence comprehension and math computation but not on word reading or spelling. Interestingly, and unlike Flynn et al.'s findings, the outcomes of Harper and Schmidt's (2016) randomised trial of group direct instruction with foster children found significant gains in maths, spelling and reading decoding but improvement that was not statistically significant in sentence comprehension. Their randomised trial evaluated a direct instruction literacy and math programme Teach Your Children Well, with university students undertaking the tutoring in a small-group format with children in foster care. Harper and Schmidt suggest that the difference in instructional mode – group in their study rather than individual – and the addition in Flynn et al.'s study of one-to-one reading with the foster carer, might account for the difference in findings on sentence comprehension.

Hickey and Flynn (2019) evaluated the impact of an individualised, home-based tutoring programme, known as TutorBright, (which uses one-on-one, in-home tutoring in reading language and maths provided by trained graduates), on the reading and mathematics skills of children in foster care. Those in the intervention group demonstrated statistically significant positive gains on reading fluency, reading comprehension and maths calculation, and statistically non-significant but positive gains on maths fluency and broad maths. However, despite these gains, the children continued to perform at below-average levels in reading and maths. Hence, we should be realistic in recognising that while interventions during school years might help children in OOHC to progress, the assumption should not be made that they will 'catch up' with their peers.

Mentoring

Rogers and Apps (2013) evaluated a mentoring programme in five London Boroughs for children in OOHC in which the mentors were university students/graduates who themselves had been in care. While findings cannot be attributed to the programme confidently, given the lack of a control group, differences in children's ages and in the model of mentoring implemented, the researchers concluded that engagement in the programme led to gains in children's confidence. The mechanisms by which this occurred included: the provision of someone with similar experiences to talk to and the use of positive role models. This appeared to enhance motivation for learning and to continue their education. Improvements in attainment and attendance occurred in some areas.

Reading interventions

Paired Reading in which an adult, the carer or a volunteer, reads together with the child has been used with children in OOHC. Studies by Osborne, Alfano & Winn (2010) replicated by Vinnerljung et al. (2014) found some positive improvements amongst the children in OOHC involved in paired reading groups. However, these studies lacked a control group, making attribution of the improvements to the paired reading difficult.

Book-gifting programmes targeted specifically at children in OOHC have also been widely used. *The Letterbox Club* (Griffiths 2012) used in many parts of England, Wales and Northern Ireland, involves the delivery of personalised parcels to 7–11-year-old children at home monthly for six months. The parcels include reading books, stationery and a mathematics game. Evaluations by the designers (e.g. Griffiths 2012) using a pre- and post-test design reported statistically significant improvements. Winter et al. (2011) in Northern Ireland also found statistically significant improvements in literacy and numeracy scores and Forsman (2019) in Sweden noted improvements in literacy using *Letterbox*. However, there was no control group in these studies, limiting the potential attribution of improvements directly to the programme.

A randomised controlled trial of *The Letterbox Club* involving 116 foster children, aged 7–11 years in Northern Ireland (Mooney, Winter & Connolly 2016), found no evidence of programme effects on reading skills or attitudes to reading. However, the process evaluation that accompanied the trial (Roberts, Winter & Connolly 2017), concluded that it was well received by the children and the carers, who reported wanting more support on how to use the materials. A major randomised controlled trial is under way in England combining both book-gifting and paired reading to support foster carers[12] and is due to report in 2020.

Foster carer/family-focused interventions

Caregiver involvement in schools occurs less for children in OOHC compared to their peers (Pears, Kim & Brown 2018) which for some might reflect carers' own negative school experiences, schools failing to 'reach out' to foster carers or short duration placements making relationships between school and carer more challenging. Pears, Kim and Brown review interventions designed to support better educational outcomes of children in OOHC, including their own KITS programme which teaches school readiness skills to preschool children and engages foster carers in workshops to improve their contact with the school and support for the child. A randomised trial of this approach demonstrated improved literacy, self-regulation and teacher-rated behaviour in the children in OOHC.

Tilbury et al.'s (2014) Australian study comparing 202 young people in care with a matched control group concluded that the school environment and levels of support influenced school engagement. For the in-care group, support from carers and their caseworker most strongly predicted school engagement, whereas in the control group, academic achievement, parental support and friends who like school were the predictors. Further evidence comes from Cheung, Lewin and Jenkins' (2012) Canadian study in which more caregiver support for education and a more positive literacy home environment were associated with greater academic success of children in OOHC, whereas caregiver school-based involvement was not significantly associated with academic achievement. Higher levels of caregiver expectations were also associated with greater academic success. This highlights the crucial role of foster carers in the education of children in OOHC.

In the evaluation of London Fostering Achievement (Sebba et al. 2016) designed to improve the education of children in OOHC across London, one component of the intervention was 'Education Champions'. These were experienced foster carers, usually with prior education experience, who were recruited by five local authorities for four hours per week. The Champions worked with foster carers to boost their confidence around supporting educational needs by, for example, attending PEP meetings with them, working with them and their foster child at home on reading or maths, or helping them to navigate the educational system.

The evaluation suggested that the Education Champions had reached many carers and were regarded by them, the social workers and teachers as having made a significant difference, in particular, to the knowledge about education and the confidence to address it. They provided training and workshops and identified and organised different types of educational activities that foster carers and children could undertake together. Education Champions were characterised by foster carers as listening to, and understanding other foster carers' concerns and experiences from a position of sympathy rather than judgement. They taught carers to be more proactive regarding their foster child's education, in particular about the purpose of the PEP meetings, what they should achieve, who should be there and how they should be run. Ten carers reported specific impact on children including increased engagement in reading and maths activities, allocation of resources (laptops, tutoring, music lessons) through greater assertiveness at the PEP meetings and more engagement with school. The model is being extended to other areas.[13]

Case Study 2: Education Champions supporting foster carers to engage in educational support

A key improvement target in one area for children in care was to improve attainment in maths at 16 years of age because although one-to-one tuition had been employed, the progress being made was insufficient. The Education Champions supported foster carers in a maths project to raise basic skills and self-esteem, and help the carers accept that maths was not as complicated as some people suggest. The Virtual School Head described it:

> the programme is called Fifteen a Day ... because the idea was the foster carers would spend 15 minutes a day working alongside the student, not teaching but engaging equally in the activities. ... Working together on the pages in this workbook ... Each page has sums, some games, some dice games, a race around the clock game, space to write their tables, timed tasks, in all, 20 pages ... The staff at the Virtual School produced a list of students they thought would benefit from doing this ... at the moment 10 are doing it ... we feel our foster carers should give some time every day to education and this is one of our key aims for next year.

Many children increased their rate of progress, one child achieved a much higher grade in maths than predicted, representing an additional two terms of progress above expectations. This local authority continued with the Champions beyond the project.

Adapted from Sebba et al. (2016).

Policy and Practice implications

This chapter has reviewed the evidence on interventions that aim to improve educational outcomes for children in OOHC. These fall broadly into four areas: systemic interventions, liaison roles between schools and social care, child-focused interventions and foster carer focused interventions. The following implications for policy and practice emerge from this selective review of the evidence:

- Ensure appropriate school placements, progress between grades and reduction in school exclusion will all be likely to contribute to better outcomes for those in OOHC. This means considering continuity in the same school when placement disruptions occur.

- School climate is critical to supporting the educational outcomes of children in OOHC. There is a need to invest in whole school staff development to ensure that the behaviours of children who have experienced neglect, abuse or adversity are better understood and responded to appropriately.
- Facilitate the relationships between children in OOHC and a significant adult in school to whom they can turn when they need support as well as providing 'safe spaces' in which to calm down will contribute to both the attendance and better outcomes of children in OOHC.
- Consider the provision of Virtual Schools as in England and Victoria, Australia or education liaison personnel who are sited alongside social work teams as in parts of the US, in order to maximise understanding across services and help make decisions that take into account both the well-being and educational aspects for children in OOHC.
- Provide tutoring using either trained tutors or foster carers to support the education of children in OOHC, in particular in literacy and mathematics.
- Assess the options for providing books to children in OOHC and training for foster carers in supporting their reading.
- Provide support for foster carers to navigate the education system, to provide ongoing support to the children they foster and to benefit from the experience of other foster carers.

Discussion questions

Some questions that arise from this chapter for further discussion:

1 How can schools take a flexible approach to meeting the specific needs of children who have experienced trauma or neglect while simultaneously maintaining whole school rules for all children? Do children and staff understand that some other children need to be 'treated' differently?

> I do feel that it does become a bit more difficult, because it feels like we're running parallel rules. And I'll give you an example, for instance, one student that I know in my Maths class, I have been told has attachment disorder, and she's sworn at me, she's used bad language with me, 'I don't want to get out of this class, you can't do anything' … I do feel that then other students are looking on this and thinking 'well, she can get away with it' and they do try.
>
> (Secondary teacher, interview)[14]

2 How do we prioritise both emotional well-being and high academic progress and are these sometimes in conflict?

3 What should the role of social workers be in promoting better educational outcomes for children in OOHC?

Notes

1 In England, the term 'children looked after' is used to describe children in the care of a local authority if a court has granted a care order to place a child in care, or has cared for the child for more than 24 hours.

2 The adoption statistics are experimental as they only include the 30% or so parents that declare that the child is adopted.
3 www.education.vic.gov.au/about/programs/Pages/lookout.aspx
4 https://assets.publishing.service.gov.uk/government/uploads/system/uploads/attachment_data/file/683556/Promoting_the_education_of_looked-after_children_and_previously_looked-after_children.pdf
5 A Special Guardianship Order is made by the Family Court which places a child or young person to live with someone other than their parent(s) on a long-term basis.
6 Fostering Connections to Success and Increasing Adoptions Act 2008.
7 https://assets.publishing.service.gov.uk/government/uploads/system/uploads/attachment_data/file/683556/Promoting_the_education_of_looked-after_children_and_previously_looked-after_children.pdf
8 www.thriveapproach.com
9 www.bathspa.ac.uk/projects/attachment-awareness/
10 http://reescentre.education.ox.ac.uk/research/evaluation-of-attachment-aware-schools/
11 www.emotioncoachinguk.com
12 www.qub.ac.uk/sites/readingtogether/
13 www.thefosteringnetwork.org.uk/policy-practice/projects-and-programmes/improving-educational-outcomes/fostering-potential
14 http://reescentre.education.ox.ac.uk/research/evaluation-of-attachment-aware-schools/

References

Australian Institute of Health and Welfare (AIHW), 2015, Educational outcomes for children in care, Canberra: AIHW.

Australian Institute of Health and Welfare (AIHW), 2016, Child protection Australia 2014–15: Child welfare series no 63, Canberra: AIHW.

Become, 2018, *Teachers who care: How to help teachers and schools support looked after children*, London: Become.

Berridge, D., Henry, L., Jackson, S. & Turney, D., 2009, *Looked after and learning: Evaluation of the Virtual School Head pilot*, London: Department for Education, Schools and Families.

Brännström, L., Vinnerljung, B., Forsman, H. & Almquist, Y.B., 2017, 'Children placed in out-of-home care as midlife adults: Are they still disadvantaged or have they caught up with their peers?', *Child Maltreatment*, vol. 22, no. 3, pp. 205–214.

Cheung, C., Lwin, K. & Jenkins, J.M., 2012, 'Helping youth in care succeed: Influence of caregiver involvement on academic achievement', *Children and Youth Services Review*, vol. 34, no. 6, pp. 1092–1100.

Courtney, M.E. & Hook, J.L., 2017, 'The potential educational benefits of extending foster care to young adults: Findings from a natural experiment', *Children and Youth Services Review*, vol. 72, pp. 124–132.

Delfabbro, P., Fernandez, E., McCormick, J. & Kettler, L., 2013, 'Reunification in a complete entry cohort: A longitudinal study of children entering out-of-home care in Tasmania, Australia', *Children and Youth Services Review*, vol. 35, no. 9, pp. 1592–1600.

DfE, 2018a, Outcomes for Children Looked After by local authorities in England, 31 March 2017 SFR 20/2018.

DfE, 2018b, Children Looked After in England (including adoption), year ending 31 March 2017 SFR 50/2017 and associated tables.

Drew, H. & Banerjee, R., 2018, 'Supporting the education and well-being of children who are looked-after: What is the role of the Virtual School?', *European Journal of Psychology of Education*, vol. 34, no. 1, pp. 101–121.

Dube, S. R. & McGiboney, G. W., 2018, 'Education and learning in the context of childhood abuse, neglect and related stressor: The nexus of health and education', *Child Abuse & Neglect*, vol. 75, pp. 1–5.

Evans, R., Brown, R., Rees, G. & Smith, P., 2017, 'Systematic review of educational interventions for looked-after children and young people: Recommendations for intervention development and evaluation', *British Educational Research Journal*, vol. 43, no. 1, pp. 68–94.

Farmer, E. & Wijedasa, D., 2012, 'The reunification of looked after children with their parents: What contributes to return stability?', *British Journal of Social Work*, vol. 43, no. 8, pp. 1611–1629.

Flynn, R.J., Marquis, R.A., Paquet, M.P., Peeke, L.M. & Aubry, T.D., 2012, 'Effects of individual direct-instruction tutoring on foster children's academic skills: A randomized trial', *Children and Youth Services Review*, vol. 34, no. 6, pp. 1183–1189.

Font, S.A., Berger, L.M., Cancian, M. & Noyes, J.L., 2018, 'Permanency and the educational and economic attainment of former foster children in early adulthood', *American Sociological Review*, vol. 83, no. 4, pp. 716–743.

Forsman, H., & Vinnerljung, B., 2012, 'Interventions aiming to improve school achievements of children in out-of-home care: A scoping review', *Children and Youth Services Review*, vol. 34, no. 6, pp. 1084–1091.

Forsman, H., 2019, 'Exploring the Letterbox Club programme's impact on foster children's literacy: Small effects, larger implications?', *Oxford Review of Education*, vol. 45, no. 4, pp. 502–518.

Griffiths, R., 2012, 'The Letterbox Club: An account of a postal club to raise the achievement of children aged 7 to 13 in foster care', *Children and Youth Services Review*, vol. 34, no. 6, pp. 1101–1106.

Harrison, N., 2017, *Moving on Up*, London: NNECL.

Harvey, A., McNamara, P., Andrewartha, L. & Luckman, M., 2015, Out of care, into university, Report for the National Centre for Student Equity in Higher Education (NCSEHE), Perth: Curtin University.

Harper, J. & Schmidt, F., 2016, 'Effectiveness of a group-based academic tutoring program for children in foster care: A randomized controlled trial', *Children and Youth Services Review*, vol. 67, pp. 238–246.

Hickey, A.J. & Flynn, B., 2019, 'A randomised trial on the effectiveness of a one-to-one tutoring program (TutorBright) to improve mathematics and reading skills for children in care in Canada', *Oxford Review of Education* vol. 45, no. 4, pp. 519–537.

Höjer, I., Lindberg, H., Nielsen, B., Gustafsson, J.E. & Johansson, H., 2018, 'Recognition of education and schooling in case files for children and young people placed in out-of-home care', *Children and Youth Services Review*, vol. 93, pp. 135–142.

Liabo, K., Gray, K. & Mulcahy, D., 2013, 'A systematic review of interventions to support looked-after children in school', *Child & Family Social Work*, vol. 8, no. 3, pp. 341–353.

Luke, N. & O'Higgins, A., 2018, 'Is the care system to blame for the poor educational outcomes of children looked after? Evidence from a systematic review and national database analysis', *Children Australia*, vol. 43, no. 2, pp. 135–151.

Mannay, D., Staples, E., Hallett, S., Roberts, L., Rees, A., Evans, R.E. & Andrews, D., 2015, Understanding the educational experiences and opinions, attainment, achievement and aspirations of looked after children in Wales, Project Report, Cardiff: Welsh Government.

Mooney, J., Winter, K. & Connolly, P., 2016, 'Effects of a book gifting programme on literacy outcomes for foster children: A randomised controlled trial evaluation of the Letterbox Club in Northern Ireland', *Children and Youth Services Review*, vol. 65, pp. 1–8.

Ofsted, 2012, The impact of virtual schools on the educational progress of looked after children, Manchester: Ofsted.

O'Higgins, A., Sebba, J. & Luke, N., 2015, *What is the relationship between being in care and the educational outcomes of children*, Oxford: The Rees Centre.

Okpych, N.J., & Courtney, M.E., 2014, 'Does education pay for youth formerly in foster care? Comparison of employment outcomes with a national sample', *Children and Youth Services Review*, vol. 43, pp. 18–28.

Osborne, C., Alfano, J. & Winn, T., 2010, 'Paired reading as a literacy intervention for foster children', *Adoption and Fostering*, vol. 34, no. 4, pp. 17–26.

Pears, K.C., Kim, H.K. & Brown, K.L., 2018, 'Factors affecting the educational trajectories and outcomes of youth in foster care', in E. Trejos-Castillo & N. Trevino-Schafer (eds), *Handbook of foster youth*, London: Routledge, pp. 208–222.

Riitano, D. & Pearson, A., 2014, 'The effectiveness of interventions designed to improve academic outcomes in children and adolescents in out-of-home care: a systematic review protocol', *JBI Database of Systematic Reviews and Implementation Reports*, vol. 12, no. 1, pp. 13–22.

Roberts, J., Winter, K. & Connolly, P., 2017, 'The Letterbox Club book gifting intervention: Findings from a qualitative evaluation accompanying a randomised controlled trial', *Children and Youth Services Review*, vol. 73, pp. 467–473.

Rogers, R. & Apps, J., 2013, 'Final evaluation report of the Greater London Authority "Near Peer Mentoring Project"', London: Greater London Authority.

Scherr, T.G., 2007, 'Educational Experiences of Children in Foster Care: Meta-Analyses of Special Education, Retention and Discipline Rates', *School Psychology International*, vol. 28, no. 4, pp. 419–436.

Scottish Government, 2018, *Education Outcomes for Looked After Children 2016/17*, Edinburgh: Scottish Government Statistics.

Sebba, J., Berridge, D., Luke, N., Fletcher, J., Bell, K., Strand, S., Thomas, S., Sinclair, I. & O'Higgins, A., 2015, *The educational progress of looked after children in England*, Oxford/Bristol, UK: The Rees Centre/University of Bristol.

Sebba, J., Luke, N., Rees, A., Plumridge, G., Rodgers, L., Hafesji, K. & Rowsome-Smith, C., 2016, *Evaluation of the London Fostering Achievement Programme*, Oxford: The Rees Centre.

Sebba, J. & Berridge, D., 2019, 'The role of the Virtual School in supporting improved educational outcomes for children in care', *Oxford Review of Education*, vol. 45, no. 4, pp. 538–555.

Tilbury, C., Creed, P., Buys, N., Osmond, J. & Crawford, M., 2014, 'Making a connection: School engagement of young people in care', *Child & Family Social Work*, vol. 19, no. 4, pp. 455–466.

Vinnerljung, B., Tideman, E., Sallnäs, M. & Forsman, H., 2014, 'Paired reading for foster children: results from a Swedish replication of an English literacy intervention', *Adoption and Fostering*, vol. 38, no. 4, pp. 361–373.

Wiegmann, W., Putnam-Hornstein, E., Barrat, V.X., Magruder, J. & Needell, B., 2014, *The invisible achievement gap, Part* 2, Berkeley, CA: Stuart Foundation.

Weinberg, L.A., Oshiro, M., & Shea, N., 2014, 'Education liaisons work to improve educational outcomes of foster youth: A mixed methods case study', *Children and Youth Services Review*, vol. 41, pp. 45–52.

Winter, K., Connolly, P., Bell, I. & Ferguson, J., 2011, *Evaluation of the effectiveness of the Letterbox Club in improving educational outcomes among children aged 7–11 years in foster care in Northern Ireland*, Belfast: Centre for Effective Education, Queen's University Belfast.

Zetlin, A.G., Weinberg, L.A., & Shea, N.M., 2006, 'Improving educational prospects for youth in foster care: The education liaison model', *Intervention in School and Clinic*, vol. 41, no. 5, pp. 267–272.

Zinn, A. & Courtney, M.E., 2014, 'Context matters: Experimental evaluation of home-based tutoring for youth in foster care', *Children and Youth Services Review*, vol. 47, pp. 198–204.

Chapter 14

Reunification in out-of-home care

Elizabeth Fernandez and Paul Delfabbro

Overview and policy content

Reunification is the cornerstone of meaningful child welfare practice and a humane response to families involved in the child welfare system. Jill Berrick has argued

> When children can no longer live at home, child welfare agencies have an obligation to support parents' efforts at reunification ... Parents should be offered reasonable opportunities to reunite with their children, and children should be offered a 'last best chance' to go home.
>
> (Berrick 2009: 10)

In a similar vein Richard Barth comments

> Children's services programs recognise – at least by assertion that if not by program design or funding – that all parents should have reasonable services to allow them to resume the care of children removed from them and that children also deserve the chance to go home to homes to which they typically want to return.
>
> (Barth 2013: vii)

Reunification is defined as the return of children placed in out-of-home care to the home of their birth or first family. The term is used interchangeably with 'restoration'. Reunification is regarded widely as the as the primary goal of child welfare systems and the most common decision in the permanence continuum (Fernandez 2017). While the prevention and protection agendas are important, for children in out-of-home care, reunification and other routes to permanence are a significant part of the mission of child welfare. This is reinforced in international, national and State-based statutes and guidance which require children to be reunified with parents when in their best interests (COAG 2009; UN 1989). Yet, rather than being centrally important to child welfare policy and practice, reunification has remained an invisible and under-prioritised area of practice. It is commonly suggested that children are best served by returning to their original carers in a safe environment that meets their needs (Wulczyn 2004). Safe reunification is also in the interests of welfare agencies, accomplishing their child protection goals and reducing the burden on their resources. However, in practice, the decision to remove children from their primary carer(s) as a response to an unsafe or inadequate care environment as well as to return them to that care is likely to be a complicated process

(McDonald, Bryson & Poertner 2006). Over the last five decades research and commentary have highlighted the challenges entailed in reunification, acknowledging that it is an overlooked component of child welfare services.

A consistent problem faced by many child protection systems around the world is that of growing numbers of children in out-of-home care (e.g. Thomas 2018). In Australia, for example, the number of children in care has risen steadily over the last decade and currently (2017–2018) it is estimated at 45,800 children. This is not because a larger number of children are necessarily being referred to care, but because children are staying in care for long periods which means that exit rates are consistently lower than entry rates, 10,200 and 11,200 children respectively (Australian Institute of Health and Welfare (AIHW) 2019). Given the cost of supporting a large volume of placements as well as concerns about the consequences of separating children from their birth families, family reunification or restoration is a strong policy imperative in many jurisdictions. Many jurisdictional child protection laws will require reunification to be a part of children's case-plans and there may be dedicated services or roles directed towards this area. In this chapter, we review the academic evidence that is currently available concerning reunification. We commence by defining what is meant by family reunification as well as what is known about reunification patterns. This is followed by a discussion of the conceptual and methodological issues that need to be considered in relation to this topic. A third section then examines the factors that appear to facilitate or reduce the likelihood of reunification. A final section is directed towards current knowledge of the practical issues and principles that should guide service delivery in this area as well as the limited range of dedicated service models that are available to facilitate reunification attempts.

Nature of reunification: definition and statistical patterns

Family reunification or restoration is usually defined as the safe return of a child or young person to their birth families. It usually assumes that young people have been placed into out-of-home care for at least some extended period and that on reunification the child will stay at home for an extended period or indefinitely. In this sense, reunification needs to be distinguished from other situations where children might come into care and go home quite frequently or quickly. Examples might include respite care arrangements where children are placed into care for short periods to provide parents with a break from caring responsibilities, or where children in care might spend some time at home as part of shared-care arrangements or other similar arrangements. Reunification instead refers to situations where there is the intention for young people to exit the care system and return to their family of origin. Internationally, a range of studies have been undertaken to elucidate the processes and predictors of reunification, the findings of which are documented in a number of scoping reviews (Biehal 2006; Farmer 2018; Fernandez & Maplestone 2006; Thoburn, Robinson & Anderson 2012).

In general, studies show that the likelihood of reunification is generally inversely related to how long children have been in care. Reunification rates tend to be much higher in the first 4 to 6 months after entry into care, with the probability falling very rapidly after this point (Delfabbro et al. 2013, 2015; Fernandez & Lee 2011; Fernandez et al. 2019). For example, in a study that tracked 468 children coming into care in the Australian State of Tasmania, Delfabbro et al. (2013) found that 50% of children had gone home after two years, but that 79% of these returns had occurred within the first four months. Similar results were reported in analyses conducted by Delfabbro et al. (2015) for two other Australian States. Another study conducted by Fernandez and Lee (2011) in the Australian State of New South Wales tracked 168 children who had come into care for the first time. The results showed that half of the same had gone home by 71 weeks in care with the fastest rates of exit in the first 13 weeks. These Australian figures mirror the patterns observed elsewhere. Courtney and Wong (1996), for example, tracked the progress of 8000 children entering care in the US and found that 50% returned home within the first six months. Wulczyn (2004), reporting findings drawn from a multi-state study, showed a pattern of decreasing probabilities over successive years, with reunification rates starting at 28% for the first year in care and then declining to 16% in year 2 and then successively lower thereafter. These findings align with studies conducted in the US (e.g. Cheng 2010; Courtney 1994; Fanshel & Shinn 1978; Goerge 1990; Wells & Guo 1999) as well as in Australia (Delfabbro, Barber & Cooper 2003; Fernandez 1999) and the UK (Bullock, Gooch & Little 1998; Farmer et al. 2009; Sinclair et al. 2007.) Some explanations for these trends are described presently in this chapter.

Conceptual and methodological issues

Although the concept of reunification would appear to be self-explanatory, there are a number of important conceptual and methodological issues that need to be taken into consideration when researching this topic and in interpreting the findings.

(a) Destination after exit from care

The first issue is where a young person goes when they exit the care system. Common sense would dictate that a young person would return home to the place from whence they came. However, it is possible that reunification would sometimes be said to have occurred if a young person returned home to relatives or other family members. For example, a not uncommon situation to occur is for children to return to their fathers who were not originally resident in the home from which they entered care. Such a situation might arise if the parents had separated some years before and the child had been living with his or her mother at the time of the child protection intervention. Some time later, the father may reappear in the child's life and be considered a suitable carer. Although the child has been reunited with a parent it is not the same parent and so the child has not strictly speaking been restored to their home. However, such situations would usually be considered a form of reunification (Delfabbro, Barber & Cooper 2003).

(b) Reunification vs exit from care

As indicated above, it is also important to differentiate between situations where children return home on an ongoing basis from those where there is an intention for children to go home. In some jurisdictions, children may be allowed to spend short periods of time with their birth families (e.g., overnight stays on weekends) while they are still in care. Each of these returns home represents a form of short-term reunification, but we would not usually consider these to be restorations because the child would still be placed under a child protection order and be under the guardianship of the State. Such situations would usually be considered a form of contact arrangement (Farmer 2018).

(c) Duration of the reunification

An issue which follows on from point (b) is the duration of the return home. For reunification to have occurred, it is not merely enough to say that the child has gone home, but that the child has managed to stay at home for a reasonable period. Although different studies might appraise this duration in different ways, it would be reasonable to argue that a child would need to be at home continuously for approximately six months before a reunification could be confirmed.

(d) Legal status

Some researchers might argue that the time at which a child protection order expired and the child was no longer under the guardianship of the State might also be a reasonable point at which to consider reunification to have occurred in a legal sense. However, this might occur soon after a child returns home, so that even short periods at home might be considered reunifications.

These situations do, however, bear some resemblance with the broad definition of reunification put forward by Maluccio, Fein and Olmstead (1986) which describes reunification as the process of helping children in out of home care attain the optimum level of reconnection with their birth family.

(e) What is a reunification outcome?

Another important consideration is to distinguish between reunification as merely an objective system outcome as opposed to an outcome that promotes the wellbeing of children and families. Thus, for reunification to be considered a success and 'achieved' in the outcome sense it would be good to be able to show that the child has returned to a relatively stable and nurturing environment and that there have been improvements in the relationship between children and their parents on their return home.

(f) Timing of the reunification

Another important issue is the timing of the reunification. Some reunifications may occur very quickly (e.g., in the first six months) after a child entered care. Others may occur between 1–2 years (medium term), whereas others might only occur after some years in care (long term). The practice issues associated with these different types of reunification might be quite different, so it may make sense to draw a clear distinction between different types of reunification. For example, identification of a program which helps children go home quickly after they enter care might not necessarily be relevant for understanding the more complex issues that might arise if reunification is attempted after a child has been in long-term care. Short-term reunification programs might share more in common with what are termed 'family preservation' programs in that the relationships are still largely intact and the circumstances and challenges associated with living at home are well known to both the child and parent. In circumstances where a longer period has gone by, there may be different changes in that the child may be older; the composition of the house may have changed; and the child and parent may have different needs or challenges.

(g) Reunification: passive vs. active process

It is important to recognise that many children who go home were often on shorter- or medium-term orders or in voluntary placements. In such cases, there was never an intention for the child to stay in care very long. The problems faced by the parent might have been of a transitory nature (e.g., parent got out of prison, had a serious short-term illness, was moving into new accommodation, a perpetrator of domestic violence moved away). Such families usually require short-term support and so reunification can sometimes occur without a large amount of casework. In other cases, where the problems were even less serious, the return home is almost a passive process in that the child simply goes home when the order expires. Such situations need to be distinguished from those in which a large amount of practice work is required to make the reunification possible. Such work might involve therapeutic components involving both the child and parent, preparation, transition and some ongoing support. Here, reunification becomes an 'active' process and, in effect, an area of service delivery that involves the application of time, skill and resources by child protection services. It must also be acknowledged that in some cases reunification might occur by default rather than by design.

(h) Statistical and research issues

There are differences in the focus of methodologies used in studies conducted in different countries. Some countries, illustratively North America and, to a degree, Australia have used large-scale longitudinal studies and quasi experimental methods with advanced statistical techniques to follow up children entering care and reunifying with parents. Some studies have used mixed methods approaches to capture the views of parents, foster carers and children. Fewer studies focus on child wellbeing outcomes. Studying reunification patterns often requires specific methodological approaches because reunification is a process which occurs over time. For example, if one were to compare the characteristics of children who went home with those who stayed in care, one might find that there are differences, but this would not tell you very much about what factors predict which children in a given cohort go home or how long this takes. To study reunification most effectively requires the use of longitudinal methods. One takes a group of children who are coming into care at the same time (e.g., over a 12-month period in a previous year) and then one tracks them over time to see how many and which children go home. To do this, usually requires setting what is called a 'censoring date', i.e., the point at which the researcher stops tracking and sees how many have gone home (e.g., this might be +2 years after the start of the baseline year). Any child who came into care early in the 12-month data collection year will, of course, have a better chance of going home than one who came in later in that 12 months because more time has elapsed. Analysis is often conducted using specialised statistical techniques such as survival analysis (which shows the probability of being in care after a certain amount of time has elapsed) and proportional hazard models which enable researchers to develop models that identify which variables predict the occurrence of reunification in the tracking period and how fast the event of reunification occurs (Courtney 1994; Delfabbro, Barber & Cooper 2003; Delfabbro et al. 2013; Fernandez 1999; Goerge 1990). Models such as this allow censoring dates to be included to capture the fact that not all children will have experienced the critical event (going home) by the time the tracking period ends.

Reunification: predictors, risk and protective factors

A large number of studies have been undertaken to examine the factors which contribute to understanding which children are more likely to go home and how quickly this occurs. As Thomas, Chernot and Reifel (2005) point out, these factors can usually be divided into different categories and can be categorised as risk or protective factors.

Child-level factors: Reunification might be more difficult if children are older; if they have disabilities, learning problems, mental health or behavioural problems. However, reunification might be easier if they have good relationships with their parents, display factors associated with resilience (e.g., better self-esteem, good social skills, intelligence, a sense of direction and a greater ability to deal with negative experiences).

Familial factors: Reunification may be less likely if families experience considerable disadvantage (e.g., inadequate housing, homelessness, lower incomes, poverty); if there is substance abuse and domestic violence, or if the entry into care involved severe forms of abuse. On the other hand, parents who have some stability and cohesiveness, good communication and relationships, informal supports and networks and better housing and financial resources are likely to have better prospects.

System factors: A range of system variables could potentially reduce the likelihood of reunification. For example, children who have been in care for a long time, had little contact with their parents, experienced a high level of placement instability and been exposed to negative peer influences in care are probably less likely to go home. Other potential inhibiting factors might be a lack of services to assist families and children, a lack of culturally appropriate services for particular groups (e.g. Aboriginal or First-nations peoples) and poor case-planning or resources that allow little time for working with families.

A number of these factors have been subject to systematic research and, on the whole, there is evidence for a number of hypothesised risk factors that militate against reunification. Some of this literature is summarised below.

Demographic risk factors

Age is often an important variable. Children who enter care at a young age tend to stay in care longer (Akin 2011; Connell et al. 2006; Farmer et al. 2009; Fernandez et al. 2019; Kortencamp, Green & Stagner 2004). In the Australian study by Fernandez et al. (2019), younger children took an average of 34.5 weeks longer to be restored than older children. This is because early entries can often be associated with long-term orders and complex familial factors that are not often resolved in one or two years. In particular, children in middle childhood (5–12 years) as well as teenagers are more likely to return than under-five-year-olds (Fanshel & Shinn 1978; Harris & Courtney 2003; Kortenkamp, Geen & Stagner 2004). In terms of gender, Harris and Courtney (2003) note that males are less likely to reunify than females.

It is noted that the longer children stay in care, the greater the likelihood of them losing contact with their parents, and this contact is known to be a strong predictor of subsequent reunification (Bullock, Gooch & Little 1998; Davis et al. 1996; Delfabbro, Barber & Cooper 2002; Fanshel & Shinn 1978; Sen & Broadhurst 2011; Wulczyn, Chen & Courtney 2011). These studies have found a strong association between consistent and regular contact. Bullock et al. note that contact in conjunction with other variables including the child's retention of a role in the family and inclusiveness of care plans was predictive of reunion. This may be explained by the possibility that contact reflects parental attachment and motivation to reunify as well as the presence of casework support to parents in the visitation process.

Another important factor is minority status (Akin 2011; Courtney 1994; Delfabbro et al. 2009; Farmer et al. 2009; Fernandez et al. 2019; Harris & Courtney, 2003; Seaberg & Tolley 1986; Wells & Guo 2004). Studies in the US show that African-American children usually stay in care much longer than other children. Similar findings have been obtained in relation to Aboriginal children in Australia. For example, in a longitudinal study, Fernandez (1999) tracked the five-year reunification patterns of 294 children who entered care during 1980 and 1984. The results showed that Aboriginal children generally returned home at a slower rate than other children. In another study, Delfabbro, Barber and Cooper (2003) and Barber and Delfabbro (2004) tracked the progress of over 100 children in OOHC in South Australia for a period of two years. Aboriginal children who had come into care because of neglect were more likely to have returned home after three months (42%) than non-Aboriginal children who had been neglected. However, this effect reversed when Aboriginal children had entered care for other often more serious forms of abuse; in those circumstances, Aboriginal children only had a 12% chance of going home compared with 58% for non-Aboriginal children (Fernandez & Delfabbro 2010).

The importance of Aboriginal status in reunification rates was also investigated in a national study that examined patterns of reunification in several different Australian States (Delfabbro et al. 2012a, b, c, 2015). In each of these studies a large cohort of children entering care for the first time in 2006–2007 were tracked for at least two years up to a maximum of almost 50 months (4 years) to study their trajectory through the OOHC system. In each study, models were developed that included Aboriginal status as one of the variables. When the data from South Australia, Victoria and Tasmania were combined as part of a single national analysis involving over 1300 cases, Aboriginal status was not a significant predictor of reunification when it was included in multivariate models. This lack of significance was also observed in Victoria and Tasmania, whereas a marginally significant result was observed in South Australia (in that State, Aboriginal children took on average 39 months to go home as compared with 36 for non-Aboriginal children). In all three States, however, survival functions nonetheless revealed a trend towards Aboriginal children staying in care for longer periods. A component of the same study focusing on the State of Queensland yielded similar trends of disproportionality wherein 54.5% of indigenous children achieved reunification compared with 68.6% of non-indigenous children (Fernandez et al. 2019). A similar result was observed in NSW in a sample of 2071 children tracked from 2006 until the end of 2010. By the end of 2010 (around 2.5 to 3 years after children had entered care), 24.9% of Aboriginal children had gone home compared with 32.1% of non-Aboriginal children (Fernandez & Ramia 2013).

Familial factors

Reunification is generally more difficult when families are affected by significant poverty in its various forms. For example, an absence of good quality and stable housing and financial problems mean that families are unable to provide a safe and nurturing home environment (Courtney 1994; Courtney & Wong 1996; Esposito et al. 2017; Fernandez et al. 2019; Goerge 1990; Lee et al. 2017; Wells & Guo 2004). Jones (1998) noted that poor accommodation in particular was an important predictor, with this being the most damaging aspect of poverty and deprivation. Residency in public housing, marginal and transient accommodation have been predictors of lower rates of reunification in some Australian studies (Fernandez 1999). Parental employment at the time of placement increased the likelihood of reunification, and loss of benefits following placement decreased its likelihood (Kortencamp, Geen & Stagner 2004). In terms of family structure, children from single parent families experience a slower rate of return – in some studies they are three times less likely to return (Wells & Guo 1999). Jones (1998) who found similar results applied statistical controls and concluded that economic deprivation rather than the structure of the single-parent household was associated with reunification and re-entry outcomes.

Exposure to single or multiple forms of abuse also decreases the likelihood that a child can be returned safely home, but the findings here are less consistent because studies usually (because of their reliance on administrative data) are often unable to distinguish the severity, causes and chronicity of abuse. In an Australian study cluster analysis conducted on reasons for entry to care found children in care from families affected by co-occurring domestic violence, substance misuse and emotional abuse experienced the least likelihood of restoration (Fernandez et al. 2019). Severe physical and sexual abuse is typically associated with a reduced likelihood of reunification, particularly if the abusive individual remains in the household (Farmer et al. 2011; Wade et al. 2011). Although some studies suggest that neglect is associated with an increased likelihood of reunification (Courtney 1994), other evidence has found a negative association (Goerge 1990; Fernandez 2012; Delfabbro, Barber & Cooper 2003) which suggests that the definition of this variable remains important. More passive neglect, perhaps arising from parental illness, poverty or other factors may not necessarily lead to a reduction in the likelihood of reunification, whereas active rejection and abandonment of children may make returns home much more improbable (Courtney 1994; Delfabbro et al. 2013). Other important family risk factors that appear to reduce the likelihood of reunification include serious mental health problems, substance abuse (Choi & Ryan 2007; Doab, Fowler & Dawson 2015; Maluccio & Ainsworth 2003) and ongoing physical illnesses in birth parents (Shaw 2010). Substance abuse, in particular, has received considerable attention because of its association with mental health problems and domestic violence, both of which have been found to be highly prevalent and associated within Australian out-of-home care populations (Delfabbro et al. 2009; Fernandez 2012).

Type of placement

The likelihood of reunification from relative/kinship care vs foster care has been examined in a number of studies (e.g. Akin 2011; Connell et al. 2006; Delfabbro et al. 2013, 2015; Testa 2001; Wells & Guo 1999). In Winokur, Holtan and Valentine's (2009) Cochrane review, reunification was examined using a simple dichotomous approach. Children were classified as reunified if they went home at any time and not reunified if they remained in care. Using this measure and a small set of studies, they found no convincing evidence of any difference between the two types of care. This inconsistency is reflected in studies conducted since their review. For example, Akin (2011) found that children initially placed into 'kinship care' were more likely to go home faster, whereas Connell et al. (2006) found that reunification was 1.16 times more likely if children had been placed into foster care.

In a very large study of reunification in Australia, Delfabbro et al. (2015) found that the evidence was generally in favour of children going home more slowly from relative/kinship care. These inconsistencies may relate to the fact that the Cochrane review used only a very broad indicator for its comparisons and that it was unable to detect more subtle differences in the rate of reunification within specified time intervals. The reason for slower reunifications for kinship care placements is generally thought to be related to the fact that these placements are considered the 'next best thing' to going home and so perhaps less case-planning is directed towards reunification. These differences between the two types of care might also explain why Aboriginal children go home more slowly. In both Australia and Canada, for example, policies are designed to keep Indigenous or First Nations people within their birth communities and so kin are often favoured over strangers in placement decision making.

System factors: case-planning and practice issues

Given that relatively few children appear to go home once they have been in care for some time, it is not surprising to find that active practice work relative to reunification is not that common. For example, as Pokempner, Mikell and Rodriguez (2018) point out, in the US only around 50% of teenagers will have a case-plan which identifies reunification as a goal. It is generally assumed that young people will soon age out of the system and that reunification is not a high policy and practice priority. In the US, for example, 20,000 children age out of the care system to live independently. The situation is likely to be similar in Australia, although current national data collection by the AIHW does not allow detailed insights into the long-term trajectories for children in out-of-home care. Despite this, there is some practice-based research which has been conducted as well as systematic tools which have been developed to assist the reunification process. In the US, for example, the extent to which families are considered suitable for family preservation services is often assessed using standardised instruments.

A good example of one of these tools is the North Carolina Family Assessment Scale (NCFAS) (Reed-Ashcraft, Raymond & Fraser 2001) that has been used in the US and also been applied in Australia as part of several studies of reunification. As indicated in Figure 14.1, this measure has been used in NSW studies and was also for a period used as the assessment tool in the South Australian Adolescent Reunification Program (ARP). The NCFAS scores families on a range of dimensions, including: the environment in the house; parenting capacity; family safety; family interactions; child wellbeing; ambivalence towards the child; and readiness for reunification. Each domain of the NCFAS has 3–10 items and is scored from 3 (clear strength) to –3 (serious problems).

This tool was used, for example, in Australia by Fernandez and Lee (2011) who report the results of a study conducted with Barnardo's in NSW in which 145 children who had entered care were tracked over an 18-month period. In their study, they showed that 53% of children had gone home after 18 months. There were virtually no reliable predicator(s) of NCFAS scores at intake, whereas closure scores were positively related to: (a) the mother's level of education, with more educated mothers (more than year 11) found to have higher scores across nearly all of the domains; (b) the mother's age: mothers under the age of 25 tended to provide safer environments and were more committed to the child and to reunification; and (c) whether siblings were returned as well. In other words, reunification seemed to be more likely when mothers were younger, better educated and when the siblings went home together. The authors do not, however, provide analyses that

Parental capabilities	**Environment**	**Family safety**	**Family interactions**	**Child wellbeing**	**Caregiver/Child Ambivalence**	**Readiness for Reunification**
• Supervision of child(ren) • Disciplinary practices • Provision of developmental/ enrichment opportunities • Parent(s')/ caregiver(s') mental health • Parent(s')/ caregiver(s') physical health • Parent(s')/ caregiver(s') use of drugs/ alcohol	• Housing stability • Safety in the community • Habitability of housing • Income/ employment • Food and nutrition • Personal hygiene • Transportation • Learning environment	• Absence/ presence of physical abuse of child(ren) • Absence/ presence of sexual abuse of child(ren) • Absence/ presence of emotional abuse of child(ren) • Absence/ presence of neglect of child(ren) • Domestic violence between parents/caregivers	• Bonding with the child(ren) • Expectations of child(ren) • Mutual support within the family • Relationship between parents/ caregivers	• Child(ren's) mental health • Child(ren's) behaviour • School performance • Relationship with parent(s)/ caregiver(s) • Relationship with sibling(s) • Relationship with peers • Cooperation/ motivation to maintain the family	• Parent/caregiver Ambivalence towards child • Child Ambivalence towards caregiver • Ambivalence exhibited by substitute care Provider • Disrupted Attachment • Pre-reunification home visitations	• Resolution of significant CPS risk Factors • Completion of case service Plans • Resolution of legal Issues • Parent/ caregiver understanding of child's treatment needs • Established Back-up supports or service Plans
Overall Parental Capabilities	**Overall Environment**	**Overall Family Safety**	**Overall Family Interactions**	**Overall Child Wellbeing**	**Overall Caregiver/Child Ambivalence**	**Overall Readiness for Reunification**

Figure 14.1 North Carolina Family Assessment Scale
Source: Adapted from Reed-Ashcraft et al. (2001).

control for the circumstances which led to the entry into care when examining the demographic predictors of NCFAS scores, so there may be other factors which relate to the mother's age and education which can explain the relationships observed. Nevertheless, the NCFAS scores at closure were found to be good predictors of reunification which suggests that the use of structured tools of this nature can be useful in reunification.

The Fernandez and Lee (2011) study generally involved reunification for children who had spent a relatively short period in care (between 2 weeks and 18 months) and received a high level of casework support and parental contact during the care episode. The broader literature as well as their own work points to a number of service delivery factors that are likely to make reunification more likely and more successful. These factors include:

- The early identification of reunification potential and provision of services to address problems that precipitated care;
- In-depth assessments of risks and strengths, of parenting capabilities and parenting capacity to change and sustain changes based on data from multiple sources (Fernandez 2012);
- Assessment of the extent to which the family structure or configuration and family interactions have changed since the entry into care (e.g., whether abusive, disruptive family members or partners have exited the home) (Farmer et al. 2011);
- Assessment of the size and quality of the parents' social network informal supports (Festinger 1996);
- The development of clear and purposeful case-plans and proactive case management (Fernandez 2016);
- Relationship-based work with parents to address their difficult emotions around removal and engage them in reunification planning (Fernandez 2012; Ruch, Turney & Ward 2010);
- Monitoring the child's reactions to separation from foster/residential carers and reattachment to parents;
- Ensuring children's wishes and preferences are heard and providing an advocate to represent their views in reunification planning (Fernandez 2012);
- Facilitated and well-managed contact that fosters and sustains the parent–child relationship;
- Professional support for parents and children during the process of reunification. Open, collaborative and dependable social-worker and family relationships to identify assistance they need and challenges they confront (Berrick, Cohen & Anthony 2011; Maltais et al. 2019);
- The provision of concrete support (e.g., help with transport, preparing the home);
- Education and training for parents (Fraser et al. 1996; Lewis 1994; Pine et al. 2009);
- Identifying disability and mental health and substance abuse problems as barriers to reunification and assisting access to appropriate services (Akin 2011);
- Advocacy to ensure that children's educational, practical and therapeutic needs are met post reunification – continuation of educational support, therapy and other interventions that supported their wellbeing in care (Fernandez 2012);
- Support, monitoring and review post return (Kimberlin, Anthony & Austin 2009).

Another screening tool to assist decision making about reunification and inform practice comes from the UK. In collaboration with local authorities, the University of Bristol and the NSPCC have developed a research informed Framework for Reunification (Wilkins & Farmer 2015) to support practitioners in their assessment and decisions about feasibility of reunification. The framework provides a structure for analysing risks and protective factors associated with child maltreatment recurrence and addresses services that are likely to ensure reunification stability.

An evaluation of the framework and its implementation in three local authorities in England endorses its usefulness and accessibility to practitioners in making reunification decisions in the stages leading up to reunification and post return home (Farmer & Patsios 2016). The Practice Framework is available on the websites of the University of Bristol and NSPCC.

Core principles of the framework include recognition of child-centred timescales, respectful engagement with families and acknowledgement of diversity. Key components and stages of the framework include:

- Assessment of risk and protective factors and parental capacity to change
- Deciding potential for reunification using a risk classification template and communicating decisions to child, parents and relevant professionals and stakeholders
- Negotiating parental agreements and continuing assessment of parenting capacity
- Providing relationship-based social work support and packages of services and supports for parents
- Establishing a multi-agency reunification plan
- Increased contact and gradual return accompanied by support to parents and children, and post return monitoring and review (Wilkins & Farmer 2015).

Reunification services

Inspection of the existing literature indicates that there are very few dedicated services designed to focus on reunification once children have been in care for some time (Pokempner, Mikell & Rodriguez 2018). Instead, most of the programs fall into the category of what is termed 'family preservation'. This is essentially a service that focuses on keeping families together and preventing children from entering care (Lewis 1994). Various controlled studies have been conducted to assess the impact of intensive family preservation services on reunification and have produced generally robust evidence of effectiveness. For example, in the Family Reunification Service (FRS) study 93% from the experimental group were reunified with parents at the three-month intensive service period in contrast to 28% of the control group. At 12 months after the service ended, 75% of the experimental group compared to 49% of the control group remained with their families (Fraser et al. 1996; Walton et al. 1993). Among other specialist reunification programs evaluated is the Family Centred Out of Home Care Program, an intensive service which involved families in planning for reunification at the time of entry to placement (Lewandowski & Pierce 2002) and the Casey Family Services Demonstration project (Fein & Staff 1993). The latter program which targeted families with multiple and serious problems and used the Homebuilders model achieved returns of 38% of the children – 3.8% of them re-entered care within the study time frame. Fuller reviews of preservation and specialist programs are available in Schuerman, Rzepnicki and Littell (1994).

These services are characterised by strong worker–parent relationships, parent-focused services, parenting skills training, counselling, substance use rehabilitational services, meeting practical needs such as transport, housing and financial assistance, joint goal setting and parental agreements. Some important interventions used include: Multi-systematic Therapy or MST (Henggeler et al. 1997) which was developed in the late 1970s. This program focuses parent management and skills training to empower parents with the skills and resources needed to address the difficulties that may arise in the home with the youth and also enable the youth to cope with the family, peer, school and neighbourhood problems (Burns et al. 2000). Another well-documented family preservation programme is *Families First*. As discussed by Osborn (2006), this model has been in existence for many decades and several studies have shown that programs that use the HOMEBUILDERS model safely prevent placement in foster care. The HOMEBUILDERS program uses a cognitive behavioural framework to explain the variety of behavioural dysfunctions. The model uses individualised in-home application of a variety of cognitive and skill-building strategies that target specific problems in the family that make their children at-risk of out-of-home placement.

A program which represents a genuine reunification service is Parent Partner Program in the US (Chambers et al. 2019). This program involves the identification of former parents who were involved in the child welfare system (e.g. their children were brought into care) and who have successfully addressed the obstacles to reunification. These potential 'partners' are formally trained as mentors and then begin to work with parents whose children have been taken into care. These partners act as role models, offer advice and support, liaise with child welfare agencies and other services and help parents become more involved in the community. An evaluation of over 500 parents who were involved with this program and a matched sample of 500 parents who were not (the control group) showed that the program significantly reduced the likelihood of children remaining in care and whether they re-entered care after going home. It did not, however, influence how long they stayed in care which may have been related to child welfare authorities wanting to allow more time for services and partnering relationships to be established. A related reunification initiative is the Partnering with Parents Program (Berrick, Cohen & Anthony 2011).

Challenge of re-entry to care

At the intersection of reunification research is a subgroup of studies investigating the factors that influence children's return after reunification with their families. McDonald, Bryson and Poertner (2006) found that children who were reunified within six months of entry to care had higher rates of re-entry to care following reunification. Trends on re-entry are reflected in similar research. Evidence from various studies in the US reveal a re-entry rate of 19–24% within 1–3 years of reunification (Courtney 1994; Well & Guo 1999; Wulczyn 2004; McDonald, Bryson & Poertner 2006). The UK research of Bullock, Gooch and Little (1998) found 28% of restored children returned to care. Older children, maltreated children, those with unstable care histories, and children with challenging behaviours are found to be most vulnerable to instability in returns. A recent UK study which analysed trajectories of 2208 children over a 10-year period retrospectively found that, of the 802 reunified children, 75% had stable reunifications (stability of return being defined as not re-entering care within two years of reunification) (Neil, Gitsels & Thoburn 2019).

It must be noted that estimations of re-entry of reunified children may vary based on research methodologies, time frames for follow up, study samples and the focus of particular studies. Re-entry to care after reunification is attributed to several factors – primarily lack of adequate interventions and services to support parents and children post reunification (Jones 1998; Sinclair et al. 2007), social isolation and lack of informal supports (Festinger 1996) and severity of parental problems including substance use (Bullock, Gooch & Little 1998; Maluccio & Ainsworth 2003), recurrence of abuse (Fuller 2005; Wade et al. 2011) family poverty (Courtney 1994; Pelton 1989). The question of whether the occurrence of re-entry should deter child welfare practitioners from reunifying children with their families is sometimes posed. Given that the families served by the child welfare system come from the most disadvantaged sections of society, and experience high levels of stress and social isolation and entrenched difficulties, parents and children may benefit from brief re-entries to care within a framework of family support.

Conclusions

Reunification or restoration is a major policy imperative in most child welfare systems in recognition of children's rights and the pressures on agencies in managing the large number of children in care. Despite this, there is relatively less attention paid to the issue of reuniting children with their families in contrast to the attention given to entry to protective care. Reunification must be recognised as an integral part of the continuum of child welfare services and practice to achieve it should be prioritised and adequately resourced. Focused and proactive planning for reunification is as important as it is for children while in care. There are relatively few dedicated services around the world which work with families and children to achieve reunification once children have been in care for some time. Instead, most reunifications occur relatively soon after children come into care and this may be more of a function of the nature of the order which applied or the problems which led to the children coming into care. Although the factors that increase the risk of coming into care or going home are well known, more practice-based research needs to be undertaken. Such work should look at the role of structured decision-making frameworks to allow for guided practice, consistency and better scrutiny of case-planning to ensure that reunification remains a part of a child's case-plan, irrespective of how long they remain in care (where this is viable and safe for the child). Equally important is research into practice approaches in reunification that have demonstrated positive outcomes with respect to stability of reunions and child wellbeing in order to build knowledge on 'What Works'. Research into reunification must be conducted in ways that take the different methodological and conceptual complexities of this area into account so as to allow valid comparisons between different studies and practice outcomes. Given that particular groups of children have been identified in studies as being vulnerable to slower and or unsuccessful returns, the underlying reasons for this and strategies to address their needs are worthy of investigation. Mixed methods and longitudinal research that follow up children post return and that incorporate wellbeing outcomes and children's voices would offer a further valuable contribution.

Questions

- What is reunification or restoration and what are some of the different ways in which this might be defined?
- What are some of the methodological and conceptual issues that need to be taken into account when studying reunification?

- Why has long-term reunification not been strongly researched or been a strong part of existing practice?
- What are of the some of the important features of any program that might attempt to reunify children with their families? What are some of the post reunification supports parents and children need to sustain reunification?

References

Akin, B.A., 2011, 'Predictors of foster care exits to permanency: A competing risks analysis of reunification, guardianship and adoption', *Children & Youth Services Review*, vol. 33, pp. 999–1011.

AIHW, 2019, *Child protection Australia: 2017–18, Child welfare series no. 70, Cat. no. CWS 65*, Canberra: Australian Institute of Health and Welfare.

Barber, J.G. & Delfabbro, P.H., 2004, *Children in foster care*, London: Taylor & Francis.

Barth R.P., 2013, 'Foreword', in E.A. Fernandez, *Accomplishing permanency: Reunification pathways and outcomes for foster care children*, New York: Springer.

Berrick, J.D., 2009, *Take me home: Protecting America's vulnerable children and families*, Oxford: Oxford University Press.

Berrick, J.D., Cohen, E. & Anthony, E., 2011, 'Partnering with parents: Promising approaches to improve reunification outcomes for children in foster care', *Journal of Family Strengths*, vol. 11, no. 1, pp. 1–13.

Biehal, N., 2006, *Reuniting looked after children with their families: A review of the research*, London: National Children's Bureau.

Bullock, R., Gooch, D. & Little, M., 1998, *Children going home: The reunification of families*, Aldershot, UK: Ashgate.

Burns, B.J., Schoenwald, S.K., Burchard, J.D., Faw, L. & Santos, A.B., 2000, 'Comprehensive community-based interventions for youth with severe emotional disorders: Multisystemic therapy and the wraparound process', *Journal of Child & Family Studies*, vol. 9, pp. 283–314.

Chambers, J.M., Lint, S., Thompson, M.G., Carlson, M.W. & Graef, M., 2019, 'Outcomes of the Iowa Parent Partner program evaluation: Stability of reunification and re-entry into foster care', *Children & Youth Services Review*, vol. 104, 353–364.

Cheng, T.C., 2010, 'Factors associated with reunification: a longitudinal analysis of long-term foster care', *Children & Youth Services Review*, vol. 32, no. 10, pp. 1311–1316.

Choi, S. & Ryan, J.P., 2007, 'Co-occurring problems for substance abusing mothers in child welfare: matching services to improve family reunification', *Children & Youth Services Review*, vol. 29, no. 11, pp. 1395–1410.

Connell, C.M., Katz, K.H., Saunders, L. & Tebes, J.K., 2006, 'Leaving foster care: The influence of child and case characteristics on foster care exit rates', *Children & Youth Services Review*, vol. 28, pp. 780–798.

Council of Australian Governments, 2009, *Protecting Children is Everyone's Business National Framework for Protecting: Australia's Children 2009–2020*, Canberra: Commonwealth of Australia.

Courtney, M.E., 1994, 'Factors associated with the reunification of foster children with their families', *Social Service Review*, vol. 68, 81–108.

Courtney, M.E. & Wong, Y.I., 1996, 'Comparing the timing of exits from substitute care', *Children & Youth Services Review*, vol. 18, pp. 307–334.

Davis, I., Landsverk, J., Newton, R. & Ganger, W., 1996, 'Parental visiting and foster care reunification', *Children & Youth Services Review*, vol. 18, no. 4/5, pp. 363–382.

Doab, A., Fowler, C. & Dawson, A., 2015, 'Factors that influence mother-child reunification for mothers with a history of substance use: A systematic review of the evidence to inform policy and practice in Australia', *International Journal of Drug Policy*, vol. 26, pp. 820–831.

Delfabbro, P.H., Barber, J.G. & Cooper, L.L., 2002, 'The role of family contact in substitute care', *Journal of Social Service Research*, vol. 28, pp. 19–39.

Delfabbro, P.H., Barber, J.G. & Cooper, L.L., 2003, 'Predictors of short-term reunification in South Australian substitute care', *Child Welfare*, vol. 82, pp. 27–51.

Delfabbro, P.H., Borgas, M., Rogers, N., Jeffreys, H. & Wilson, R., 2009, 'The social and family backgrounds of infants in care and their capacity to predict subsequent abuse notifications: A study of South Australian out-of-home care 2000–2005', *Children & Youth Services Review*, vol. 31, pp. 219–226.

Delfabbro, P.H., McCormick, J., Kettler, L. & Fernandez, E., 2012a, Reunification patterns in South Australia: An analysis of social and demographic correlates, Adelaide: South Australian Department for Families and Communities.

Delfabbro, P.H., McCormick, J., Kettler, L. & Fernandez, E., 2012b, Reunification patterns in Tasmania: An analysis of social and demographic correlates, Adelaide: South Australian Department for Families and Communities.

Delfabbro, P.H., McCormick, J., Kettler, L. & Fernandez, E., 2012c, Reunification patterns in Victoria: An analysis of social and demographic correlates, Adelaide: South Australian Department for Families and Communities.

Delfabbro, P.H., Fernandez, E., McCormick, J. & Kettler, L., 2013, 'Reunification in a complete entry cohort: A longitudinal study of children entering out-of-home care in Tasmania, Australia', *Children & Youth Services Review*, vol. 35, pp. 1592–1600.

Delfabbro, P.H., Fernandez, E., McCormick, J. & Kettler, L., 2015, 'A comparative analysis of factors predicting reunification from out-of-home care in Australia', *Child Indicators Research*, vol. 8, pp. 259–273.

Esposito, T., Delaye, A., Chabot, M., Trocme, N., Rothwell, D., Heile, S. & Robichand, M-J., 2017, 'The effects of socioeconomic vulnerability, psychological services, and social service spending on family reunification: A multilevel longitudinal analysis', *Environmental Research and Public Health*, vol. 14, pp. 1–15.

Fanshel, D. & Shinn, E.B., 1978, *Children in foster care: A longitudinal study*, New York: Columbia University Press.

Farmer, E. & Patsios, D., 2016, *Evaluation report on implementing the reunification practice framework*, Bristol, UK: University of Bristol.

Farmer, E.M.Z., Southerland, D., Mustillo, S.A. & Burns, B.J., 2009, 'Returning home in systems of care: Rates, predictors and stability', *Journal of Emotional & Behavioral Disorders*, vol. 17, pp. 133–146.

Farmer, E., Sturgess, W., O'Neill, T. & Wijesada, D., 2011, *Achieving successful returns from care: What makes reunification work?*, London: BAAF.

Farmer, E., 2018, *Reunification from out-of-home care: A research overview of good practice in returning children home from care*, Bristol, UK: University of Bristol.

Fein, E. & Staff, I., 1993, 'Last best chance: Findings from a reunification services program', *Child Welfare: Journal of Policy, Practice, and Program*, vol. 72, no. 1, pp. 25–40.

Fernandez, E., 1999, 'Pathways in substitute care: Representation of placement careers of children using event history analysis', *Children & Youth Services Review*, vol. 21, pp. 177–216.

Fernandez, E. & Maplestone, P.H., 2006, *Permanency planning*, Literature Review commissioned by Department of Community Services (DoCS), Sydney: University of New South Wales.

Fernandez, E. & Delfabbro, P.H., 2010, 'Reunification in Australia: Insights from South Australia and New South Wales', in R. Barth & E. Fernandez (eds), *How does foster care work?*, London: Jessica Kingsley, pp. 111–129.

Fernandez, E. & Lee, J-S., 2011, 'Returning children in care to their families: Factors associated with the speed of reunification', *Child Indicators Research*, vol. 4, pp. 749–765.

Fernandez, E., 2012, *Accomplishing permanency: Reunification pathways and outcomes for Foster children*, New York: Springer.

Fernandez, E. & Ramia, I., 2013, Reunification patterns of children entering out-of-home care in New South Wales, Report to NSW Department of Family and Community Services, Sydney: Department of Family and Community Services.

Fernandez, E., 2016, 'Case management in child protection: Challenges, complexities and possibilities', in E. Moore (ed.), *Case management inclusive community practice*, Oxford: Oxford University Press.

Fernandez, E., 2017, 'Pathways to protection and permanency: Getting it right for children, young people and families', *Developing Practice: The Child Youth and Family Work Journal*, vol. 47, pp. 2–12.

Fernandez, E., Delfabbro, P., Ramia, I.O. & Kovacs, S., 2019, 'Children returning from care: The challenging circumstances of parents in poverty', Special Issue, *Children & Youth Services Review*, vol. 97, pp. 100–111.

Festinger, T., 1996, 'Going home and returning to foster care', *Children & Youth Services Review*, vol. 18, pp. 383–402.

Fraser, M.W., Walton, E., Lewis, R.E., Pecora, P.J. & Walton, E.K., 1996, 'An experiment in family reunification: Correlates of outcomes at one-year follow up', *Children & Youth Services Review*, vol. 18, pp. 335–362.

Fuller, T., 2005, 'Child safety at reunification: A case-control study of maltreatment recurrence following return home from substitute care', *Children & Youth Services Review*, vol. 27, no. 12, pp. 1293–1306.

Goerge, R.M., 1990, 'The reunification process in substitute care', *Social Service Review*, vol. 64, pp. 422–457.

Harris, M.S. & Courtney, M.E., 2003, 'The interaction of race, ethnicity, and family structure with respect to the timing of family reunification', *Children & Youth Services Review*, vol. 25, no. 5/6, pp. 409–429.

Henggeler, S.W., Melton, G.B., Brondino, M.J., Scherer, D.G. & Hanley, J.H., 1997, 'Multisystemic therapy with violent and chronic juvenile offenders and their families: The role of treatment fidelity in successful dissemination', *Journal of Consulting & Clinical Psychology*, vol. 65, pp. 821–833.

Jones, L., 1998, 'The social and family correlates of successful reunification of children in foster care', *Children & Youth Services Review*, vol. 20, no. 4, pp. 305–323.

Kimberlin, S.E., Anthony, E.K. & Austin, M.J., 2009, 'Re-entering foster care: Trends, evidence, and implications', *Children & Youth Services Review*, vol. 31, no. 4, pp. 471–481.

Kortenkamp, K., Geen, R. & Stagner, M., 2004, 'The role of welfare and work in predicting foster care reunification rates for children of welfare recipients', *Children & Youth Services Review*, vol. 26, no. 12, pp. 577–590.

Lee, J.S., Romich, J., Kang, J-Y, Hook, J. & Marcenko, M., 2017, 'The impact of income on reunification among families with children in out-of-home care', *Children & Youth Services Review*, vol. 72, pp. 91–99.

Lewandowski, C.A. & Pierce, L., 2002, 'Assessing the Effect of Family-Centered Out-of-Home Care on Reunification Outcomes', *Research on Social Work Practice*, vol. 12, no. 2, pp. 205–221.

Lewis, R.E., 1994, 'Application and adaptation of intensive family preservation services to use for the reunification of foster children with their biological parents', *Children & Youth Services Review*, vol. 16, no. 5/6, pp. 339–361.

Maltais, C., Cyr, C., Parent, G. & Pascuzzo, K., 2019, 'Identifying effective interventions for promoting parent engagement and family reunification for children in out-of-home care: A series of meta-analyses', *Child Abuse & Neglect*, vol. 88, pp. 362–375.

Maluccio, A.N., Fein, E. & Olmstead, K.A., 1986, *Permanency planning for children: Concepts and methods*, London & New York: Routledge, Chapman & Hall.

Maluccio, A.N. & Ainsworth, F., 2003, 'Drug use by parents: A challenge for family Reunification practice?', *Children & Youth Services Review*, vol. 25, no. 7, pp. 511–533.

McDonald, T., Bryson, S. & Poertner, J., 2006, 'Balancing reunification and re-entry goals', *Children & Youth Services Review*, vol. 28, no. 1, pp. 47–58.

Neil, E., Gitsels, L. & Thoburn, J., 2019, 'Returning children home from care: What can be learned from local authority data?', *Child & Family Social Work*, vol. 25, no. 3, pp. 1–9.

Osborn, A., 2006, A national profile and review of services and interventions for children and young people with high supports in Australian out-of-home care, Unpublished PhD Thesis in Psychology, University of Adelaide.

Pelton, L., 1989, *For reasons of poverty: A critical analysis of the public child welfare system in the United States*, New York: Praeger.

Pine, B., Spath, R., Werrbach, G., Jenson, C. & Kerman, B., 2009, 'A better path to permanency for children in out-of-home care', *Child & Youth Services Review*, vol. 31, pp. 1135–1143.

Pokempner, J., Mikell, D. & Rodriguez, J., 2018, Making reunification possible for older youth, https://jlc.org/news/making-reunification-possible-older-youth, accessed 4 September 2019.

Reed-Ashcraft, K., Raymond, K. & Fraser, M., 2001, 'The reliability and validity of the North Carolina Family Assessment Scale', *Research on Social Work Practice*, vol. 11, pp. 503–520.

Ruch, G., Turney, D. & Ward, A., 2010, *Relationship based social work: Getting to the heart of practice*, London: Jessica Kingsley.

Schuerman, J.R., Rzepnicki, T.L. & Littell, J.H., 1994, *Putting families first: An experiment in family preservation*, New York: Aldine de Gruyter.

Seaberg, J.R. & Tolley, E.S., 1986, 'Predictors of length of stay in foster care', *Social Work Research & Abstract*, vol. 22, pp. 11–17.

Sen, R. & Broadhurst, K., 2011, 'Contact between children in out-of-home placements and their family and friends networks: A research review', *Child & Family Social Work Online*, vol. 16, no. 3, pp. 298–309.

Shaw, T.V., 2010, 'Reunification from foster care: Informing measures over time', *Children & Youth Services Review*, vol. 32, no. 4, pp. 475–481.

Sinclair, I., Baker, C., Lee, J. & Gibbs, I., 2007, *The pursuit of permanence: A study of the English care system*, London: Jessica Kingsley.

Testa, M.F., 2001, 'Kinship care and permanency', *Journal of Social Service Research*, vol. 28, pp. 25–43.

Thoburn, J., Robinson, J. & Anderson, B., 2012, *Returning children from public care*, London: Social Care Institute for Excellence.

Thomas, C., 2018, *The care crisis review: Factors contributing to national increases in looked after children and applications for care orders*, London: Family Rights Group.

Thomas, M., Chernot, D. & Reifel, B., 2005, 'A resilience-based model of reunification and reentry: Implications for out-of-home care services', *Families in Society*, vol. 86, pp. 235–243.

United Nations, 1989, Convention on the rights of the child, New York: United Nations.

Wade, J., Biehal, N., Farrelly, N. & Sinclair, I., 2011, *Caring for abused and neglected children: Making the right decisions for reunification or longterm care*, London: Jessica Kingsley.

Walton, E. Fraser, M.W. Lewis, R.E. & Pecora, P.J., 1993, 'In-home family-focused reunification: An experimental study', *Child Welfare*, vol. 72, no. 5, pp. 473–487.

Wells, S. & Guo, S., 1999, 'Reunification and reentry of foster children', *Children & Youth Services Review*, vol. 21, pp. 273–294.

Wells, S. & Guo, S., 2004, 'Reunification of foster children before and after welfare reforms', *Social Service Review*, vol. 78, pp. 74–95.

Wilkins, M. & Farmer, E., 2015, *Reunification: An evidence-informed framework for return home practice*, London: NSPCC.

Winokur, M., Holtan, A. & Valentine, D., 2009, 'Kinship care for the safety, permanency, and wellbeing of children removed for maltreatment', *The Cochrane Collaboration*, pp. 1–122.

Wulczyn, F., 2004, 'Family reunification', *The Future of Children*, vol. 14, pp. 94–113.

Wulczyn, F., Chen, L. & Courtney, M., 2011, 'Family reunification in a social structural context', *Children & Youth Services Review*, vol. 33, pp. 424–430.

Chapter 15

Creating a family life for a child through adoption

John Simmonds

Adoption has had a long-standing presence in the UK and over the last 20 years has been firmly embedded in government policy as an option for children who have come into State Care and cannot safely return to the birth parents or other family members within the child's timescale. The child's urgent need to establish a strong relational world centred on the adults who they experience as their parents cannot be underestimated. However, the enforced termination of the legal and experiential relationship between the birth parents and child creates a powerful set of experiences for the birth parents – a strong sense of mistrust, disempowerment, coercion, injustice and conflict. This has resulted in various challenges to the adoption sector including an inquiry and report from the British Association of Social Workers into the ethical and human rights position of social workers when it comes to adoption (Featherstone, Gupta & Mills 2018). Other challenges focus on the morality of government setting targets for local authorities in the number of children they must place for adoption or the consequences of government policy in removing core support services from vulnerable families and creating poverty and deprivation in the process with the solution to place children with 'middle class' parents. There have a number of protests or campaigns about 'stolen babies' or children ripped from the arms of their parents by social workers. Adoption is a powerfully conflictual and conflicted area of policy and practice.

The development of adoption over time

The origins of adoption in the UK were somewhat different to the place it now occupies. History clearly indicates the significant risks to babies when parents cannot provide them with the care they need, including being abandoned and left to die. There may have been other options in providing care – informal arrangements in the local community or placing the child in an orphanage or institutional care. These issues were highlighted in the early 1900s with the large number of UK families who lost their husbands/fathers in the First World War – the overall number of deaths was 700,000 but the exact numbers who had families is not identified. These losses were then immediately amplified by the Spanish flu epidemic in the UK where 228,000 people died, although again the number of men who had a family is not identified specifically. Apart from the huge numbers of families who were affected by loss and grief as a result of both of these tragedies, there was specific concern about the maintenance of social and moral order in a society where husbands and fathers were in the dominant position in both day to day matters but especially when it came to the inheritance of title and/or estate. There was no legalised resolution of this issue until the Adoption of Children Act 1926 came into law where adopted children were given a legal status as though they had 'been born into lawful wedlock'. This applied to those children who were born with the legal status of 'illegitimate' but were then placed typically through religious-based organisations with married couples identified as being of good 'social and moral standing'. Adoption was the only option for infertile couples at that time and the legalisation addressed the complex issue of 'baby farming' by giving couples a lawful pathway to having children.

The growth in babies being placed for adoption reached its peak in the UK in 1968 when just under 25,000 placements were made. Thirty years later in 1998 this had fallen to just under 5,000. This reflected significant changes in the society's perspective on single parenthood with a general acceptance that where mothers wanted to keep their babies, even if they were single or without a partner, they could do so and would be entitled to State-funded services such as housing and income. At the same time, the availability of effective forms of contraception – the 'birth pill' and the legalisation of abortion reduced the risk of unwanted pregnancies. But throughout that time, the potential for adoption to be a solution for other groups of children was being explored – particularly those children who were disabled, from black and minority ethnic backgrounds or were older. Uncertainty about the motivation of prospective adopters to adopt these children was a key question but the focus on seizing the opportunity to do so was at the heart of a number of adoption agencies and this resulted in very positive outcomes in placing these children. At the same time, the emergence of 'permanence' as key concept in addressing the needs of children who could not live with their birth parents or birth family contributed to this drive to explore the potential for adoption to enable children to have a stable, secure, loving and safe family life, as it needs to be for every child. As the identification of various forms of child maltreatment became a major issue of concern (Kempe et al. 1962), the potential for adoption to address the need for some of those children became a viable and important option. However, the challenge in obtaining parental consent to the placement of those children was and remains a contentious issue. It was partly solved in some countries, notably the USA by the legal option to dispense with the consent of the parents where this was authorised in the due process of law by the courts. The other option was the placement of children through international adoption – again a contested option although international treaties and agreements have come to regularise this option.

Lifelong impact

A very significant part of the adoption story has been its impact on the child over their childhood, adolescence and into adulthood. It is a lifelong intervention with profound consequences for the child and all of those other individuals involved – many of which are positive but some of which have been seen as problematic. However, while the exploration of these issues has become an accepted part of adoption, that was not recognised in the early stages of adoption or indeed for most of the first 50 years following the first adoption legislation in 1926. During that time there was a strong view that adoption was a 'fresh start' for the child where their birth parents were insignificant alongside the reasons why they were placed for adoption. As such, active secrecy was one recommendation, accessing the child's birth records not legally possible and confusion, uncertainty and unhappiness a consequence of all of this. However, the views and perspectives of adopted adults came to have a huge influence as their need to know, the questions that arose about their identity and their drive to make contact with their birth parents became articulated (Howe, Feast & Coster 2000).

Adoption came to significantly change as a result of these challenges and experiences. Some of this has been reflected in adopted adults having legal access to their birth records and this has typically involved access to counselling to inform this process. Other developments have included identifying the benefits and/or risks for the adoptive person, the adoptive parents and the birth parents in making contact. And others have introduced a new set of concepts such as 'grafting a child onto a new family tree'. This gives recognition to the significance of the transition from one family to a new family and what that might come to mean for the individual in their construction of an adoption narrative. An important part of this has been the recognition of grief and loss both in the short and longer term (Verrier 2009). In turn, these have come to be seen as impacting on the development of an individual's identity – 'who am I and what do I feel about that?'. All of these questions could be exacerbated by observable physical differences between the child and the adopters, especially in the case of 'trans-racial adoption'. Other differences could also be exacerbated such as questions to adopted children at school – both from peers and as a part of classroom projects. Others could be raised during typical family encounters such as complying with daily routines – 'You wouldn't say that if I wasn't adopted?' or 'You are not my real mum and dad!'. In some circumstances, this might be reversed – 'You don't realise how lucky you are that we adopted you?'

All of these issues have come to be integrated into a wide-ranging set of adoptive parenting and adoptive family issues. These range from the need that every adopted child has to know that they were adopted, why they were adopted and who their birth parents and other family members were. And this then includes a recognition of the lifelong questions that will arise from this. And over time, these have expanded into other associated questions such as:

- Is the development of adopted children similar to non-adopted children of the same age?
- What are the specific developmental issues that impact on adopted children?
- If the child experienced early forms of adversity, how do they recover or adapt following their placement for adoption?
- Do adopted children feel fully integrated into their adopted family with all the positive consequences this would be expected to have on their emotional and social well-being?
- Are there any specific issues that are adoption related that needed to be addressed?
- What were the experiences of the adoptive parents and other members of the family?
- Did the adoptive placement endure over time? And how does that compare to children raised by the birth parents?

The answers to these questions are complex but research over the years gives a generally positive or very positive picture. This is so in three broad areas:

- the stability, security, quality and enduring nature of adoptive placements (Palacios et al. 2019; Selwyn, Wijedasa & Meakings 2015)

- the positive development of the child over time over all domains – physical, emotional, behavioural, cognitive and social (Aarons, Hurlburt & Horwitz 2011; Juffer et al., 2011; Schoenmaker et al. 2014; Van IJzendoorn & Juffer 2006)
- the overall satisfaction of adoptive parents and adopted children.

At the same time, a number of risk factors have also been identified:

- Genetic and epigenetic factors which influence the child's development.
- Poor antenatal care resulting from foetal malnourishment, exposure to alcohol and prescribed and illegal drugs and the absence of appropriate health care.
- The age of the child at placement. There is strong evidence that the younger the child when placed, the better the outcomes for the child. This typically means under 1 year but there is some variation in this depending on the study.
- Exposure to early adversity such as maltreatment and instability in the early care of the child such as moving between family members or foster carers.
- The emergence of externalising behavioural issues in the child such as aggression, child-to-parent violence and sexualised behaviour.

The rapid progress in the identification and understanding of children's development over the last 75 years has generally and undoubtedly had a significant impact on our understanding of what matters in their development. Two aspects of this have had significant exploration. The first is the nature and quality of parenting specifically. The second are those factors that are embedded in the relational world of the family including siblings, grandparents and other family members and then the connections this creates with the community around them. This includes the developmental opportunities that come from school and education, play with other children whether this is focussed such as sport, art or music or more general such as play dates. These will evolve and change as the child grows older and specific age-related issues and opportunities emerge. Adoption creates and enables all of these opportunities but it emerges out of one core issue that cannot be ignored – the breaking and disruption of the child's relationship with their birth parents and the fundamental connections and circumstances that they were born into. Where this results from State intervention to protect the child from maltreatment and the significant risks associated with this, the advantages to the child including their survival cannot be under-estimated. But the breaking of the originating relationship cannot be ignored either. Adoptive parenting and family life are adoption and family life plus plus.

The contribution of the framework of attachment

One of the most significant concepts that has had a positive impact on child development and then adoption specifically is that of attachment. Bowlby (Bowlby 1975; Bowlby & Fry 1961) articulated in a profoundly influential way the child's fundamental need for their primary carers, usually parents, to be sensitive, responsive, child centred and readily available. While some of this will directly focus on the basic provision of food, warmth, routine and a healthy home environment including the active management of risk – all factors which enable the child's survival and promote their development – the interactive emotional components of this are critically important. They create an internal sense in the child's mind and body of a secure basis that is readily available and reasonably predictable. And that internal sense is heavily influenced by what is active in the mind and body of the carer/parents – drawing on their own individual lifetime experience and the way this has become represented and embedded in their minds and bodies – their 'internal working model' (Bretherton & Munholland 1999). Bowlby's extensive articulation of the concept of attachment came to set out its core features, along with key collaborators such as Ainsworth and colleagues (2015) in their development of the secure/insecure patterns. Main and Solomon (1986) added the disorganised pattern of attachment and over time much of this basic framework has been explored, added to and evolved. Overall attachment has enabled and prioritised the importance of early relationships as being key to the child's emotional development over time and in many respects over the course of their lifetime (Sroufe 2005). The concept of attachment is one of the most influential child, adolescent and adult concepts even where there continue to be specific challenges and further development in our understanding of significant factors over the life course. The focus on the baby's response to the experience and stress of separation from the person/s who have come to be the secure base in the baby's mind have also emphasised the significant risks that result when babies do not have the ready availability of a relational secure base. This is amplified even more when parenting is a direct threat to the child's safety. This might be a threat from the general environment the child lives in – domestic violence and/or drug and alcohol use and misuse or a direct threat to the child – physical, sexual or emotional abuse or neglect. Whatever form these threats might take specifically, the capacity of human beings to adapt to survive will become significant. But those adaptations may result in patterns of thinking, feeling and behaviour that do not promote the positive engagement of the individual in the world around them or the ability to recognise opportunity. A significant part of this as children grow older is the development of their capacity to learn how to problem solve over a wide range of issues – day to day routines, playing with toys, forming relationships with other adults and children and participating in education. Positive problem solving depends on the nature of the problem to be solved but invariably includes exploring the nature of the problem, learning from past experience, seeking help when required, taking turns, understanding how to work cooperatively with others including setting appropriate boundaries, planning and having access to resources. There are emotional, cognitive, cultural and social aspects to problem solving as well as the potential and the likelihood of things going wrong.

The impact of maltreatment

The key features of a child's development as briefly set out above, quickly lead to recognising that the developmental pathway for many children is influenced by a range of challenges, disadvantages and deprivations, some of which are outside of the control of the child and parents and some of which directly come from the child or their parents. The impact of early adversity through the experience of maltreatment has come to be strongly identified as a key factor in influencing child developmental health and social outcomes (Cicchetti & Toth 2005; Cicchetti & Valentino 2015). Another powerful example comes from a substantial study by Gilbert and colleagues (2009) who identified maltreatment as a primary factor in the emergence of mental health difficulties. This has been identified for both adolescents and adults, extends across a wide range of symptoms including physical health and impacts on a diverse range of individual outcomes – educational, personal relationships, employment and income. The study identifies maltreatment as not only increasing the chances of mental health difficulties, but also likely to amplify them with more severe symptoms that are more difficult to treat and more persistent over time. It is also important to note that, as important as this picture is, the association between maltreatment and mental health is probabilistic – it increases the likelihood of poor mental health and its consequences rather than predicting it. Other developments such as the concept of adverse childhood experiences have provided another important perspective on these issues (Felitti et al. 1998; Rosenman & Rodgers 2004). The challenge associated with maltreatment is also of significant concern when looking at the number of individuals whose lives are affected by maltreatment. In 2015/16 Australia reported 164,987 child protection investigations out of 355,935 notifications with 60,989 of those children identified to be at risk of harm. In the USA, 674,000 children were identified out of 3.5 million children who were referred to State services where there was concern about maltreatment. Of these, the largest group were under 1-year-olds at 25.3 per 1000. While these significant rates of maltreatment have become well known, they also need to be set within the broader exploration of the factors that generate these risk factors – multi-dimensional individual, family and community factors. This includes those State factors such as the availability of universal support services to families such as finance, housing, health and education. There is also the need for specific services such as early parenting interventions and child protection services that are focussed on enabling parents to address the issues that have created the risk factors associated with maltreatment such as mental health problems, drug and alcohol misuse and domestic violence. There are also significant issues associated with the generational transmission of adversity and maltreatment. Again, Adverse Childhood Experiences is one such framework that has enabled a deeper understanding of these issues over the life course with many other informative and supportive frameworks (National Center for Injury Prevention: Division of Violence Prevention 2014).

As a part of the services designed to address the risks associated with maltreatment, each country will develop a specific policy, practice and legal framework that directly protects children where they have been identified as at risk and under threat from maltreatment where continuing to live with their parents is not an option in the short or longer term. This can range from institutional care, support to enable the child to be cared for by their extended family, 'stranger' foster care or in a minority of countries, adoption. The primary aim of these services is to protect the child but also to enable them as far as is possible to recover and resume as close to a 'normal' developmental pathway as possible. As noted above, lawful adoption is a significant model designed to enable this with a lifelong perspective that encompasses both the creation of a new family life for the child, adolescent and adult, but also the breaking of the legal link with the birth family even if some form of a relational link continues through 'contact'. The focus of the rest of this article is addressing the question of developmental recovery – how should we or how can we come to think about recovery in a way that is informed by the best of what we have come to know about human development.

The contribution of neuroscience

Over recent years, developments in neuroscience have enabled a more systematic formulation of the primary processes that operate within the individual from birth onwards that maximises their chances of both survival and development into adulthood. As a part of that, the environment that babies are born into needs to be immediately, regularly and appropriately responsive to those needs. The best of what attachment theory and evidence has told us is that this is primarily in the hands of sensitive, responsive and available parents where they can draw on practical and emotional and social support in that challenging task. However, there are always likely to be degrees of challenge in this process where the response of the parents is complicated through lack of experience, preoccupation with other matters and the absence of resources. Babies typically respond to these issues through degrees of flexibility in their bodily systems but, where this reaches the trigger points in those systems, they will then come to adapt to ensure survival even if that results in degrees of adjustment that are not in their longer-term best interests. Every individual has bodily systems that will respond to heightened degrees of threat – immunological systems when it comes to infections or bodily adjustments when it comes to significant environmental temperature changes. Where the perceived threat is a direct physical threat from other people, then the immediate psychological and physical responses will drive what we have come to know as 'Fight', 'Flight' or 'Freeze' and the system in place that facilitates the response – the HPA – hypothalamic-pituitary-adrenal Axis (Heim et al. 2008; Tarullo & Gunnar 2006). As important as these advances have been, it is also essential to note that for every individual child and adult, their adaptations over time to the challenges in their physical and social environment and the individual systems that enable this need are fundamental to what we generally call learning. The rapid emergence of a baby's capacity to engage in the environment around them, learn from that experience and incorporate it into who they are and what they do could not be more significant. And that will grow as various bodily systems create opportunities to do so – physical maturity, language, social relations enabled and sustained by an appropriate combination of emotional, cognitive, behavioural and social processes. The overarching concept of 'executive functioning' has been an important development in bringing these dimensions together (Best & Miller 2010). These systems enable the growing child to be able to exercise control over their approach to problem identification, planning and finding a workable solution. The experience of 'reward' will be a very important part of this whether this means the feeling of hunger disappearing after a meal, feeling more comfortable after a nappy change, feeling excited during a play date or loved after a cuddle. The presence and involvement of parents, teachers, siblings and a wide range of other people will be highly significant in generating these reward experiences. And the readiness of bodily systems to incorporate the experience of reward as learning and then become activated when further experience and circumstance indicate that this should be so is fundamental. And so the cycle of *experience – reward – learning – experience* is key to the child's development, including their engagement with others and more generally the world around them. Learning how to interact with the physical and social environment in a positive and rewarding way is of huge significance in the development of children and adults, both in ensuring their survival, enabling problem solving and directly experiencing the rewards in doing so.

There are also a wide range of stressors and risks in all of these activities, whether they are common daily activities or specific and unusual activities. There may be a misunderstanding in the nature of the problem and hence what might help solve it – are you hungry or tired or missing your daddy? Are you not feeling well – your tooth is coming through or you have a bit of a temperature? Or the child goes on a play date which they are very excited about but then another child is angry and wants all the toys to themselves. Or the child is trying to build a tower with bricks and another child comes and knocks them down. These are all standard stressors and the child will feel degrees of unhappiness about them and will react accordingly. It is at these times that, hopefully, mummy or daddy will calm them down, reassure them and try to find a solution. The impact on the child's core systems that regulate stress and the absence of sufficient reward will depend very much on prior learning, current reassurance and on-going support, and then identifying alternative solutions to problem solving. Learning to survive in difficult circumstances is one of the core issues in human and individual development but this will always create degrees of stress where the capacity to engage and learn in complex and challenging circumstances is heavily compromised by the past.

The impact that various forms of maltreatment have on the capacity and development of the child to engage in the process of learning and adaptation is likely to be serious. But the detail of this must always be explored, taking into account the multi-dimensional factors that set out what influences what and with what consequences – both in the short and over the longer term. For the child, the adaptation and learning of their bodily systems will be focussed on responding to the risks that their parents/s or family circumstances create. This might include the significant absence of food or warmth and particularly the absence of daily routines where parents typically communicate to their child that 'all is well' and 'will be well'. These threat and stress factors will be heightened when there is a significant absence of sensitive, child centred, loving and readily available direct interaction with the child – the basis for the development of attachment. This one set of issues can run alongside many other sources that are a threat to the child – direct aggression and physical threat, including the observation or the direct experience of domestic violence or being attacked and injured, including sexual abuse. The consequences of this wide range of threats will be specific systemic adaptations by the bodily and psychological systems, including establishing a heightened perception of potential and actual threat in order to take immediate action to survive (McCrory & Viding 2015). These heightened levels of anxiety can be identified through maladaptive changes in the normal cortisol patterns (Dozier et al. 2006). They can also be identified as bodily trauma responses (Herringa 2019; Weems et al. 2019). These adaptations as a heightened 'threat response' will have an impact on the systems described above that 'ordinarily' facilitate a child's engagement, learning and development. The subsequent impact of symptomatic and systematic adaptations to a neglecting or abusive family environment over the immediate and longer term are likely to be profound across many developmental dimensions.

Adoption needs to be seen within this critical set of child development issues, both understanding the impact on the child's growth and capacity to develop and responding to the challenges that might emerge after the child is placed. It is also one option across the range of potential interventions to keep children safe and promote their optimal development. An understanding of child development is also significant in other types of family placement such as kinship care or fostering. And the impact on a child's development can be facilitated or exacerbated by the child's journey from removal from their birth parents to final permanence placement. That intermediate period is one of uncertainty – what will the final plan be, will the local authority get approval from the court, can we find suitable adoptive parents? And what happens to the child in the meantime when they are placed with temporary carers (Hardy et al. 2013; Meakings & Selwyn 2016) who, at best, the child will come to experience as parental figures but whom they also may experience as a threat. And then what happens when we remove the child from their foster parents when they will have developed a relationship with them, hopefully in a meaningful and positive way? And how will they adapt to a new set of parents – with all the positive expectations that accompany the act of 'placing a child' for adoption?

Developmental recovery in adoption: the need for support services

The placing of a child for adoption is a hugely significant step in the process of enabling recovery from a set of early experiences that are the very opposite of what a child needs. The child will have adapted to those early experiences to maximise their chances of survival. But those adaptations will continue to be risk factors in the present and into the future. The settling of the child into their adoptive family will hopefully enable new learning that readjusts those adaptations with the child coming to know and trust their new parents to provide a more facilitative and enabling set of experiences. This is significantly dependant on their bodily systems having the capacity to positively respond to allow those new experiences to be actually experienced for what they are. A friendly face and appropriate bodily movement in the adopter that is meant to reassure and comfort if experienced by the child as a frightening face and a threat, because of heightened sensitivity in the perceptual system, will be a challenge for the adopter and a problem for the child. Over time, adaptations may take place as the adopter's friendly face and their bodily movement continues and the child's perceptual systems become less threat sensitive. But there is always a challenge in the degree to which new learning can take place when past experience is embedded and a driver in the opposite direction. There is significant evidence about the degree of developmental recovery adopted children do make (Juffer et al. 2011; Van IJzendoorn & Juffer 2006) but we cannot ignore the on-going challenges of persistent developmental issues (Selwyn et al. 2015; Selwyn & Meakings 2016; Sonuga-Barke et al. 2017) where this reflects the child's experience of significant adversity through maltreatment. Adoptive parenting and adoptive family life in these circumstances need to be framed to take into account that there may be an on-going series of challenges, not because the adopters or child have failed in some way but because the child's adaptation to early adversity needs to be understood as their way of survival and that learning does not suddenly evaporate. New experiences are critically important in positively realigning the child's systems, with parenting and family life at the top of the list. Alongside this is the importance of ensuring that an evidence-informed adoption support framework is available. This would include ensuring that the adopters or the child/adolescent or other relevant people could ask for an assessment of their current needs and circumstances when they have concerns about problems that are persistent and/or troubling. These may be happening in the context of the family, at school, in the social network or with the birth family. They may also present themselves in a variety of ways – physical or mental health, learning, behaviour or emotional issues or in combination with the child, the adoptive parents, siblings or others directly experiencing this. The evidence base for the effectiveness of interventions offered as a part of that service should be embedded within the design of the service. That must also include a service that is a wrap-around to enable adoptive families to support one another through social media, meetings, play dates, mentoring and the provision of information.

The evolution of adoption is complex, challenging and conflicted. In many ways it is easier to avoid it altogether, given its history. But for some children in the most difficult of circumstances, it is an option that fundamentally focusses on their rights, needs and circumstances in the long term and that means where it is recognised as a lifelong intervention of the most profound kind. As such though, it must not be constructed as a one-off intervention with a 'happy ever after' perspective. The child's significant adaptation to maltreatment affects all of their bodily systems and these become deeply embedded. Adoptive family life must be seen as a therapeutic intervention where the best of parenting and family life needs to be combined with the best of evidence-based interventions delivered in a comprehensive child- and family-centred system. Children and their adopters deserve no less.

References

Aarons, G.A., Hurlburt, M. & Horwitz, S.M., 2011, 'Advancing a conceptual model of evidence-based practice implementation in public service sectors', *Administration and Policy in Mental Health and Mental Health Services Research*, vol. 38, no. 1, pp. 4–23.

Ainsworth, M., Blehar, M., Waters, E. & Wall, S., 2015, *Patterns of attachment*, New York: Psychology Press.

Best, J. & Miller, P., 2010, 'A developmental perspective on executive function', *Child Development*, vol. 81, pp. 1641–1660.

Bowlby, J., 1975, *Attachment and loss*, Harmondsworth, UK: Penguin.

Bowlby, J. & Fry, M., 1961, *Child care and the growth of love* (2nd edn), Harmondsworth, England: Penguin Books.

Bretherton, I. & Munholland, K., 1999, 'Internal working models in attachment relationships: A construct revisited', in J. Cassidy & P. Shaver (eds), *Handbook of attachment: Theory, research, and clinical applications*, New York: The Guilford Press, pp. 89–111.

Cicchetti, D. & Toth, S.L., 2005, 'Child maltreatment', *Annual Review of Clinical Psychology*, vol. 1, pp. 409–438.

Cicchetti, D. & Valentino, K., 2015, 'An ecological-transactional perspective on child maltreatment: Failure of the average expectable environment and its influence on child development', in D. Cicchetti & D. Cohen (eds), *Developmental psychopathology: Risk, disorder, and adaptation* (2nd edn, Vol. 3), Hoboken, NJ: John Wiley & Sons.

Dozier, M., Manni, M., Gordon, M.K., Peloso, E., Gunnar, M.R., Stovall-McClough, K.C., Eldreth, D. & Levine, S., 2006, 'Foster children's diurnal production of cortisol: An exploratory study', *Child Maltreatment*, vol. 11, no. 2, pp. 189–197.

Featherstone, B., Gupta, A. & Mills, S., 2018, *The role of the social worker in adoption - ethics and human rights: An Enquiry*, Birmingham: BASW.

Felitti V., Anda R., Nordenberg, D., Williamson, D., Spitz, A., Edwards, V., Koss, M.P. & Marks, J., 1998, 'Relationship of childhood abuse and household dysfunction to many of the leading causes of death in adults. The Adverse Childhood Experiences (ACE) Study', *American Journal of Preventive Medicine*, vol. 14, no. 4, pp. 245–258.

Gilbert, R., Spatz, C., Browne, K., Fergusson, D., Webb, E. & Janson S., 2009, 'Burden and consequences of child maltreatment in high-income countries', *The Lancet*, vol. 373, no. 9657, pp. 68–81.

Hardy, C., Hackett, E., Murphy, E., Cooper, B., Ford, T. & Conroy, S., 2013, 'Mental health screening and early intervention: Clinical research study for under 5-year-old Children in Care in an inner London borough', *Clinical Child Psychology and Psychiatry*, vol. 20, no. 2, pp. 261–275.

Heim, C., Newport, D. J., Mletzko, T., Miller, A.H. & Nemeroff, C.B., 2008, 'The link between childhood trauma and depression: Insights from HPA axis studies in humans', *Psychoneuroendocrinology*, vol. 33, no. 6, pp. 693–710.

Herringa, R., 2019, 'Commentary: Paediatric post-traumatic stress disorder from a neurodevelopmental network perspective: reflections on Weems et al', *Journal of Child Psychology and Psychiatry*, vol. 60, no. 4, pp. 409–411.

Howe, D., Feast, J. & Coster, D., 2000, *Adoption, search & reunion: The long term experience of adopted adults*, London: Children's Society.

Juffer, F., Palacios, J., Le Mare, L., Sonuga-Barke, E.J., Tieman, W., Bakermans-Kranenburg, M.J., Vorria, P., Van Ijzendoorn, M.H. & Verhulst, F.C., 2011, 'II. Development of adopted children with histories of early adversity', *Monographs of the Society for Research in Child Development*, vol. 76, no. 4, pp. 31–61.

Kempe, C.H., Silverman, F.N., Steele, B.F., Droegemueller, W. & Silver, H.K., 1962, 'The battered-child syndrome', *Journal of the American Medical Association*, vol. 181, pp. 7–24.

Main, M. & Solomon, J., 1986, 'Discovery of an insecure-disorganized/disoriented attachment pattern', in *Affective development in infancy*, Westport, CT: Ablex Publishing, pp. 95–124.

McCrory, E.J. & Viding, E., 2015, 'The theory of latent vulnerability: Reconceptualizing the link between childhood maltreatment and psychiatric disorder', *Development and Psychopathology*, vol. 27, no. 2, pp. 493–505.

Meakings, S. & Selwyn, J., 2016, '"She was a foster mother who said she didn't give cuddles": The adverse early foster care experiences of children who later struggle with adoptive family life', *Clinical Child Psychology and Psychiatry*, vol. 21, no. 4, pp. 509–519.

National Center for Injury Prevention: Division of Violence Prevention, 2014, Essentials for childhood – Steps to create safe, stable, nurturing relationships and environments. www.cdc.gov/violenceprevention/pdf/essentials_for_childhood_framework.pdf, accessed 12 August 2019.

Palacios, J., Rolock, N., Selwyn, J. & Barbosa-Ducharne, M., 2019, 'Adoption breakdown: Concept, research, and implications', *Research on Social Work Practice*, vol. 29, no. 2, pp. 130–142.

Rosenman, S. & Rodgers, B., 2004, 'Childhood adversity in an Australian population', *Social Psychiatry and Psychiatric Epidemiology*, vol. 39, no. 9, pp. 695–702.

Schoenmaker, C., Juffer, F., van IJzendoorn, M.H. & Bakermans-Kranenburg, M.J., 2014, 'Does family matter? The well-being of children growing up in institutions, foster care and adoption', in A. Ben-Aryeh, F. Casas, I. Frones & J.E. Korbin (eds), *Handbook of child well-being: Theories, methods and policies in global perspective*, Dordrecht: Springer, pp. 2197–2228.

Selwyn, J., Wijedasa, D. & Meakings, S., 2015, *Beyond the adoption order: Challenges, interventions and adoption disruption*, London: British Association for Adoption and Fostering.

Selwyn, J. & Meakings, S., 2016, 'Adolescent-to-parent violence in adoptive families', *British Journal of Social Work*, vol. 46, no. 5, pp. 1224–1240.

Sonuga-Barke, E., Kennedy, M., Kumsta, R., Knights, N., Golm, D., Rutter, M., Selwyn, J., Meakings, S. & Kreppner, J., 2017, 'Child-to-adult neurodevelopmental and mental health trajectories after early life deprivation: The young adult follow-up of the longitudinal English and RomanianAdoptees study', *The Lancet*, vol. 389, 1539–1548.

Sroufe, L.A., 2005, *The development of the person: The Minnesota study of risk and adaptation from birth to adulthood*, New York: Guilford Press.

Tarullo, A.R. & Gunnar, M.R., 2006, 'Child maltreatment and the developing HPA axis', *Hormones and Behavior*, vol. 50, no. 4, pp. 632–639.

Van IJzendoorn, M. & Juffer, F., 2006, 'The Emanuel Miller Memorial Lecture 2006: Adoption as intervention. Meta-analytic evidence for massive catch-up and plasticity in physical, socio-emotional, and cognitive development', *Journal of Child Psychology and Psychiatry*, vol. 47, pp. 1228–1245.

Verrier, N., 2009, *The primal wound: Understanding the adopted child*, London:British Association for Adoption and Fostering.

Weems, C., Russell, J., Neill, E. & McCurdy, B., 2019, 'Pediatric posttraumatic stress disorder from a neurodevelopmental network perspective', *Journal of Child Psychology and Psychiatry*, vol. 60, pp. 395–408.

Chapter 16

Beyond care

Identities, transitions and outcomes

Philip Mendes and Jade Purtell

This chapter examines the policy and practice challenges associated with leaving care. It is recognised that many young people are not well prepared to leave care and that effective preparation, transition and ongoing support services are essential to facilitate better life outcomes. Studies have shown that many young people struggle when they leave care due to the sudden end to formal networks of support that usually occurs at 18 years of age. Many experience difficulties in accessing stable housing, participating in ongoing education or employment, and developing supportive social connections. The most vulnerable young people are those involved in substance abuse and/or offending, or those with mental health problems and developmental disabilities. This chapter draws on a recent evaluation of the Berry Street Stand By Me leaving care program in the State of Victoria to highlight principles for effective leaving care policy and practice.

Introduction

Young people transitioning from out-of-home care (often called care leavers) are universally a vulnerable group whose needs often have been neglected not only by their biological parents, but also in some cases by their substitute parent, the state (Stein 2016). Leaving care is formally defined as the cessation of legal responsibility by the state for young people living in out-of-home care, which generally occurs at no later than 18 years of age. In practice, however, leaving care is a major life transformation, and a process that involves transitioning from dependence on state accommodation and supports (notwithstanding their inherent and considerable limitations) to so-called independence and self-reliance (Cashmore & Mendes 2015). Care leavers often face significant barriers to accessing educational, employment, housing and other development and transitional opportunities that are readily available to their non-care peers. This social exclusion seems to be particularly harsh for those who have developmental disabilities or mental health concerns (McDonald, Ellem & Wilson 2016); those involved in substance abuse or criminal justice systems (Carr & McAlister 2016); those who transition from residential care; Indigenous young people; those who become early parents; and unaccompanied asylum seekers (Mendes, Pinkerton & Munro 2014).

Care leavers are not a homogeneous group and have varied backgrounds and experiences in terms of the structure and capacity of their families, the type and extent of abuse or neglect as well as the age at which they entered care. They also differ in relation to their cultural and ethnic backgrounds; their in-care experiences including length of stay and level of placement stability; their developmental stage and needs when exiting care;

and, the quantity and quality of professional and community supports available to them (Cashmore & Mendes 2015).

The leading English researcher Mike Stein (2012) has broadly classified care leavers into three categories. The first he terms the 'moving-on group'. Young people in this group are likely to have experienced secure and stable placements, be highly resilient, welcome independence, and be able to make effective use of leaving and aftercare supports. The second group he terms 'survivors'. They have experienced significant instability and discontinuity. Outcomes for this group tend to reflect the effectiveness of post-care supports provided. The 'strugglers' are the third group. They are likely to have had the most negative pre-care experiences, and are most likely to experience significant social and emotional challenges. Stein's (2012) research found that after-care support was unlikely to alleviate these problems, but was still viewed as important by them. It is important to remember that outcomes for care leavers are fluid (as indeed, the quality of post care support and resources differs across localities and governments), and some may have poor initial transitions and fall into the survivor or struggler group, but later will be able as they mature (and with the availability of ongoing supports at 20 or 21 years old) to 'move on' into the mainstream. They need to be able to access second or third chances, just as ordinary parents in the community stand by their own children as they test limits and learn from their mistakes.

In summary, it has generally been accepted that successful outcomes for care leavers result from:

- Secure and stable placements;
- Educational support and progress whilst in out of home care;
- Planned and gradual transitions from care that reflect individual levels of maturity and skill development; and
- The provision of stable accommodation and a range of ongoing relationship and material supports after leaving care including a dedicated caseworker or personal adviser till at least 21 years of age (Cashmore & Mendes 2015). The outcomes for care leavers reflect the connection between two key factors: one is their Individual Agency or resilience (within a social context), and the second being the availability of ongoing positive relationships via what we call Social Capital through professional and informal support networks (Dinisman & Zeira 2011).

The reasons for the vulnerability of care leavers are arguably threefold. First, many come from highly chaotic and disadvantaged families characterised by poverty, relationship breakdown, substance abuse, violence, disability and mental illness. Such pre-care experiences of abuse and neglect often result in long-term trauma that contributes to global and chronic developmental delays. Many children enter care with significant emotional and behavioural problems, and physical health deficits. Additionally, the sudden separation from birth parents, extended family, friends and community connections as well as often, siblings, that occurs on entry to care can be highly debilitating and hugely disruptive to education and employment (Jackson & Cameron 2014).

Second, some young people experience inadequacies in state care including poor quality caregivers, and constant shifts of placement, carers, schools and workers. In Australia, the most disadvantaged group of adolescents in care are mostly placed in residential care facilities which operate on a rostered worker model. This is typically said to be because these young people have been deemed unsuitable for foster or kinship placements. Residential care workers are generally low paid and poorly trained, and may lack the skills to understand behavioural manifestations of trauma exposure and to engage and support the young people. Nevertheless, many children and young people in out-of-home care experience supportive and stable placements including an ongoing positive relationship with carers and workers, which enable them to overcome adversities resulting from their pre-care experiences.

Third, many care leavers can call on little, if any, direct family support or other social and community networks to ease their transition into independent living. They may not have access to the opportunities or have the broader social connections that other young people use: to attain part-time work; to develop pathways into further and higher education; to access shared and affordable housing; and, to form supportive relationships.

In addition to these major disadvantages, care leavers currently experience an abrupt end at 16–18 years of age to the formal support networks of state care, including the funding of their core housing, education or training, and health needs. That is, the state as corporate parent usually fails to provide the ongoing financial, social and emotional support and nurturing offered by most families. Most other young people, at least in countries such as Australia now live at home until 21 or even 25 years of age, and even those who leave home may still call on their families for ongoing financial, practical and emotional assistance. In contrast, care leavers, who as a result of their background experiences are the group least likely to be developmentally ready for independence at 18 years of age, are expected to almost instantaneously transform into self-sufficient adults without any safety net (Mendes & Snow 2016).

Conversely, there is increasing evidence from a number of jurisdictions that extending care till at least 21 years of age results in improved outcomes. This is because it offers: continuity and stability; a nurturing environment; help for engagement in education, employment and training; and empowers young people and gives them greater choice and control over the timing and process of their transition (Matheson 2018; Mendes & Rogers 2020).

For example, Mark Courtney and his colleagues in California, USA cite specific benefits of extended care such as: enhanced educational outcomes, improved earnings and less economic hardship, fewer early pregnancies, lower levels of homelessness, reduced mental health difficulties or involvement in the criminal justice system, and greater involvement of noncustodial fathers with their children (Courtney & Hook 2017; Courtney & Okpych 2017).

Similarly, Emily Munro and colleagues in England cite systemic benefits of the Staying Put extended foster care program such as: stable and supportive relationships providing ongoing emotional support to young people who are not developmentally ready for adulthood at 18 years; and housing and associated stability which facilitates engagement in employment, education and training, and enables young people to undertake a gradual transition that mirrors the pathways of their peers in the general population. Specific positive outcomes included: greater housing stability, and higher engagement in education or training and employment including greater access to higher education which should lead to higher future earnings and less reliance on public benefits (Munro et al. 2012).

Australian and Victorian policy and practice context

A total of 47,915 children were in out-of-home care (OOHC) in June 2017 including 17,664 Indigenous children – a rate ten times that of non-Indigenous children. Total spending annually is $3.1 billion. The vast majority of children in OOHC (93 per cent) had been placed in either foster or relative/kinship care or other types of home-based care. Only about 5 per cent reside in residential care which is generally reserved for older adolescents with complex needs (AIHW 2018). About 3,130 young people nationally in Australia aged 15 to 17 years transition from OOHC each year (AIHW 2017: 48). But no specific figures are provided for those who leave care at 18 years of age, or what percentage of care leavers come from each care category.

OOHC in Australia is the responsibility of the community services or child welfare department in each State and Territory, and each has its own legislation, policies and practices. Consequently assistance to care leavers is inconsistent and fragmented, although the national out-of-home care standards, introduced in December 2010, suggest minimum benchmarks such as the requirement for each care leaver to have a transition from care plan commencing at 15 years of age (Department of Families, Housing, Community Services and Indigenous Affairs 2010). Additionally, the latest National Child Protection Framework Action Plan for 2015–18 identifies improved outcomes for care leavers as one of the three key strategies to be implemented, and refers to improved housing supports as a priority in order to prevent youth homelessness (Department of Social Services 2015a). There is also some Commonwealth funding available to care leavers through the Transition to Independent Living Allowance (TILA) which provides financial assistance up to $1,500 for young people aged 15–25 years who have departed OOHC within the past 24 months (Department of Social Services 2015b). Access is limited to a once-off payment and a young person must have a caseworker to apply for the payment.

But neither the National Standards or Child Protection Framework provide any specific funding incentives to jurisdictions to assist the introduction of additional supports, nor do they impose any accountability measures to enforce action by the states and territories (Beauchamp 2016). To date, all legislative provisions are discretionary, not mandatory. This optional duty compares unfavourably with the mandatory obligation contained in the English Children (Leaving Care) Act 2000 to assist care leavers via a formal Pathway Plan and supportive Personal Adviser until at least 21 years of age, and a similar obligation via the Staying Put Bill (2013) in Scotland to provide care leavers with advice, guidance and assistance until 26 years of age (Baidawi 2016).

The state of Victoria legislated via the Children, Youth and Families Act 2005 for the provision of leaving care and after-care services for young people up to 21 years of age. The Children, Youth and Families Act 2005 appears to oblige the government to assist care leavers with finances, housing, education and training, employment, legal advice, access to health and community services, and counselling and support depending on the assessed level of need, and to consider the specific needs of Aboriginal young people. However, Section 16(2) of the Act emphasises that these responsibilities 'do not create any right or entitlement enforceable at law', suggesting that leaving care programs are in fact discretionary, and care leavers do not actually have any legal right to seek or demand support services from government (Mendes, Johnson & Moslehuddin 2011).

To be sure, the government has established mentoring, post-care support and flexible funding support for young people transitioning from care or post care in all eight regions. These services, which cost approximately 11 million dollars a year, include discrete Indigenous support, education and employment, and housing assistance programs (DHHS 2017). But the service system retains significant limitations. A considerable proportion of the funding is allocated to young people aged 16 or 17 years who are still in the care system, rather than to those aged 18 years and over. Also, many young people seem to find the myriad of programs with their discrete age and eligibility criteria complicated and confusing.

Not surprisingly, a number of independent research studies have documented that many care leavers experience poor outcomes because they:

- Are not developmentally ready at 18 years to live independently;
- Have poor emotional regulation and difficulties in establishing social relationships;
- Experience limited ongoing participation in education;
- Often exit care directly into homelessness and/or endure ongoing housing instability;
- Are at risk of spending time in the youth justice system.

In addition, those young people who are Indigenous often experience estrangement from culture and community, on top of all these other issues listed (Harvey et al 2015; Johnson et al. 2010; McDowall 2008; Mendes, Saunders & Baidawi 2016; Muir & Hand 2018).

Six official public inquiries by governments and parliamentary committees over the past seven years (five at state and territory level in Victoria, New South Wales, South Australia, Queensland and the Northern Territory; and one by the Commonwealth Senate, see Community Affairs References Committee 2015) have identified similar concerns. These inquiries concur that care leavers are vulnerable to poor outcomes as evidenced by homelessness, offending and minimal progress in education, and that legislative and policy reform is required to ensure enhanced support till at least 21 years of age (Mendes & McCurdy 2019).

The Stand By Me program

Berry Street is the largest child and family welfare organisation in Victoria. Their programs include foster and kinship care, residential care, family violence services, education and training programs, therapeutic services, youth services, family services and community (development) programs. In 2011, Berry Street undertook a scoping study of leaving care supports in the State of Victoria. The study highlighted the very poor long-term outcomes for some young people when they leave state care, particularly those who are likely to have had the most negative pre-care experiences (Whyte 2011).

As a result of these findings, Berry Street introduced the Stand By Me (SBM) pilot program in its Northern Regional Office in early 2013 for a three-year period with funding from the Ian Potter Foundation and the Lord Mayors Charitable Foundation. The pilot concluded in December 2015. SBM was an intensive case support service for young people transitioning from the out-of-home care system. Two workers were appointed to each work with six young people totalling 12 young people. SBM aimed to promote a successful transition by utilising an early intervention approach that involved engaging and developing relationships with the young person and their support workers whilst they were still in care, and continuing to work with them more intensively post care.

The program targeted 16–21-year-olds who were on a child protection guardianship or custody order and who were likely to be more vulnerable leaving care in areas such as being at risk of homelessness; presenting with complex behaviours and intensive support needs related to disability, substance use, mental health issues, exclusion from education and training, and limited community networks; having a history of unresolved trauma; and having limited skills or capacity to live in shared accommodation (Berry Street 2012a).

The SBM program was developed as an adaptation of the Personal Adviser (PA) model introduced in the UK via the Children (Leaving Care) Act 2000. The Personal Adviser provides continuous support for care leavers from 16 to 21 years or until 24 years if they are still in education or training, and coordinates the resources and services required to meet their Pathway Plan. The Plan identifies the young person's needs for support and assistance in core areas such as health and mental health, housing, financial support, living skills, education and training, employment and family and social relationships, and how these needs will be addressed (Department of Health 2001).

The aims and objectives of the Stand By Me program were informed by an extensive review of the leaving care research literature (Whyte 2011), as well as Berry Street's practice experience supporting young people in OOHC, transitioning from care and post care. Several service and support gaps were identified in the current leaving care system for young people with complex support needs, particularly those lacking family support during the transition from care. This group of young people are particularly vulnerable to falling through service gaps in a fragmented leaving care system, often resulting in unsafe and unstable accommodation, and isolation in the absence of a supportive network. Consequently, the SBM worker roles included the following:

- Working with the case managers and care teams to identify young people who are likely to need ongoing support with the leaving care transition and post care;
- Working alongside the case manager, whilst the young person is still in care, to promote assessment, planning and skill development;
- Post care, assuming a more assertive role up to the age of 21, providing a continuity of relationship with a view to establishing and maintaining the young person with an ongoing community-based support network;
- Facilitating community connections;
- Mediating in family and relationship difficulties;
- Adapting to the needs of the young person as they develop over time (Berry Street 2012b).

Notably, one of the principal aims of SBM was to assist a group of young people at high risk of homelessness to identify, secure and maintain affordable and stable housing options.

Stand By Me evaluation

The evaluation of the SBM program was undertaken by Monash University, and overseen by an SBM Steering Group including Berry Street senior management, policy staff and

SBM workers, with representation from the Department of Health and Human Services Leaving Care policy staff (Purtell et al. 2016).

The evaluation aimed to:

- Understand to what extent the UK Personal Adviser model could be translated to the Australian and Victorian child, youth and family welfare service system context;
- Identify the most effective aspects of the SBM model;
- Understand clients' experience of SBM support;
- Understand how time and financial resources were utilised by the SBM program;
- Assess whether the program delivered the short, medium and longer term benefits and outcomes intended;
- Identify the areas in which the program was most successful in improving young people's outcomes; and
- Identify any necessary modifications to improve program efficacy.

Ethics approval to conduct the evaluation was attained from the Monash University Human Research Ethics Committee in 2012. Evaluation methods included qualitative semi-structured interviews with a range of Victorian leaving care stakeholders both within and external to the SBM pilot. The SBM cohort were referred mainly from residential care and lead tenant placements, and the program was only open to those most at risk of homelessness and other negative outcomes. The semi-structured interview schedule for the SBM supported group (nine young people, three of the 12 were not available for interview) was based around what support young people reported receiving through the program, and how they evaluated that support.

The evaluation also conducted interviews with non SBM supported young people (eight) focusing on their leaving care experiences including leaving care planning, post-care housing, relationships with family and social networks, physical and mental health, education, employment and training, and community connections. The alternate group in the SBM evaluation was recruited through existing post care programs, and those interviewed were receiving significant supports and mostly living in stable and supported accommodation which included significantly subsidised rents. These young people were described as having a slightly lower level of complexity than the SBM cohort. However, two of them had either a physical or intellectual disability, and one was already a parent.

The evaluation also interviewed and conducted focus groups with a range of professionals and carers – including the four Stand By Me workers and management and eight non-SBM staff from the various residential care, home-based care, lead tenant and post-care support programs – who had worked either with clients in the SBM program or other young people exited from care without SBM support. These stakeholders provided a system-centric perspective on differences they noticed between the two groups of young people.

Thematic content analysis was performed with all data generated from interviews with staff and young people. Specifically, categories of housing pathways, family relationships, independent living skills, education, employment and training, income/brokerage, mental health, alcohol and other drugs, social supports and networks, disability, and pregnancy and parenting were coded. Thematic analysis of coded data identified commonalities and differences in respondents' perspectives on issues for care leavers, and the impact of the SBM program. Additionally, thematic analysis identified effective program elements of

SBM, as described by young people, as well as SBM and broader Berry Street leaving care and post-care services staff.

Key findings

The evaluation found that a number of key elements of the SBM program were conducive to promoting positive outcomes for young people in areas such as housing, family relationships, education, employment, income, physical and mental health, social supports and social networks, early pregnancy and parenting, and living skills. They were as follows:

The Stand By Me worker–client relationship

Most of the young people were able to develop close working relationships with their workers whilst still in care. The SBM-supported young people who participated in the evaluation experienced the worker–client relationship as a central and reliable adult support, which appeared to constitute a therapeutic relationship in itself. These relationships delivered both emotional and practical assistance to young people, as well as a vehicle for accessing wider services and supports.

Reduction of leaving care and post-care anxiety

The period of pre-discharge engagement appeared to alleviate an identified period of 'leaving care anxiety', during which many care leavers typically disengage from supports and exhibit escalating challenging behaviours. The availability of a key support person throughout the transition from care appeared to enhance engagement with services in both the leaving and post care periods.

Enhanced leaving care planning and implementation

Although Australian studies typically report low rates of leaving care plan completion, leaving care planning was able to be completed and implemented for all SBM supported young people, and SBM workers facilitated access to available brokerage and supports.

Holistic support, flexible brokerage and funding advocacy

The intensive case management provided by SBM workers enabled the delivery of wrap-around support, including practical assistance. SBM workers provided transport to and support with essential appointments, informal counselling, and emotional support for young people's aspirations, concerns, ongoing stress and anxiety and achievements. SBM workers assisted young people in purchasing household, employment and education-related goods, as well as personal necessities such as medication and clothing. There were also opportunities for supporting competence in independent living skills. Additional financial support assisted SBM supported clients to develop social networks and community connectedness, for example by supporting access to recreational activities. SBM workers were also available to respond to crises, which were occasional for some young people and more ongoing for others. SBM clients were also referred to other support services, and staff advocated for their access to welfare services and programs in the broader community, with a view to promoting greater social inclusion.

Case study of Stand By Me participant: Jessica

Jessica is a 20-year-old woman who first entered residential care at the age of 13 years, having moved from a foster family following her refusal to attend high school in year 7. Her foster family was unable to accommodate Jessica remaining at home throughout the day. Jessica enjoyed primary school but experienced bullying and teasing from other students at high school, who laughed at her difficulties with spelling and made fun of her second-hand uniform. Jessica continued to refuse to attend high school in residential care, and was not eligible for alternative education programs until she turned 15.

During this period Jessica routinely arose at midday, smoked marijuana at a friend's house in the afternoon, and returned to the unit in the evening to watch television and sleep. Staff searched for educational options for Jessica during this time, taking her to the library to identify her interests. Jessica often selected books on different exotic animals, and was familiar with a range of species, often impressing her residential workers. Unit staff helped Jessica to enrol in a Certificate II in Animal studies with a local TAFE provider, a major achievement after Jessica's hiatus from education. Unfortunately, Jessica did not enjoy the study.

At 16 years of age Jessica was introduced to the Stand By Me program. Staff at her residential unit informed Jessica that her SBM worker would support her planning and preparation to transition from care. Barbara arrived at the unit to take Jessica out for a milkshake, and was warned that Jessica was agitated following a phone call with her mother. Jessica emerged, swearing and yelling that her mother, whose boyfriend was a drug dealer, shouldn't be permitted to have custody of her two siblings. Barbara said she could see this was a stressful time and she could come back another day, but offered to take Jessica out if she wished. Jessica took this up.

In the car, Barbara asked if Jessica was familiar with the local area and if she spent much time with friends. She described spending a lot of time around Flinders St Station, starting trouble with a group of friends. Barbara changed the subject and asked if she preferred the eastern suburbs where she had grown up. Jessica snapped back, indicating that was where she had lived with her mum and dad who were dealing heroin, stating that she did not miss it, and was glad to be away from 'all those junkies'. Just as Barbara was wondering if Jessica's mood would improve at all, she noticed a dog being walked and remarked 'Aww. Look at that Staffy. What an awesome dog!'

Barbara quickly established Jessica's passion for animals and discussed this with unit staff. Together they explored the Certificate II in Animal Studies at the RSPCA instead of TAFE. Jessica progressed to enrolling in the course and thoroughly enjoyed it, citing the hands-on nature of the course as very motivating. Following her completion of the certificate she wanted to stay on as a volunteer to develop her work experience.

Jessica's motivation for her course meant that she was fully engaged with Leaving Care planning with her Stand By Me worker. She accessed Leaving Care brokerage for a computer, mobile internet, various educational tools and resources. She also received a yearly Myki ticket to travel to and from her course and elsewhere. When Jessica was 17, a Lead Tenant vacancy became available, and Barbara supported Jessica to select and purchase furniture and household goods Jessica would require upon leaving care. They also looked for extra storage options since it remained uncertain where Jessica would move to after exiting the Lead Tenant placement.

While discussing leaving care plans, Jessica mentioned that the prospect of being alone when she turned 18 was frightening. Barbara emphasised that the preparation being undertaken would help to ensure Jessica was well prepared and could look forward to becoming more independent. Barbara targeted youth foyers and supported housing programs to register Jessica for vacancies but they were rare and had lengthy waiting lists.

Barbara also maintained familiarity with Jessica's friendship circumstances to identify potential housemates; however, Jessica's friends studying at the RSPCA seemed to live with family. Her other friends from Flinders St seemed to live with older people who supplied with drugs, cigarettes and food and had lots of parties. Barbara encouraged Jessica to find more positive friendship networks.

No suitable housing vacancies had been found by Jessica's eighteenth birthday. She was anxious about losing the Department's support, and indicated a desire to just smoke bongs and ignore the problem. Barbara explained that Stand By Me was able to work with Jessica for another year and a half, and that they could fund emergency housing if needed and would continue to look for safe and suitable housing options with Jessica.

Just prior to her eighteenth birthday Jessica met someone at the RSPCA who lived in a three-bedroom student house and was looking for a tenant. Jessica was scared to live with other people without workers being in charge, but was equally scared of going to a refuge, or having to stay with her friends from Flinders St. Barbara explained that if it did not work out Stand By Me could help, so there was a back-up.

Barbara worked closely with Jessica over the subsequent six-month period, supporting her to deal with share house frustrations and at times, strained relationships with housemates. During this time they also worked on finding employment, and Jessica eventually secured part-time work in a pet store. Jessica found this improved her confidence and social skills, as she gained significant practice speaking to strangers. When Stand By Me ended, Jessica was working up to 25 hours a week in the pet shop, and was happy with both the job and her employer. She had been able to pay her rent and bills at the share house for two months prior to the end of the program and felt more confident about confronting household issues with her housemates who were also good friends now.

Jessica's great progress through SBM was enabled through the gradual building of trust and the consistency of emotional support provided by the SBM worker. This slow process involved encouragement, guidance and the setting of incremental goals and evolving levels of support to match Jessica's motivation and capability. Where other workers before her had tried and given up in the face of Jessica's complexity, Barbara had the benefit of time to build a positive, safe and durable relationship and to provide the plethora of supports required to create the right conditions for assisting Jessica to make progress in her educational re-engagement, her housing and her other achievements over time.

Case study questions

1 What does Jessica's experience tell us about the importance of a stable and supportive relationship with an adult providing ongoing emotional support for facilitating positive transitions from care?
2 How significant for care leaver outcomes are the availability of pro-social friendship networks?

Specific findings regarding strengthened housing assistance

The provision of safe, secure and affordable accommodation is a crucial component in the transition from care to independent living, and is closely linked to positive outcomes in health, social connections, education and employment. Yet research suggests that, compared to their non-care peers, care leavers are at much greater risk of homelessness (Mendes, Johnson & Moslehuddin 2011).

The 12 SBM clients were provided with housing support including advocacy and access to brokerage funds from the time of exiting care. This included renegotiating continued arrangements with existing foster or kinship carers; providing emotional support to those who moved in with family or partners and assistance in maintaining these housing arrangements; supporting young people whilst they moved into independent living including in one case funding private rental or hotel accommodation; and/or identifying alternative options where the situation became untenable.

Nine of the 12 SBM supported young people were in stable, ongoing housing at the end of the three year SBM support period in December 2015. This outcome was notable, given that the program targeted care leavers at high risk of homelessness. The housing assistance provided by SBM seems to have played a key role in enabling care leavers to move from OOHC to other secure accommodation without experiencing the trauma of not knowing where they would stay.

A number of workers from the Berry Street post-care support information and referral program noted why SBM had been influential in preventing homelessness. One of them commented:

> We've had some young people who have accessed post care brokerage who are SBM clients. So what I noticed is that most of those young people, who are quite complex, that have SBM workers are able to survive those really difficult crisis-driven events. For example, if they become homeless and they've got someone who is actually able to do that advocacy with them, they go with them to access points.

SBM workers supported young people with different housing options depending on their preferences. Where young people's preferences were not considered to be in their interest by workers, they were helped to consider other possibilities, for example:

> Without [my SBM worker], I wouldn't have known about all my funding. I wouldn't be in a proper house at the moment. I'd probably be staying in my Nan's little spare room, which is dust-filled, and falling apart and stacked with mass amounts of stuff that she's storing. Or going from house to house, crashing at people's places or something. Whereas now, I actually have a place to be, I have my own room, I have my own bathroom, there's a kitchen and everything. It makes so much difference because without having one set place, I would have been too stressed to get into school.
>
> (Caine, SBM supported young person)

Two SBM supported young people commented that without access to SBM their post-care trajectories could have been terrible:

> We talked about this the other day. I reckon I could have probably been dead ... Then if I was homeless all the time, and I didn't have any food or shelter or anything, I would be sleeping on the street. I probably would have got pneumonia. I couldn't afford any food or something, I was starved. So yeah, I probably would be dead.
>
> (Jarrod, SBM supported young person)

> Like, pretty much, if I didn't have SBM, I'd probably still be on drugs out in the gutter with nothing, because that's what happens. They [the government Department of Human Services] kick you out a couple of months before you're 18 with nowhere to go, no money, no job, no schooling. And how are you meant to get schooling? How are you meant to get a job? How is someone meant to give you a go when you're on drugs and you have no idea? You have no previous work experience, so you don't have a reference. You know what I mean? Like, how are you meant to go out, and how are you going to get a job when you're on the street? That was half my problem. I've only just been able to get into a course and start looking for work now because I have a stable address.
>
> (Stacey, SBM supported young person)

In contrast, the eight young care leavers not supported by SBM each described pathways from care which included housing instability within six to 18 months of leaving care. These young people required assistance from specialist homelessness services to access emergency accommodation such as refuges, or subsidised and supported accommodation as in transitional and public housing (Purtell et al. 2016).

Specific findings regarding family relationships

Care leavers face independence alone, without the benefit of a safety net of extended family, friends and wider community supports. Yet family members can be a key source of support. Those young people who are able to establish positive relationships with their family in care and/or when transitioning from care are more likely to enjoy a positive self identity and self-confidence, and overall better outcomes. Conversely, those who lack family support may find it harder to establish other relationships (Mendes, Johnson & Moslehuddin 2012).

A clear theme throughout the interviews conducted concerned the importance of family of origin to young people. Many young people spoke about feeling connected to their families, but also described stress and conflict in these relationships, or an inability to rely on family support. Difficulties with family members were common across the SBM supported and non-supported groups.

A number of the young people talked about the process of negotiating those relationships and the work involved in doing so. For some, it took some time for them to get along with family members and form boundaries for themselves along the way. For example, one young man left care to live with his mother which lasted about six months. But then the placement broke down, and he no longer had the safety net of his residential care bed to return to:

> It was heartbreaking that it did because I was enjoying it at home, but it was for the better that I left ... Support with mum now is really good. Like when I did move into the place I'm in we didn't speak for a month because she didn't want me to leave but also she was telling me to leave when she was in anger and when I did up and go and I said that's it, I'm gone and moved in, we didn't speak at all and it was like I had to try and rebuild what we had and it was very hard. It took time to do it. There was times where it felt alright but there was just times where it felt like I just gave up on it.
>
> (Pete, non SBM supported young person)

Interviews with SBM clients suggested family relationships were also important to them in terms of building personal identity:

> I have a better relationship with my mum now. I know more about my heritage and everything and my family, which is good. I find it important to know where you come from and everything, which I didn't really before ... It's really important to know who your family is for so many reasons, I mean there's medical reasons, there's just so much ... With my mum's help I started going on Ancestry.com and building a family tree and everything. It's really interesting to find out things about my family.
>
> (Caine, SBM supported young person).

Many of the non SBM young people interviewed attempted reunification with family members post care because this was their only housing option. But many of these parents or families still had the same mental health or substance abuse problems or disabilities that had provoked child protection interventions in the first place. Consequently, these placements did not offer safe environments for vulnerable young people, and their breakdown resulted in the care leaver becoming homeless. Conversely, the SBM program worked with clients to test family relationships while there was a safety net prior to leaving care, in an attempt to strengthen the positivity and resilience of these relationships.

Young people supported by the SBM program were then able to reside with family post care, with the safety net of SBM support in the event of a relationship breakdown. During their time with family (which also frequently ended due to strained relationships), SBM clients were supported to reflect on their expectations and their experiences of returning to family, to help facilitate more positive outcomes. This occurred whether the young person continued to live with family, remained in regular contact with them, or did not.

To be sure, family reconnection work can be complicated and required more intensive interventions than the SBM program had originally anticipated, including areas in which workers were relatively inexperienced. It may be useful for workers in any roles similar to SBM, to have specific supervision around family reconnection work. Access to secondary consultations with relevant professionals may also be helpful where young people are not willing to be referred to family or relationship counselling themselves.

Discussion

The SBM program targeted a group of vulnerable young people with complex needs who were considered to be at high risk of poor long-term outcomes. Most had exited from residential care, and held few positive family or community connections. Yet, the combination of relationship support and structural assistance provided by SBM seems to have been effective in facilitating positive outcomes for most of the SBM cohort in key areas such as housing, health, education and family relationships. The major elements of the SBM model that contributed to these outcomes included: a long engagement period prior to exiting care that enabled workers to develop a good rapport with young people; ongoing holistic support accompanied by flexible brokerage funding that avoided siloing and assisted young people in their broader family, social and community contexts; effective leaving care planning and strong independent advocacy that encouraged the active participation of young people in key processes; and specific housing support that provided a safety net to avoid the trauma of homelessness.

The outcomes of the SBM program are consistent with international research findings that construct effective transition programs as approximating the ongoing supports offered to non-care young people by their natural parents. Transitions from care need to be based on maturity, rather than chronological age; respect the individual experiences and choices of care leavers and encourage their participation; offer ongoing assistance as required usually till at least 21 years of age; and provide both material resources and emotional/relationship supports. Policy makers need to display the same duty of care to care leavers that they would demand for their own children in terms of facilitating their access to core life opportunities (Beauchamp 2016; Cashmore & Mendes 2015).

Discussion Questions

1. Why are care leavers universally a vulnerable group?
2. How important is it for leaving care practice and policy to be informed by the experiences and knowledge of care leavers? In what ways?
3. Do governments have a responsibility to provide ongoing supports beyond 18 years of age particularly in areas such as housing and education, training and employment? If Yes, in what ways?

References

Australian Institute of Health and Welfare, 2017, Child protection Australia 2015–16, Canberra: AIHW.

Australian Institute of Health and Welfare, 2018, Child protection Australia 2016–17, Canberra: AIHW.

Baidawi, S., 2016, *Continuing care in Australia: An analysis of State and Territory legislation and policy*, Melbourne: Anglicare Victoria and Home Stretch.

Beauchamp, T., 2016, 'Young people transitioning from care in Australia: A critical but neglected area of policy development', in P. Mendes & P. Snow (eds), *Young people transitioning from out-of-home care*, London: Palgrave Macmillan, pp. 265–284.

Berry Street, 2012a, Stand By Me program logic statement, Melbourne: Berry Street.

Berry Street, 2012b, Stand By Me: A Berry Street leaving care preliminary proposal February 2012, Melbourne: Berry Street.

Carr, N. & McAlister, S., 2016, 'The double-bind: Looked after children, care leavers and criminal justice', in P. Mendes & P. Snow (eds), *Young people transitioning from out-of-home care*, London: Palgrave Macmillan, pp. 3–21.

Cashmore, J. & Mendes, P., 2015, 'Children and young people leaving care', in A. Smith (ed.), *Enhancing children's rights: Connecting research, policy and practice*, Basingstoke, UK: Palgrave Macmillan, pp. 140–150.

Community Affairs References Committee, 2015, Out of home care, Canberra: Commonwealth of Australia.

Courtney, M. & Okpych, N., 2017, *Memo from CalYouth: Early findings on the relationship between extended foster care and youths' outcomes at age 19*, Chicago, IL: Chapin Hall, University of Chicago.

Courtney, M. & Hook, J., 2017, 'The potential economic benefits of extending foster care to young adults: Findings from a natural experiment', *Children and Youth Services Review*, vol. 72, pp. 124–132.

Department of Families, Housing, Community Services and Indigenous Affairs, 2010, An outline of National Standards for Out-of-Home Care, Canberra: Australian Government.

Department of Health, 2001, Children (Leaving Care) Act 2000. Regulations and Guidance, London: Department of Health.

Department of Health and Human Services, 2017, Housing assistance to young people transitioning from care, Melbourne: Victorian Government.

Department of Social Services, 2015a, Driving change: Intervening Early, National Framework for Protection Australia's Children 2009–2020, Canberra: Commonwealth of Australia.

Department of Social Services, 2015b, Review of the Transition to Independent Living Allowance (TILA): An analysis of the 1 January 2014 reforms to TILA, Canberra: Department of Social Services.

Dinisman, T. & Zeira, A., 2011, 'The contribution of individual, social support and individual characteristics to perceived readiness to leave care in Israel: An ecological perspective'. *British Journal of Social Work*, vol. 41, pp. 1442–1458.

Harvey, A., McNamara, P., Andrewatha, L. & Luckman, M., 2015, *Out of care, into university: Raising higher education access and achievement of care leavers*, Melbourne: La Trobe University.

Jackson, S. & Cameron, C., 2014, *Improving access to further and higher education for young people in public care*, London: Jessica Kingsley.

Johnson, G., Natalier, K., Mendes, P., Liddiard, M., Thoresen, S., Hollows, A. & Bailey, N., 2010, *Pathways from out of home care*, Melbourne: Australian Housing and Urban Research Institute.

McDonald, S., Ellem, K. & Wilson, J., 2016, 'Supporting young people with an intellectual disability transitioning from out-of-home care to adult life in Queensland, Australia', in P. Mendes & P. Snow (eds), *Young people transitioning from out-of-home care*, London: Palgrave Macmillan, pp. 265–284.

McDowall, J., 2008, *Report card: Transitioning from care*, Sydney: CREATE Foundation.

Matheson, I., 2018, '*Extending care from 18 to 21: Towards an international evidence base*', Paper presented to EUSARF Conference, Porto, 2–5 October.

Mendes, P., Johnson, G. & Moslehuddin, B., 2011, *Young people leaving state out-of-home care*, Melbourne: Australian Scholarly.

Mendes, P., Johnson, G. & Moslehuddin, B., 2012, 'Young people transitioning from out-of-home care and relationships with family of origin: an examination of three recent Australian Studies', *Child Care in Practice*, vol. 18, no. 4, pp. 357–370.

Mendes, P., Pinkerton, J. & Munro, E., 2014, 'Guest Editorial: Young people transitioning from out-of-home care: An issue of social justice', *Australian Social Work*, vol. 67, no.1, pp. 1–4.

Mendes, P., Saunders, B. & Baidawi, S., 2016, *Indigenous care leavers in Victoria*, Melbourne: Monash University.

Mendes, P. & Snow, P., 2016, 'Introduction', in P. Mendes & P. Snow (eds), *Young people transitioning from out-of-home care*, London: Palgrave Macmillan, pp. xxxi–xli.

Mendes, P. & McCurdy, S., 2019, 'Policy and practice supports for young people transitioning from out- of-home care: An analysis of six recent inquiries in Australia', *Journal of Social Work*, vol. 20, no. 5, pp. 599–619.

Mendes, P. & Rogers, J., 2020, 'Young people transitioning from out-of-home care: What are the lessons from extended care programs in the USA and England for Australia?', *British Journal of Social Work*, vol. 50, no. 5, pp. 1513–1530.

Muir, S. & Hand, K., 2018, *Beyond 18: The longitudinal study on leaving care, wave 1 research report*, Melbourne: Australian Institute of Family Studies.

Munro, E., Lushey, C., Maskell-Graham, D. & Ward, H., 2012, *Evaluation of the Staying Put: 18 Plus Family Placement programme: Final report*. Loughborough, UK: Centre for Child and Family Research.

Purtell, J., Mendes, P., Baidawi, S. & Inder, B., 2016, *Evaluation of the Berry Street Stand By Me program: Wraparound support to smooth the transition from out-of-home care*, Melbourne: Monash University Department of Social Work.

Stein M., 2012, *Young people leaving care: Supporting pathways to adulthood*. London: Jessica Kingsley.

Stein, M., 2016, 'Foreword', in P. Mendes & P. Snow (eds), *Young people transitioning from out-of-home care*, London: Palgrave Macmillan pp. v–vii.

Whyte, I., 2011, *Just beginnings: The report of Berry Street's Leaving Care Scoping Project*, Melbourne: Berry Street.

Part 4

Children, parents and carers as stakeholders

Chapter 17

Child protection and child participation

Jan Mason and Tobia Fattore

Introduction

Child protection, as a system of care, and child participation, as a process of involving children in decision making that concerns them, are linked through the codification of both *protection* and *participation*, as principles which apply to the rights of children in the United Nations Convention on the Rights of the Child (UNCRC) of 1989, along with a third principle – that of *provision*. Historically, child protection policy has been a key discourse[1] for the way in which childhood and child–adult relations are structured (Mason 2005). Therefore, the contemporary conjunction of child protection with child participation practices has a significance that extends beyond those children and families whose lives are the focus of child protection policy and practices. This significance was acknowledged by Bardy (2000), who describes the Convention as a 'suggested "contract" between the child and adult generations, as a desired model where children have access to resources, they are protected and they are allowed to participate'.

The focus of this chapter is the conjunction between: the *protection* and *participation* rights of the 'suggested "contract" between child and adult generations'; the tensions inherent in this conjunction when translated into child protection policy; and the potential to mitigate these tensions through examining the role power plays in child participatory practices.

We first analyse the meanings of *protection* and *participation* of children, as codified in the principles in the Convention and their intersection in child protection practices. We then identify different constructions of the child and associated discourses that characterize advocacy for protection and participation of children, with particular attention directed to issues of risk, vulnerability and agency. We then identify some of the practice strategies and issues that are at the centre of discourses relating to children's participation in child protection, taking child protection policy in Australia as an example. We extend beyond conventional notions of participation by framing participation around the concepts of relational participation, advocacy coalitions and deliberative democracy, taking into account the role of power in participation and the relationship between participation and provision in child protection processes.

Children's 'right' to protection

Advocacy for children's right to protection through state intervention can be traced back to the 19th century, to policies framed in terms of the mechanics of governing childhood towards state approved social goals. In contemporary Western society these social goals are framed by the widespread risk, anxiety and ontological insecurity[2] about the future described by Beck (1992). Childhood as a separate life stage, with the notion of 'becoming' central to its social construction, has been a vehicle 'readily available for mobilization around moral panics and the definition of social ills' (Katz 2008: 7). Within this paradigm children, because of their construction as incomplete and becoming adults, are targeted as 'an economic and psychic investment in the future' (Katz 2008: 9–10). Policies to protect vulnerable children are influenced by concerns, not only to prevent harm to children, but also by concerns to ensure that children fulfil their potentials and become skilled and productive workers in the future (Parton 2006: 1–2). In child protection policy and practice the focus on risk of harm to children is framed by an increasing individualization of the child, within a 'profitable' or 'social investment' orientation (see Gilbert, Parton & Skivenes 2011; Lister 2015) that is directed at the child (and society) in the future.

Since the 1970s, in England and other Western countries, children and indeed childhood have increasingly been conceptualized, in public forums, the media and state-initiated inquiries as vulnerable and 'at risk' (see Parton 2006). Constructed as both passive and innocent, children are considered 'unequipped to manage the threats and challenges of the adult world and so they are in need of protection' (Collings & Davis 2008: 183). In statutory child protection practices threats of risk to children are defined in terms of acute and chronic forms of harm and can denote both 'the likelihood of abuse occurring and the likelihood of harm resulting from abuse' in the future (Daniel 2010: 234). In the process by which, as Pinkney notes, for the UK, 'protectionism has become institutionalised, normalised and "taken for granted"' (Pinkney 2013: 274), immaturity and vulnerability, as spelt out in the UNCRC, constitute the rationale for strategies directed at protecting society's future adults, from risk. This concept of vulnerability is articulated in the Preamble of the UNCRC, in terms of child immaturity, thus: 'the child, by reason of his (sic) physical and mental immaturity, needs special safeguards and care, including appropriate legal protection, before as well as after birth'. In Article 19, the response to these needs is defined by the principle of the right to protection from specific harms of physical and emotional violence, neglect and abuse.

Children's 'right' to participation and its significance for children in the protection and care system

Advocacy for child participation generally and for child participation in child protection and care systems specifically, typically constructs children as having agency, as having the capacity to make a difference to their worlds and the worlds of others. In the following discussion we define four broad streams of advocacy for children's right to participate, highlighting the significance of different ideological perspectives for their relevance to child participation in child protection practice, particularly as they relate to concepts of competence, vulnerability and empowerment. We then identify the extent to which these differing ideologies are reflected in the participatory principles in the Convention.

The first stream of advocacy has roots in the longstanding liberalist emphasis on individuals as active participants in their own lives. Its application explicitly to children is traceable to the writings of the 17th-century philosopher John Locke, albeit in a constrained way, as he believed the rights children have can be overridden by parents (Caplan 1997). This stream in its contemporary neo-liberal form is characterised by an emphasis on the 'self' in modernity. The constraints Locke and neo-liberal proponents of child agency place on children as agents, pertain, as Ruddick (2007, p. 514) argues, to a construction of the child, whereby 'the child is a limit condition to the liberal subject: it is, de jure, an impossible subject since, by liberal definition, the child cannot speak for him or herself without adult authorization'. In quoting this statement by Ruddick (2007), Hartung (2011) reminds us that this liberal conceptualization of the child's right to voice, whilst seemingly liberatory continues to confine children 'to a predetermined identity, one dependent upon adults' (p. 90).

More radical roots of advocacy can be seen in the arguments of child liberationists, strong in the 1970s in the United States. Key amongst these advocates was the educationalist, John Holt (1974). He and other child rights advocates argued against the child protectionist or 'caretaker' movement of the era, challenging the appropriateness of aligning age with competence and arguing that children, regardless of age, should be able to participate where interest and knowledge motivates them to do so. Even if derided at the time, such demands contributed an impetus for examining the nature of childhood and children's rights (see Archard 2014; Smith 2014).

A third stream of advocacy, gaining momentum since the 1980s, has been the 'new childhood studies' or 'new sociology of childhood'. Advocates in this stream, through their research, have acknowledged children as agents, while reminding us that children have lives that are important not just in the future, but also in their present (e.g. Alanen 2014; Mayall 2002). In furthering what Alanen describes as the 'normative' intention of contemporary childhood researchers to improve children's social position (p. 5), proponents of these theories have given a legitimacy and authority to the way children are perceived as *agentic* (see Queenerstedt & Queenerstedt 2014). An important element of the structural analysis promoted by these advocates is a focus on empowerment of children which highlights children's struggles to be heard, at both global and local levels (e.g. Ennew 1994; John 1996).

Advocacy by both adults and children, for children as service users, to be heard directly, by practitioners and policymakers in protection and care systems constitutes a fourth stream of advocacy. This stream reflects a movement sometimes spearheaded by children and sometimes in collaboration with adults, whose intent is made explicit by a 15-year-old girl in care who states 'it's my life and I deserve to have a say' (Testro 2006).

The first formal attempt to hear the views of children in the care and protection system directly was the 'Who Cares' conference, conducted by the English National Children's Bureau in 1975. Outcomes of this conference, in which children aged 12–16 talked about their experiences of care, included the production of a book on children's views of care and changes needed to the system and the launch in 1979 of the National Association of Young People in Care. A similar formal opportunity for children to voice their experiences and advocate for change was the 'Young People in Care Speakout' conducted by the NSW Association of Child Caring Agencies (1980), leading to the establishment of the Australian Association of Young People in Care. This association was consolidated with state level 'young people in care' groups in Australia, to form the CREATE Foundation in the early 1990s, whose purpose was 'representing the voices of children and young people with an out-of-home care experience'. The significance of children in care speaking out and being heard in child protection and care practices is summed up by David Hill, writing that children in the protection and care system, 'are the least represented, least protected [sic] and most vulnerable group in our community' (Hill 1996).

CREATE, in defining itself as the '(n)ational consumer body for the voices of children and young people with a care experience', is directly aligning with the broader consumer or service user movement. Oswell (2013) points to the 'often intertwined histories' of children as democratic subjects, actors with a stake in social institutions, and children as consumers (p. 4). Recognition of children as 'consumers' within the child protection and care systems has been described as having 'filtered down [sic]' from adults to children from as early as the 1960s and 1970s (Butler & Williamson 1996) and is supported by arguments that children as 'citizens and service users share the same fundamental rights to participate as others', in decisions about their welfare (Sinclair & Franklin 2000: 1). As managerialism has become more central to child protection decision making, participation influenced by this stream of advocacy has been incorporated into some out-of-home care management systems, such as that of Barnardo's Australia (see Tregeagle & Mason 2008).

The different ideologies and concepts outlined in discussion of the four streams of advocacy can be identified in the participatory-related articles in the Convention, although there is only one instance in the Convention where direct reference is made to child agency – that is, in the phrase, children's '*active* participation' (Article 23, our italics). It is the first clause of Article 12, that supports the Convention being viewed as both the expression of, and impetus for, advocacy for children's agency to be recognized (Quennerstedt 2010), in that it states: 'States Parties shall assure to the child who is capable of forming his or her own views the right to express those views freely in all matters affecting the child'. Advocates for children's rights have argued the symbolic importance of this clause as the first international expression of children's right to have a say (John 1996; Freeman 1995).

The second clause of Article 12 establishes the importance of children being provided with 'the opportunity to be heard in any judicial and administrative proceedings affecting the child'. This is significant in terms of children's direct advocacy to be heard in child protection and care decision making. In contrast, the second part of this clause, where it elaborates on the meaning of the 'capable' child ('the views of the child being given due weight in accordance with the age and maturity of the child'), reflects the liberalist stream of advocacy. As a counterpoint to the first clause, this element of the second clause embeds in the CRC the *vulnerability* discourse. It has the effect of reinforcing childhood as a time of dependency-induced vulnerability and facilitates support for the developmental paradigm's normalization of pre-convention adult–child social relations by maintaining adults' prerogative to govern children through assessments of their maturity, so that adults typically make decisions regarding children's participation in protection contexts based on children's chronological age (Pinkney 2013).

Debates which followed the codification of children's rights in the Convention were initially about the implications of taking children's rights seriously, how to effectively implement them and arguments that ratification would undermine the family, by usurping parents' rights (see Alston & Brennan 1991; Franklin 1995). By 1995 the debates had 'tended to move away from questions about whether children have a right to participate in decision making, to constructing analytical models for children's participation' (Franklin 1995: 14).

Of the various 'models', or typologies of child participation, Roger Hart's 'ladder of children's participation' (Hart 1992) is considered the most significant and influential (John 1996; Hartung 2011). This model, adapted by Hart from Arnstein's (1969) model of adult participation, conceptualizes forms of non-participation and levels of participation on eight separate rungs and, according to Hart (2008), provides professional groups and institutions with clarity in thinking about ways of engaging and working with children. Hart's ladder has been modified through application in the field by other researchers, for example Shier (2001) and Lansdown (2011). Fundamental to these models are attempts to deal with issues of adult–child power, based on assumptions that adults can give power to children to move up the rungs to various levels of social participation, implying that power resides either with children or adults and that children can, once empowered, act autonomously (see Hinton 2008; Hartung 2011). We reframe the concept of child autonomy in child protection processes in a later section of this chapter. In the following discussion we implicitly question the concept of practitioners empowering children in the child protection process, by describing the power relations in which children and practitioners are embedded, according to their social positioning in child protection processes that impact child participation.

The positioning of children and practitioners in child protection practice

Our examination in the following section of the social relations of children and practitioners in child protection practice starts from van Bijleveld, Dedding and Bunders-Aelen's (2015) 'state-of the-art' review of English language studies on children's and young people's participation 'within child welfare and child protection services' (p. 129). These findings indicate that both practitioners and children consider it important that children participate in child protection decision-making forums but experience barriers to this participation. We link these barriers with the structural social relations by which practitioners and children are differently positioned in protection meetings, as a space characterized by relations of power. These power relations are described by Ulvik (2015: 194) as reflecting 'related and binary' social categories of practitioners and children in participative protection processes. Drawing on the work of Ulvik (2015) and of Winter (2010), we identify three contrasting positionings according to which children are marginalized in child protection forums, constructed around age, knowledge and socio-economic inequalities, embedded in what Winter describes as 'taken-for-granted ways of understanding, thinking and doing which are internalized', maintaining practitioners in positions of dominance (p. 192).

The first of the social positionings is that inherent in the binary categories of adult and child, where children and professionals are 'defined by each other's negations and implying an intergenerational relation' (Ulvik 2015). Within this generational relation adults are in a structural position where they generally have more power than children and therefore are able to control and regulate children. Practitioners can assume, by virtue of their adulthood, the right to make decisions to exclude or ignore children's contributions, on the basis of notions that children lack maturity and the ability to understand what is in their own 'best interests' (see GCYP 2008; van Bijleveld, Dedding & Bunders-Aelen 2015). Both these notions bring with them multiple contested meanings. In child protection contexts where more than one practitioner is involved in decision making about a child's interests they sometimes strongly disagree concerning important judgements and decisions, based on information taken into account and biases introduced by the values and experiences of practitioners. For children to be able to trust and feel safe in their structurally subordinated position it is important for them to be able to assert some control or power (Bessell 2015; Fattore, Mason & Watson 2016; Moore, McArthur & Noble-Carr 2015; Sanders & Mace 2006) - a control clearly missing for many children in the participatory process of child protection assessments (see Bessell 2015; Mason & Gibson 2004).

In participating in child protection decisions as in other forums, children are not necessarily wanting to exercise their agency through making 'autonomous' decisions.

Rather, children understand decision making as involving compromise and negotiation. This includes wanting to understand decisions made by adults where they differ from children's preferred options (e.g. Mason & Gibson 2004). There is evidence from Bessell's research (2011) that in instances where children feel they have not been heard in participatory processes, they employ their agency in ways such as that illustrated in the following quote, ' I had to run away before anyone would listen to me ... but (even then) no-one really listened' (p. 498).

The second of the categories in which practitioner and child are 'differently positioned', is that of practitioner 'as helper' in possession of expertise and the child as 'in need of help' (Ulvik 2015: 198–199). In this positioning, the professional worker is accredited with the power of 'expert', a bearer of 'scientific' knowledge (see Freidson 1986: 4–6). As a professional, the worker is accredited with 'expert' power in the use of scientific knowledge (see Freidson 1986: 4–6). Typically, the 'scientific' language of developmentalism, employed by practitioners, has the effect of discounting the child as 'a bearer of experience'. Instead the child is constructed as 'incomplete', in a process of 'becoming' (Katz 2008: 7). The use of developmentalism to discount children's experiential knowledge, is embedded in, for example, assessment frameworks used by practitioners such as the English *Framework for the Assessment of Children in Need and their Families* (see Thomas 2010) and, as a tool can be used to discount children's views as, 'not sensible' or influenced by adults in their lives (Archard & Skivenes 2009).

A third positioning can be identified as overlaying intergenerational relations and 'expert adult–unknowing child' relations. This is a positioning based on what are typically differences in socio-economic and cultural backgrounds between practitioners and children (and parents) in child protection participatory processes. In this positioning, practitioners' 'knowledge of the child' is maintained in interactions with children and their parents, in forums such as children-in-care review meetings, through the construction of these children as bearing 'inscribed in their habitus the instability of the living conditions of their family, that of the sub-proletariat doomed to insecurity in their conditions of employment, housing, and thereby of existence' (Winter 2010: 194). While there has been strong ongoing quantitative evidence on the association between socio-economic disadvantage and child protection interventions (e.g. Doidge et al. 2017; Pelton 1978), as Pelton found in his 1978 research, the myth of 'classlessness' of child abuse and neglect 'persists not on the basis of evidence or logic, but because it serves certain professional and political interests' (p. 616). While some Australian research does not support the findings of Morris et al.'s recent English research, in this research there was evidence of the persistence of the link between socio-economic circumstances and decision making in child protection interventions. From their interviews with social workers, Morris and colleagues conclude that amongst social workers, there is a pervasive 'notion of an underclass that social work must regulate and persuade into respectability' (Morris et al. 2018: 370). While workers in interviews could recognize the link between poverty and risk of harm, when responding within the organizational culture in which they practice, their focus was on 'managing individual risk detached from socio-economic conditions' (p. 370).

The gulf, between the contexts of social workers' lives and that of children subject to child protection processes is reflected in assumptions workers make about the lack of credibility of children considered vulnerable to poor parenting. Workers reject children's contributions on, for example, the basis that children are 'ignorant of alternative ways of living' (Archard & Skivenes 2009: 398). Bessell (2015) draws attention to the way socio-economic status of children and their families combines with professionals' use of the concepts of children as 'vulnerable' or 'disadvantaged' to exclude or marginalize their contributions.

The social positioning of practitioners and children in child protection processes constitutes the framework in which the child 'participation principle' is implemented following its codification in legislation in those countries, such as Australia and other signatories to the UN Convention.

The participation principle in child protection processes – some Australian examples

Various Australian state jurisdictions enshrine participation of children and their families in child protection processes, whether in legislation, policy directives or practice guidelines. This is reflected in the first supporting outcome of the *National Framework for Protecting Australia's Children 2009–2020* (COAG 2009): that 'Children live in safe and supportive families and communities', and has as an essential dimension for achieving this outcome that 'children's right to participate in decisions that affect them is a key signal of valuing and supporting children' (p. 15).

In New South Wales, the Children and Young Persons (Care and Protection) Act 1998 has participation as one of its foundational principles. This principle extends to all aspects of the child protection process, from the point of first report to the point a young person leaves care, and to decisions made by anyone who exercises functions under the Act. Section 10 of the Act outlines the participation principle and specifies the duty of relevant agencies to provide children with adequate and appropriate information, the opportunity to express their views and to respond to a decision, and any assistance necessary to help them express their views. In circumstances where caseworkers are required to determine the intervention required, provisions in legislation and best practice guidelines specify that workers need to include children and families in decision making. For example, the *NSW Care and Protection Practice Standards* (NSW FaCS 2014) include collaboration as an essential practice standard. The Victorian Department of Human Services *Best Interests Case Practice Model* (Vic DHS 2012) instructs workers on how to engage with families, build partnerships with families and empower children and families.

Child protection processes include several distinct stages. Where an assessment is made that intervention is required, it can take a variety of forms, including provision of services to the family, supervision and monitoring of the family by a child protection authority or removal of the child from their family, on a temporary or permanent basis, with the child being placed in some alternative care arrangement. Once a decision has been made as to the intervention required, many families and children experience an ongoing interaction with the statutory child protection system, particularly where the child is placed in alternate care on a short- or long-term basis. As well as workers representing the statutory child protection agency, non-government organizations providing alternate care and/or other child protective services to the child or family are also frequently involved.

When we consider children's involvement in the child protection system we need to consider the way participation functions across these different stages or phases of the child protection system, including the kinds of participation possible and the purpose of children's participation. It is therefore helpful to differentiate modes of participation around different phases of the child protection system. We suggest a typology that relates techniques of participation with different but related purposes within the child protection system. This typology has three levels:

- At the level of direct practice with children, participation revolves around *relational participation*
- At the level of ongoing support and service provision, participation must also involve practices of *advocacy coalition building*
- At the level of policymaking and service development, participation revolves around practices of *deliberative democracy* that involve legitimate representative groups.

Relational participation

Most participation is envisaged around direct practice with individual children involved in different stages of the child protection process. In studies exploring children's experiences of participation in these child protection processes, the personal relationship between children and workers tasked with their care is frequently noted as the key facilitator for participation. van Bijleveld, Dedding and Bunders-Aelen (2015), in reviewing the research on children's participation in child protection, find that relational qualities were cited by children as being most important to them. In direct service roles, therefore, participation strategies rely on what can be described as the intrinsic qualities of the worker, whether ascribed or developed through professional training, used to develop meaningful relationships with children. We can describe this first kind of participation as involving *relational participation*. The concept of relational participation builds on Martha Fineman's work on vulnerability (Fineman 2013). Fineman argues that our dependence on the care of others, and therefore our vulnerability, is an inevitable aspect of being embodied beings. Recognizing the universality of our embodied vulnerability provides the possibility for conceiving autonomy as relational rather than individualized. MacKenzie (2013) extends upon this by arguing that autonomy requires relational skills and capacities.

Common relational qualities identified in the research that support children's participation in child protection include workers taking the time to get to know the child, having conversations, listening, learning, understanding, responding and being open to the child. These workers strive to provide appropriate choices to children, but always discuss the range of possible options and the implications of decisions with children as part of the decision-making process (Bell 2002; Bessell 2011; Jobe & Gorin 2013; Leeson 2007). Rather than engaging through formal meetings, workers make the time to engage in conversations with children over time in informal settings, in which children can feel comfortable sharing their thoughts, feelings and concerns (Bessell 2015; Testro 2006). In so doing, workers attempt to reduce power imbalances implicit in the positioning of adults and children. These attributes are often labelled informal mechanisms for participation. However, a distinction between formal and informal participation can mislead the significance of these attributes for formal processes.

Relational participation in practice: case planning processes

Case planning meetings are a mechanism through which the importance of relational participation as a basis for children's participation in child protection is demonstrated

(CREATE Foundation 2001; Sanders & Mace 2006). Case planning processes are often initiated by the statutory child protection agency or the service responsible for organizing supports for children and families. Specific examples that integrate service user participation include the Looking After Children (LAC) and Supporting Children and Responding to Families (SCARF) frameworks.

Some research indicates that case planning processes have improved possibilities for participation, for example by providing a channel through which regular communication with and accountability from workers occurs (Fernandez 2007; Kufeldt et al. 2006; Tregeagle & Mason 2008). However, for case planning processes to be successful as a participatory mechanism, they need to be characterized by the qualities that support relational participation for children as described previously. van Bijleveld, Deddingand Bunders-Aelen (2015) found that

> [f]or children, a good relationship is important to create a situation in which they feel free to say what they want and to feel that they are taken seriously. ... Children see participation as the possibility to have a say in the decisions that are important to them, not the ones chosen by the social workers. Furthermore, they want to be listened to and to feel that they are taken seriously.
>
> (pp. 136–137)

Workers commonly viewed children's participation as a means for information-gathering, as assessing the capacity of the child to provide useful information, and as a strategy to obtain compliance for decisions made by workers (Archard & Skivenes 2009; Vis & Thomas 2009).

Advocacy coalitions

The relatively benevolent way relational participation is conceived doesn't adequately accommodate how power is asserted through relationships or made invisible through the taken-for-granted ways in which institutions operate to position practitioners and children. This is especially pertinent to child protection where there are competing interests and structured power imbalances between actors that are written into the statute. Usually, decisions pertaining to the child are made by a number of adults, many of whom the child has never met. While children's best interests are at the core of child protection work, in all child protection stages, adults are the key gatekeepers of resources and it is adults who determine whether and in what ways children participate.

Recognition of the importance of resolving the interests of different stakeholders is given effect in the NSW child protection legislation, through methods of dispute resolution before a case reaches the stage of a hearing. Section 65 of the Children's Care and Protection Act states that the purpose of preliminary conferences includes identifying areas of disagreement and dispute between parties and the best ways of resolving issues in dispute (s. 65a-c). Additionally, legal proceedings are clearly an area where different interests are brought into negotiation. Section 99 of the Act provides that a legal representative may be appointed to the child in Children's Court proceedings and that the lawyer will act on the instruction of the child.

While, ideally, all parties involved in child protection processes will develop a shared understanding of the aims and objectives of the processes, the reality is that this is difficult to achieve and aims and objectives will need to be negotiated between the parties (D'Cruz & Stagnitti 2008; Healy & Meagher 2007). For participation strategies to be meaningful, we need to consider how they can be deployed strategically to serve the interests of children at the centre of child protection processes, characterized by competing interests, conflicting problem definitions and significant inequality in terms of power. If we consider participation as part of a process involving a variety of stakeholders, many of whom are responsible for providing ongoing support to children and families, then the purpose of participation is to inform processes through which a range of resources (often through case management and monitoring) can be brought together to support children and their families. Therefore, there is often a need to build coalitions of diverse interests, including those of the child, their siblings, their biological parents, other carers and critically those of the variety of service providers working with the child – what we can describe as advocacy coalitions.

This perspective draws from the Advocacy Coalition Framework developed by Sabatier and Jenkins-Smith (Sabatier 1988; Sabatier & Jenkins-Smith 1993). They argue that policymaking involves a sub-system of actors (policy researchers, advocates and lobbyists, decision makers, journalists and so on) who advocate their own conception of policy problems, explanations of causes and preferred solutions. Coalitions of actors are formed and disbanded over time. This network approach highlights the importance of building coalitions, often representing diverse interests, to meet desired outcomes in pragmatic ways.

We can usefully apply this framework to child protection practice, by understanding participation, not only as working directly with the child, but also as about building coalitions amongst stakeholders, and developing alliances which advocate for children's needs within the context of their care requirements. We can see advocacy coalitions developed between services through memorandums of understanding, interagency guidelines for child protection practice and through informal collaborations. These service level collaborations may endure as an ongoing framework for alliances. By contrast, from the perspective of the child and the family, the value of the service system resides in the degree to which their involvement in the coalition meets their needs. We can therefore evaluate the degree to which coalitions are working effectively by assessing the extent that *resources held in one part of the coalition are used to meet the needs of other coalition members*, namely children and families.

Several features of effective advocacy coalitions work in the interests of the child. These include:

Respectful engagement: Healy and Darlington (2009) argue that respect is a practitioner's ability to demonstrate to the child and their family that knowledge and experience from differing perspectives are valued and will contribute to decision making.

Information sharing: Key to decision making is the degree to which respective parties can access relevant information, deem what information is relevant to discussion, define what the problem parameters are and control information flow. Having greater information gives parties significant advantage in negotiations, and deeming what counts as relevant knowledge is a key way in which power is deployed. For example, children frequently describe having inadequate information about what was going to happen to them (Bessell 2011).

Transparency: Related to information sharing is transparency, requiring all parties to be clear about the purpose of the child protection intervention. Transparency builds trust and reduces misunderstandings between the coalition actors and helps avoid creating unrealistic expectations about what decisions can be made and what outcomes can be delivered.

Accountability: Accountability places an obligation on decision makers to take responsibility for their actions. This ensures that decisions agreed upon are followed through. Much of the research has demonstrated the far too common experience of workers acting on behalf of either the statutory or designated care agency, promising outcomes that are not delivered, whether that be a placement decision or the provision of some kind of resource.

Substantive outcomes: This relates to whether children feel they are contributing to decisions on issues considered of importance to them. An effective advocacy coalition works towards identifying effective outcomes that all parties can live with. In the context of child participation, this means that the child's interests must be represented by an agent with the authority to obtain resources needed by the child.

Advocacy coalitions in practice: family group conferences

Family group conferences are a mechanism that could be used for this kind of coalition building. They are used as a means of formally involving families in decision making about the protection and care of their children, and also as a tool through which case management can occur. All Australian states and territories have policy directives aimed at promoting family participation in child protection matters, and family group conferences are a common practice to facilitate family participation in child protection (Dillon, Greenon & Hills 2016; Polkki, Vornanen & Pursiainen 2012; Sanders & Mace 2006; Vis & Thomas 2009). These conferences often include the professionals involved with the family (caseworkers, counsellors, doctors, refuge workers, etc.). Increasingly, it is an expectation that children will participate in some way in these meetings, to ensure that they remain at the centre of case planning (for example, see the Queensland Child Safety practice Manual 2017).

A specific example is Aboriginal Care Circles that share some elements of Family Group Conferences but extend the list of participants to include community members, not just close kinship members (Best 2011). The involvement of the community members, along with family members and the child, means relevant community-based information can be included in the decision-making processes and that local resources and context-specific factors can be taken into account.

Deliberative democracy

A range of participatory mechanisms have been developed to involve children in decision making around more systemic issues in child protection, such as operations and management, service planning, policy and legislation development. These include consultation strategies, use of advisory or reference groups, networks of groups (involving a network of strategically linked groups of children meeting regularly with a support worker), parallel structures (a youth body that runs alongside adult-led decision-making processes), and the inclusion of children on committees (Testro 2006).

This literature rarely addresses the fundamentally political nature of policy development, perhaps assuming that if rigorous mechanisms are established for children's participation, then their involvement will automatically have some effect. Questions regarding the strategic use of children's participation at this level, of the way in which representation may be manipulated, the role which the contest of ideas plays in policy formation and the competing imperatives of the state in implementing change, are rarely discussed.

We would suggest that, when considering the participation of children in service development and policymaking in child protection, a framework that considers policymaking as involving deliberative democracy might be suitable, because it frames children's participation as part of a participatory political process based on deliberation between interested parties. This approach is based on work of Frank Fischer and John Dryzek, inspired by the critical theory of Jurgen Habermas (Dryzek 1990; Fischer 2003). Deliberative democracy is based on the ideal of democratic association through free public argument between citizens. For a political decision to be legitimate it requires the right of all to participate in deliberation. Decisions are legitimate when they arise out of a deliberative process where all who wish to participate can do so (Habermas 1984).

Habermas' work is important because he suggests that we can maintain communicative relationships that are non-instrumental and non-objectifying. Evidence should be used to create shared understandings of the issues and policymakers have a role of being deliberative practitioners, who facilitate dialogue within a value framework that promotes social equity. This process-oriented approach also has the potential to expand the range of issues deemed relevant for deliberation. This is because Habermas' theory broadens the meaning of participation from conventional politics, which takes place in narrowly defined arenas, to social and cultural spheres as well, so that children can express themselves politically in a variety of local and organizational settings, and opens up the range of topics which children can influence beyond the trivial, including local area service planning; service development, service organization (such as staff recruitment, developing resources for carers and staff); service review, monitoring and evaluation; policy and legislative development and evaluation.

The problem facing policy practitioners in implementing this approach is the continued existence of systemic power inequalities that stand in the way of collaborative processes. For deliberative processes to be participatory for children, requires that the skills needed to facilitate relational participation and those that characterize effective building of advocacy coalitions (respectful engagement, information sharing, transparency, accountability and meeting substantive outcomes) also characterize the deliberative process. These features would contribute to making the processes more child-oriented, so that tokenism is avoided.

In addition to these criteria, we would also add an additional requirement, that *legitimacy* is needed for participatory processes at this high level to be meaningful. One of the dangers of children's involvement in policy and service design is that they may be co-opted into the process and their involvement used to justify decisions that have already been made. For example, Australian governments have relied on the involvement of CREATE, which represents the interests of children in care, as the main means of hearing from children at this level of institutional decision making. This sole reliance leaves out the perspectives of children involved in child protection processes who have not been placed in care. Other modes of representation are required in this case, or alternatively the ambit of representation for peak groups needs to be expanded.

This means legitimate advocacy groups must drive policy agendas and be involved in policymaking processes. It is important to note that peak representative groups must constantly work to maintain their legitimacy, by showing how they have collected evidence about their constituent members' interests. Through strategies of consultation, advocacy and resource provision, peak bodies can legitimately claim that their work is based on a unique kind of expertise to represent children in deliberative processes – an *expertise based on the lived experience of being a child or young person involved in child protection.*

Deliberative democracy in practice: Co-production in child protection

An example of deliberative democracy in practice is exemplified in co-production of human services. Building on well-established principles of community development, co-production involves the delivery of public services in an equal and reciprocal relationship between professionals and service-users. It is an approach that recognizes that effective service delivery relies as much on the knowledge assets and efforts of service-users, as it does the expertise of professional providers.

Recognition of the range of skills that exist within a community is captured by the concept of the core economy, which focuses on the resources embedded in people's everyday lives – such as their time, local knowledge, skills and experience. Effective human service work utilizes the range of skills in this core economy. Professionals and service-users come together in an interdependent relationship, recognizing all are vital for effective service delivery. Service development involves engagement with peer and personal networks, as well as professional networks, to transfer knowledge and support change. Professionals facilitate change rather than primarily provide services. Rather than seeing children and families as passive recipients of child protection processes, they are potential 'knowledge experts' responsible for the co-design and delivery of services and involved in decision making.

In concluding this section we agree with Bessell who, in talking with children in out-of-home care, concluded that 'children and young people want respectful, supportive, and—crucially—ongoing relationships with the adults in their lives, including adult professionals' (Bessell 2015: 28–29). However, we also argue that there is a fundamental mismatch in the way participation is understood – as the capacity of individual children to participate in decision-making processes – and other modes of political practice which are fundamental to the operation of child protection processes at the *service* and *policy* levels and also need to be taken into account.

Conclusion

In questioning whether the conjunction of child protection and child participation is a 'risky or emancipatory conjunction' we are reflecting on the tensions which become evident in analysing the meanings of child protection and participation and discussing some of the issues that frame the implementation of these concepts. Our analysis highlights that the riskiness experienced by practitioners and children in implementing the participation principle in child protection processes involves power inequalities and organizational pressures. These contribute to a wariness by both practitioners and children towards engagement in participatory processes. Practitioners, positioned to dominate child protection decision making, implement the policy goal of protecting children as investments, not just from harm but from the implications this harm has for future adult productivity. Children from their position of limited power are often wary of, or resist, participating when they lack trust in adults they do not know, as well as of the outcomes of their engagement in the protection process.

At the same time, children and their adult collaborators, including some practitioners, continue to advocate for children participating in decision making about their lives, as underlined by official statements on the participation principle, its endorsement in legislation and in various mechanisms operating as part of child protection decision making. Our discussion of different modes of participation highlights the importance in moving towards potentially emancipatory implementation of the child participation principle in child protection processes through acknowledging modes of political practice, beyond that at the level of individual child participation, to include service- and policy-level practices. The options we have outlined for their potential contribution to improving child protection outcomes, have significance for the way they reverberate discursively with ongoing changes in child–adult relations in society, more generally.

Case study

Five children from the one Aboriginal family come into care. The children have the same mother but two different fathers. They are aged 3, 4, 6, 8 and 14. There are concerns that the 4- and 6-year-olds may have suffered neurological damage associated with foetal alcohol syndrome. Practitioners were asked to intervene in the family and remove the children, on the basis of long-term neglect of the children and emotional abuse they were experiencing due to an escalation of the domestic violence the mother was subject to, and which the children were witnessing. There also tend to be a number of male visitors on whom the mother relies for financial assistance, even though some of them are abusive to her.

The children are placed initially, while decisions are being made about their longer-term care, with two different families, the three youngest with one family and the older children with another. The younger children are with Aboriginal kin, and the two oldest with a non-Aboriginal foster carer in the city. They are confused about what is happening to them, the 4-year-old wants to be with the 14-year-old and the two other young children want to be with the 12-year-old. Most of all, all except the oldest want to be with their mother.

Two different agencies are involved with the temporary placement of these children. The first an Aboriginal agency, the second a non-Aboriginal agency because of the problems the Aboriginal agency was having in placing the two older children. Because of the heavy workload in their geographical area, at the time of entry to care it was not possible to make alternative arrangements.

Case study: Reflective questions

- Describe how you think the principles of protection and participation apply in the strategies you would employ to make longer-term arrangements for the children?
- How would the provisions principle have any relevance?
- Considering the participation strategies we have outlined in this chapter, what organizational obstacles do you think you might confront in this process?
- How would you work within the constraints these impose?

Notes

1 Discourse refers to both conversation and ways of constituting knowledge which frame social practices, subjectivity and power as articulated in the work of Michel Foucault (for example Foucault 1977).
2 Insecurity that connects with the very essence of one's being.

References

Alanen, L., 2014, 'Childhood and intergenerationality: Toward an intergenerational perspective on child well-being', in A. Ben-Arieh, F. Casas, I. Frønes & J.E. Korbin (eds), *Handbook of child well-being: Theories, methods and policies in global perspective*, Dordrecht: Springer.

Alston, P. & Brennan, G., (eds), 1991, *The UN Children's Convention and Australia*. Canberra: ANU Centre for International and Public Law.

Arnstein, S., 1969, 'A ladder of citizen participation', *Journal of the American Planning. Association*, vol. 35, no. 4, pp. 216–224.

Archard, D., 2014, *Children: Rights and childhood*, Routledge: London.

Archard, D. & Skivenes, M., 2009, 'Hearing the child', *Child & Family Social Work*, vol. 14 no. 4, pp. 391–399.

Bardy, M., 2000, 'The three P's of children's rights: Provision, protection and participation' CYC-Online. *eJournal of the International Child and Youth Care Network (CYC-net)* Issue 16. May 2000.

Beck, U., 1992, *Risk society: Towards a new modernity*, London: Sage.

Bell, M., 2002, 'Promoting children's rights through the use of relationship', *Child & Family Social Work*, vol. 7, no. 1, pp. 1–11.

Bessell, S., 2011, 'Participation in decision-making in out-of-home care in Australia: What do young people say?', *Children and Youth Services Review*, vol. 33, no. 4, pp. 496–501.

Bessell, S., 2015, 'Inclusive and respectful relationships as the basis for child inclusive policies and practice: The experience of children in out-of-home care in Australia', in T. Gal & B. Duramy (eds) *International perspectives and empirical findings on child participation: From social exclusion to child-inclusive policies*, Oxford: Oxford University Press.

Best, R., 2011, *Aboriginal Care Circles: Putting principles into practice*, Paper presented to the Australasian Institute of Judicial Administration Conference on Child Protection in Australia & New Zealand5–7 May 2011, Brisbane.

Butler, I. & Williamson, H., 1996, '"Safe"? Involving children in child protection', in I. Butler, & I. Shaw (eds), *A case of neglect? Children's experiences and the sociology of childhood*, London: Routledge, pp. 37–55.

Caplan, B., 1997, *Philosophical notes no. 45*, London: Libertarian Alliance.

Collings, S. & Davies, L., 2008, ' "For the sake of the children": Making sense of children and childhood in the context of child protection', *Journal of Social Work Practice*, vol. 22, no. 2, pp. 181–193.

Council of Australian Governments, 2009, *Protecting children is everyone's business: National Framework for Protecting Australia's Children 2009–2020*, Canberra: Commonwealth of Australia.

CREATE Foundation, 2001, Participation in Case Planning Processes: A consultation with children and young people in care about their experience in decision making, Victoria: Department of Human Services.

Daniel, B., 2010, 'Concepts of adversity, risk, vulnerability and resilience: A discussion in the context of the "Child Protection System"', *Social Policy & Society*, vol. 9, no. 2, pp. 231–241.

D'Cruz, H. & Stagnitti, K. 2008, 'Reconstructing child welfare through participatory and child-centred professional practice: A conceptual approach', *Child & Family Social Work*, vol. 14, pp. 156–165.
Dillon, J., Greenop, D. & Hills, M., 2016, 'Participation in child protection: A small-scale qualitative study', *Qualitative Social Work*, vol. 15, no. 1, pp. 70–85.
Doidge J., Higgins, D., Delfabbro, P. & Segal, L., 2017, 'Neglect risk factors for child maltreatment in an Australian population-based birth cohort', *Child Abuse and Neglect*, vol. 64, pp. 47–60.
Dryzek, J.S., 1990, *Discursive democracy: Politics, policy, and political science*, Cambridge: Cambridge University Press.
Ennew, J., 1994, 'Time for children or time for adults?', in J. Qvortrup et al. (eds), *Childhood matters: Social theory, practice and politics.*, Aldershot, Avebury Press, pp. 125–144.
Fattore, T., Mason, J. & Watson, E., 2016, *Children's understandings of well-being: towards a child standpoint*. Dordrecht: Springer.
Fernandez, E., 2007, 'Supporting children and responding to families: Capturing the evidence on family support', *Children & Youth Services Review*, vol. 29, no. 10, pp. 1368–1394.
Fineman, M.A., 2013, 'Equality, autonomy and the vulnerable subject in law and politics', in M.A. Fineman & A. Grear (eds), *Vulnerability: Reflections on a new ethical foundation for law and politics*, Ashgate, UK: Farnham, pp. 13–27.
Fischer, F., 2003, *Reframing public policy: Discursive politics and deliberative practices*, Oxford: Oxford University Press.
Foucault, M., 1977, *Discipline and punish: The birth of the prison*, New York: Pantheon Books.
Franklin B., 1995, 'The case for children's rights: A progress report', in B. Franklin (ed.), *The handbook of children's rights: Comparative policy and practice*, London: Routledge, pp. 3–22.
Freeman, M., 1995, 'Children's rights in a land of rites', in B. Franklin (ed.), *The handbook of children's rights: Comparative policy and practice*, London: Routledge, pp. 70–88.
Freidson, E., 1986, *Professional power*. Chicago, IL: University of Chicago.
Guardian for Children and Young People (GCYP), 2008, Participation of children and young people in decisions made about their care: A literature review [Unpublished manuscript]. Adelaide: Government of South Australia.
Gilbert, N., Parton, N. & Skivenes, M., 2011, *Child protection systems: International trends and orientations*, Oxford: Oxford University Press.
Habermas, J., 1984, *Theory of communicative action, volume one: Reason and the rationalization of society*, Boston, MA: Beacon.
Hart, R., 1992, *Children's participation: From tokenism to citizenship*, Florence: Innocenti Research Centre.
Hart, R., 2008, 'Stepping back from "The Ladder": Reflections on a model of participatory work with children', in A. Reid, B. Bruun Jensen, J. Nikel & V. Simovska (eds), *Participation and learning*, Dordrecht: Springer, pp. 19–31.
Hartung, C., 2011, Governing the 'agentic' child citizen: A poststructural analysis of children's participation, Doctor of Philosophy thesis. University of Wollongong.
Healy, K. & Darlington, D., 2009, 'Service user participation in diverse child protection contexts: principles for practice', *Child & Family Social Work*, vol. 14, pp. 420–430.
Healy, K. & Meagher, G., 2007, 'Social workers' preparation for child protection: revisiting the question of specialization', *Australian Social Work*, vol. 60, pp. 321–335.
Hill, D., 1996, 'Foreword', in J. Owen (ed.), *Every childhood lasts a lifetime*, Brisbane: Association of Children and Young People.
Hinton, R., 2008, 'Children's participation and good governance: Limitation of the theoretical literature', *International Journal of Children's Rights*, vol. 16, pp. 285–300.
Holt, J., 1974, *Escape from childhood*, Boston, MA: E.P. Dutton.

Jobe, A. & Gorin, S., 2013, '"If kids don't feel safe they don't do anything": Young people's views on seeking and receiving help from Children's Social Care Services in England', *Child & Family Social Work*, vol. 18, no. 4, pp. 429–438.
John, M. (ed.), 1996, *Children in charge: The child's right to a fair hearing*, London: Jessica Kingsley.
Katz, C., 2008, *Childhood as spectacle: Relays of anxiety and the reconfiguration of the child*, New York: City University of New York.
Kufeldt, K., McGilligan, L., Klein, R. & Rideout, S., 2006, 'The Looking After Children assessment process: Promoting resilient children and resilient workers', *Families in Society*, vol. 87, pp. 565–574.
Lansdown, G., 2011, *Every child's to be heard: A resource guide on the UN Committee on the Rights of the Child. General comment No.12*, London: Save the Children and UNICEF.
Leeson, C., 2007, 'My life in care: experiences of nonparticipation in decision-making processes', *Child & Family Social Work*, vol. 12, no. 3, pp. 268–277.
Lister, R., 2015, 'Investing in children and childhood: A new welfare policy paradigm and its implications', in *Childhood: Changing contexts, comparative social research*, Bingley, UK: Emerald Group Publishing, pp. 383–408.
Mackenzie, C., 2013, 'The Importance of Relational Autonomy and Capabilities for an Ethics of Vulnerability', in C. Mackenzie, W. Rogers & S. Dodds (eds), *Vulnerability: New essays in ethics and feminist philosophy*, Oxford: Oxford University Press, pp. 33–59.
Mason, J., 2005, 'Child protection policy and the construction of childhood', in J. Mason & T. Fattore (eds), *Children taken seriously: In theory, policy and practice*, London: Jessica Kingsley.
Mason, J. & Gibson, C., 2004, The needs of children in care: A report on a research project. Developing a model of out-of-home care to meet the needs of individual children, through participatory research. North Parramatta, NSW: Uniting Care Burnside, and Social Justice and Social Change Research Centre, University of Western Sydney.
Mayall, B., 2002, *Towards a sociology for childhood: Thinking from children's lives*, Buckingham, UK: Open University Press.
Moore, T., McArthur, M. & Noble-Carr, D., 2015, *Taking us seriously: Children and young people talk about safety and institutional responses to their safety concerns*. Melbourne: Institute of Child Protection Studies, Australian Catholic University.
Morris, K., Mason, W., Bywaters, P., Featherstone, B., Daniel, B., Brady, B., Bunting, L., Hooper, J., Mirza, N., Scourfield, J. & Webb, C., 2018, 'Social work, poverty, and child welfare interventions', *Child & Family Social Work*, vol. 23, pp. 364–372.
NSW Department of Family and Community Services, 2014, *Care and protection practice standards*, Sydney: Office of the Senior Practitioner.
Oswell, D., 2013, *The agency of children: From family to global*, Cambridge, UK: Cambridge University Press.
Parton, N., 2006, *Safeguarding childhood: Early intervention and surveillance in a late modern society*, Basingstoke, UK: Palgrave Macmillan.
Pelton, L., 1978, 'Child abuse and neglect: The myth of classlessness', *American Journal of Orthopsychiatry*, vol. 48, no. 4, pp. 608–617.
Pinkney, S., 2013, 'Trust relationships between children, social welfare professionals and the organisations of welfare', in H. Warming (ed.), *Participation, citizenship and trust in children's lives: Studies in childhood and youth*, Basingstoke, UK: Palgrave Macmillan, pp. 93–113.
Polkki, P., Vornanen, R. & Pursiainen, M., 2012, 'Children's participation in child-protection processes as experienced by foster children and social workers', *Child Care in Practice*, vol. 18, no. 2, pp. 107–125.
Queensland Department of Child Safety, Youth and Women, 2017, *Child safety practice manual*, Brisbane: Queensland Department of Child Safety, Youth and Women.

Quennerstedt, A., 2010, 'Children, but not really humans? Critical reflections on the hampering effect of the "3 p's"', *International Journal of Children's Rights*, vol. 18, no. 4, pp. 619–635.

Quennerstedt, A. & Quennerstedt, M., 2014, 'Researching children's rights in education: sociology of childhood encountering educational theory', *British Journal of Sociology of Education*, vol. 35, no. 1, pp. 115–132.

Ruddick, S., 2007, 'At the Horizons of the Subject: Neo-liberalism, neo-conservatism and the rights of the child Part One: From 'knowing' fetus to 'confused' child', *Gender Place and Culture*, vol. 14, no. 5, pp. 513–527.

Sabatier, P., 1988, 'An advocacy coalition framework of policy change and the role of policy-oriented learning therein', *Policy Sciences*, vol. 21, no. 2/3, pp. 129–168.

Sabatier, P. & Jenkins-Smith H. (eds), 1993, *Policy change and learning: An advocacy coalition approach*, Boulder, CO: Westview Press.

Sanders, R. & Mace, S., 2006, 'Agency policy and the participation of children and young people in the child protection process', Child Abuse Review, vol. 15, pp. 89–109.

Shier, H., 2001, 'Pathways to participation: Openings, opportunities and obligations, a new model for enhancing children's participation in decision-making, in line with Article12.1 of the United Nations Convention on the Rights of the Child', *Children & Society*, vol. 15, pp. 107–117.

Sinclair, R., & Franklin, A., 2000, 'Quality protects. Research briefing 3: Young people's participation', London: Department of Health, Research in Practice and Making Research Count.

Smith, K., 2014, *The government of childhood: Discourse, power and subjectivity*, Basingstoke, UK: Palgrave Macmillan.

Testro, P., 2006, *Listening, hearing and acting: Approaches to the participation of children and young people in decision making – a review of the literature*, Brisbane: Queensland Government Department of Child Safety.

Thomas, J., 2010, Re-Constructing Children's Identities: Social work knowledge and practice in the assessment of children's identities [Doctoral dissertation], Retrieved from Proquest Dissertations and Theses Database (UMI No. U585453).

Tregeagle, S. & Mason, J., 2008, 'Service user experience of participation in child welfare case management', *Child & Family Social Work*, vol. 13, pp. 391–401.

Ulvik, O.S., 2015, 'Talking with children: Professional conversations in a participation perspective', *Qualitative Social Work*, vol. 14, no. 2, pp. 193–208.

UN Committee on the Rights of the Child, 2009, General Comment No. 12 The Right of the Child to be Heard, Geneva: UN Committee on the Rights of the Child.

van Bijleveld, G.G., Dedding, C.W.M. & Bunders-Aelen, J.F.G., 2015, 'Children's and young people's participation within child welfare and child protection services: A state-of-the-art review', *Child & Family Social Work*, vol. 20, pp. 129–138.

Victorian Department of Human Services, 2012, *Best interests case practice model*, Melbourne: Victorian Government Department of Human Services.

Vis, S.A. & Thomas, N., 2009, 'Beyond talking – children's participation in Norwegian care and protection cases', *European Journal of Social Work*, vol. 12, no. 2, pp. 155–168.

Winter, K., 2010, 'The perspectives of young children in care about their circumstances and implications for social work practice', *Child & Family Social Work*, vol. 15, pp. 186–195.

Chapter 18

The right of Aboriginal and Torres Strait Islander children and families to effective child protection services

Clare Tilbury and Natalie Lewis

Acknowledgement: We wish to acknowledge contributions to the development of ideas presented in this chapter from colleagues at SNAICC – National Voice for our Children and the Family Matters campaign – Strong communities. Strong culture. Stronger children.

Introduction

Child welfare inequality occurs 'when children and/or their parents face unequal chances, experiences or outcomes of involvement with child welfare services that are systematically associated with structural social dis/advantage and are unjust and avoidable' (Bywaters et al. 2015: 100). This describes exactly the situation of Aboriginal and Torres Strait Islander children and families in Australia, who are disadvantaged on all social indexes of economic development, health, education, housing and employment (Commonwealth of Australia 2019). Their entrenched and increasing over-representation in the child protection system shows that government strategies aiming to address this structural social inequality have failed. New approaches are required that directly tackle inequality and, in doing so, incorporate the views of Aboriginal and Torres Strait Islander communities about directions for policy and practice.

The aim of this chapter is to:

- Describe the scale and nature of over-representation in Australia, using available administrative data
- Argue for a rights-oriented theoretical framework for Aboriginal and Torres Strait Islander child wellbeing to replace the current child protection orientation
- Set out actions that are required to enact a rights framework
- Discuss implications for child protection workers and other professionals involved in responding to the needs of Aboriginal and Torres Strait Islander children and families.

Dimensions of over-representation

In contemporary child protection systems, there is a very high level of government intrusion into Aboriginal and Torres Strait Islander family life. In 2017–18, 163.8 out of every 1000 Aboriginal and Torres Strait Islander children were subject to some form of child protection intervention (investigations, orders, or placement in out-of-home care).

Aboriginal and Torres Strait Islander children were eight times more likely to be subject to child protection interventions than non-Indigenous children in 2017–18 (AIHW 2019) and 10.2 times more likely to be living in out-of-home care (SNAICC 2019).

Child protection involvement is not just more likely for Aboriginal and Torres Strait Islander families, it is also more likely to be repeated. Recurrence refers to children who are notified, investigated, or substantiated more than once. Aboriginal and Torres Strait Islander children are over-represented in repeated contact at multiple stages of intervention. A Queensland study found that there were consistently higher rates of repeated contact for Aboriginal and Torres Strait Islander children using re-report, re-notification, re-substantiation, and subsequent protective intervention as recurrence measures (Jenkins et al. 2018). Indigenous children were 1.7 times more likely to be re-notified and 2.1 times more likely to be subject to a repeat substantiation. Indigenous status was a stronger predictor of subsequent reports and investigations than a rating of 'high risk' on the risk assessment tool. The prevalence of risk factors such as age of children, prior maltreatment, neglect, parental drug or alcohol use, or domestic violence did not account for differences in the likelihood of recurrence (Jenkins et al. 2018). Decision-making tools commonly used for risk assessment in child protection systems that use recurrence as a proxy for maltreatment, and that do not take these differences into account, can lead to inequitable and inaccurate risk assessments for Aboriginal and Torres Strait Islander children.

The types and nature of maltreatment experienced also differ between the population groups: Aboriginal and Torres Strait Islander children are more likely to be reported for chronic types of maltreatment (neglect, types of emotional harm) that may be more observable and hence more likely to be substantiated, with neglect being much more frequently the reason for placement out-of-home (AIHW 2019). These trends reveal significant levels of unmet needs within Aboriginal and Torres Strait Islander families, arising from inequalities of income, housing, employment, and health. These disparities signify the failure of government to deliver equitable, accessible, and effective health and social supports for Aboriginal and Torres Strait Islander people. In turn, the level of over-representation of Aboriginal and Torres Strait Islander children in care reflects the failure of broader social policies.

Over-representation starts at the initial contact of Aboriginal and Torres Strait Islander families with the child protection system and increases at each decision point. The greatest disparity occurs for the most intrusive intervention – placement in out-of-home care. The rate for non-Indigenous children has remained relatively stable at 5.2 per 1000 in 2018 (compared to 3.0 in 2000) whereas the rate for Aboriginal and Torres Strait Islander children was 59.4 per 1000, a much larger increase from 18.3 per 1000 children in 2000 (AIHW 2001; 2019). The rate of placement for infants is higher than for other age groups, with 41.6 per 1000 Aboriginal and Torres Strait Islander children admitted to out-of-home care in 2017–18, compared to 4.6 per 1000 non-Indigenous children (AIHW 2019). A West Australian study found that the risk factors associated with placement of Aboriginal and Torres Strait Islander children in out-of-home care included living in the most disadvantaged communities and in remote and very remote areas of Australia (O'Donnell et al. 2019). Most concerningly, the level of over-representation of Aboriginal and Torres Strait Islander children in the coercive end of the child protection system is increasing over time, rather than decreasing (SNAICC 2019).

Rights framework

The current orientation of the child welfare system in all Australian jurisdictions can be characterised as primarily 'child protection', whereby 'the primary gate-keeping threshold for determining who receives a service and is seen as a priority for response is driven by concerns about child abuse and neglect' rather than broader welfare needs (Gilbert, Parton & Skivenes 2011: 251). The child protection orientation has the following features:

- The main focus is on maltreatment rather than the family's need for support and resources;
- The State is a watchdog, leading to intervention being seen as a last resort when preventative measures are insufficient;
- Processes are legalistic, investigative, and adversarial; and
- The focus of change efforts is individual behaviour and responsibility (e.g., domestic violence, alcohol use) rather than structural factors (e.g., overcrowded housing, lack of community facilities and amenity).

This approach to child welfare means that most families who are investigated each year for suspected child maltreatment do not receive any ongoing services or assistance (55.7% in 2017–18; AIHW 2019). Families can be investigated for suspected child maltreatment multiple times without receiving any ongoing support, even if they have high levels of unmet needs that are not adequately responded to, in part due to insufficient preventative family support services. There are procedural justice implications if state intervention is repeated and intrusive, but not perceived by its recipients to be helpful. Many Aboriginal and Torres Strait Islander people feel child protection to be a continuation of unfair policies that subject them to harsh judgements with no resulting benefit to their lives. When interventions are not responsive, respectful, or supportive, this perpetuates feelings of distrust and negativity towards child protection authorities and undermines trust, compliance and cooperation (Ivec, Braithwaite & Harris 2012).

In many respects, the situation for Indigenous children and families in Australia and Canada is similar, with high levels of Aboriginal over-representation within a child protection oriented system. McKenzie and Shangreaux (2011) propose an alternative orientation more suited to Aboriginal people in Canada, termed the 'community caring' model. This involves:

- Family support with the whole community conceptualised as family and focusing on community strengthening;
- Conceptual models such as the 'healing circle' and 'medicine wheel' to signify a return to traditional processes of assessment and problem-solving that consider physical, emotional, cultural, and spiritual dimensions of child and family well-being;
- Community jurisdictional control over services rather than the State; and
- Family group conferencing to facilitate family participation and localised decision making.

Aboriginal and Torres Strait Islander community organisations in Australia have long advocated for on a child protection system that recognises their right to self-determination, to make their own decisions about their own children. The Aboriginal and Torres Strait Islander Child Placement Principle (Child Placement Principle), first agreed to by all State and Territory governments in 1984, recognised the right of connections to family, community, culture, and country in child welfare policy and practice. The principle has five elements, as follows (SNAICC 2017):

- Prevention: the right of each Aboriginal and Torres Strait Islander child to be brought up within their own family and community
- Partnership: the participation of Aboriginal and Torres Strait Islander community representatives, external to the statutory agency, in decision making about individual cases at all decision-making points (e.g., intake, intervention, placement, judicial decisions) and in the design and delivery of child welfare services
- Placement: adhering to a hierarchy of options when placing an Aboriginal and Torres Strait Islander child in out-of-home care to ensure connection with their Aboriginal and Torres Strait Islander family, community, culture, and country. Lower order placement options (e.g. with non-related, non-Indigenous carers or in residential care) should only be considered when higher order options have been exhausted. As where and with whom a child is placed is not a once-only decision, higher order options should be revisited
- Participation: the right of Aboriginal and Torres Strait Islander children, parents, and family members to participate in decision making about their lives
- Connection: the right of Aboriginal and Torres Strait Islander children in out-of-home care to maintain their connections to family, community, culture, and country.

When it was first enacted by governments, the broad intent of the principle was reduced to a one-dimensional legislative provision: a preferred hierarchy of placement options. The child placement principle came to be seen in practice as only about placement. This communicated at law that authorities were compelled to consider an Aboriginal or Torres Strait Islander child's right to cultural continuity and connection only for the purpose of making a placement decision, when removal was deemed necessary. Over time, implementation became about administrative compliance with the placement provisions, not the intent of the principle to ensure a child's connection to kin, country, and culture. Following sustained advocacy, in 2017 the Commonwealth and all jurisdictions agreed to implement all five elements of the child placement principle in the *Fourth Action Plan of the National Framework for Protecting Australia's Children* (Department of Social Services 2018).

The principle works across the continuum of the child welfare system to protect and realise the rights of Aboriginal and Torres Strait Islander children, families, and communities. It provides a framework to reconceptualise child protection practice to give effect to the intent of the Child Placement Principle as imagined in the United Nations Convention on the Rights of the Child 1990 and the United Nations Declaration on the Rights of Indigenous Peoples 2008. Importantly, rights expressed in the Child Placement Principle extend beyond individual case decisions to involvement in system design, implementation, and evaluation.

Actions

Since 2016, a national campaign, Family Matters, has been led by SNAICC – National Voice for our Children with the aim of Aboriginal and Torres Strait Islander children growing up safe and cared for in family, community, and culture. The campaign sets a goal to eliminate the over-representation of Aboriginal and Torres Strait Islander children living in out-of-home care by 2040 (SNAICC 2019). The campaign proposes a range of inter-connected actions and strategies that, if properly implemented, would tackle both the causes and consequences of over-representation.

The foundation of a new approach to child welfare is a commitment to self-determination. This is core to achieving the Family Matters campaign aim. Despite the recommendation over 20 years ago from the National Inquiry into the Separation of Aboriginal and Torres Strait Islander Children from their Families (known as *Bringing Them Home*) (Human Rights and Equal Opportunity Commission 1997, Recommendation 43), a human rights framework that confers rights on Indigenous peoples and on children and the transfer of Aboriginal and Torres Strait Islander children's welfare to community control has not been realised. It is clear from the growing body of evidence that outcomes are improved for Aboriginal and Torres Strait Islander children and families when children, families, communities, and their representatives are active participants in service design, implementation, and delivery (e.g., Chandler & Lalonde 1998; Cornell & Taylor 2000; Denato & Segal 2013). Communities are therefore entitled to adequate funding and other resources to enable them to support and provide for families and the safety and wellbeing of their children.

Action to implement the five elements of the Child Placement Principle requires attention to legislation, policy, programs, processes, and practice. Drawing on the *Guidelines for Implementing the Indian Child Welfare Act* (United States Department of the Interior 2016), the concept of 'Active efforts' has been incorporated to articulate that efforts to implement the principle must be affirmative, active, thorough, and timely (Queensland Aboriginal and Torres Strait Islander Child Protection Peak 2017). In a cross-jurisdiction commitment, governments have agreed to take active efforts to implement the five elements of the Child Placement Principle, with specific commitments initially to Aboriginal and Torres Strait Island family-led decision making and cultural support planning for children in care (Department of Social Services 2018).

Properly resourced preventative services are also necessary to tackling social inequality and address over-representation. A complex interplay of individual, family, and community level factors underpin safety and wellbeing outcomes for Aboriginal and Torres Strait Islander children and families. While Aboriginal and Torres Strait Islander peoples are over-represented in measures of disadvantage, they are under-represented in service systems that prevent unnecessary entry to out-of-home care (SNAICC 2019). Investment in both universal (e.g. early childhood education, child and maternal health) and targeted (e.g., housing, mental health) preventative measures would improve access to early intervention or earlier interventions to address concerns.

Actions should address the intergenerational trauma experienced by adults who as children were stolen from their families – members of the Stolen Generations – and their descendants. Widespread, unresolved grief and loss continue to have a profound impact on social and emotional wellbeing. Aboriginal and Torres Strait Islander children have witnessed and experienced intergenerational trauma relating to child removals and the resultant ongoing disruption to cultural identity and connections (Zubrick et al. 2005). Descendants of the Stolen Generations are, for example, 1.3 times more likely to have poor mental health than Aboriginal and Torres Strait Islander people who are not members of the Stolen Generations (AIHW & Healing Foundation 2018). Children of parents removed under forced removal policies operating from the 1860s until the 1960s were twice as likely to have clinically significant emotional or behavioural difficulties than Aboriginal and Torres Strait Islander children whose parent was not removed (Zubrick et al. 2005). Other enduring impacts on health, cultural connection, and socio-economic outcomes include a higher likelihood of experiencing discrimination, police arrest, violence, and not speaking an Indigenous language (AIHW & Healing Foundation 2018). Forced removal policies no longer exist, but very high rates of placement in out-of-home care persist, and there are multi-generations within Aboriginal and Torres Strait Islander families who have experienced being in care.

This leads to one of the grave consequences of over-representation, being the number of children who grow up in care without an understanding of their family and cultural heritage. Aboriginal and Torres Strait Islander communities have called on governments to rule out adoptions and permanent care orders for their children. There are provisions to obtain these types of orders within the child protection legislation of most jurisdictions under the guise of children achieving permanence, yet they are contrary to the recommendations of *Bringing Them Home* (HREOC 1997). True permanence and a sense of belonging for Aboriginal and Torres Strait Islander children cannot be achieved if orders are made that have the effect of separating them in childhood from their cultural heritage. There are serious implications for causing harm to those children, families, and communities and exacerbating inter-generational trauma through successive removals of children from the care of their parents and extended families.

Countering the deficit discourse in Aboriginal and Torres Strait Islander child protection is essential, and this requires Aboriginal and Torres Strait Islander perspectives to be heard. Most research on Aboriginal and Torres Strait Islander communities has focused on problems within families and communities, with a reluctance to examine or accept different cultural approaches or understanding the strengths of families (Featherstone 2017). A counter-approach was taken in an Indigenous-led study that explored what well-functioning families are doing to identify strengths and positives that contribute to effective and strong families. The concept of 'well-functioning' was found to be not the absence of difficulties, but the fight to be the best they could be for their children in spite of a family history of trauma. Characteristics of well-functioning families were identified as: physical and emotional connection between children, parents, grandmothers, and extended family; an emphasis on the child's environment; learning through play; and promoting the independence of children by allowing them to access the freedom to control their environment. Parents understood that their children would be growing up in a harsh world, so developing their spirit was therefore seen as essential (Featherstone 2017). A more positive orientation to child welfare would recognise such practices as strengthening and supportive.

An important theme of the Family Matters campaign is accountability and data sovereignty. Data sovereignty is a tool for using data to advance the self-determination and aspirations of Aboriginal and Torres Strait Islander people (SNAICC 2019: 6). It allows Aboriginal and Torres Strait Islander people to tell the story from the data in ways that counter aspects that government might downplay or interpret negatively, and to highlight gaps or issues with publicly available data that serve to limit transparency and undermine accountability. The aim is to use data to make governments accountable to the Aboriginal and Torres Strait Islander community and provide a way of recording and reporting on the status of children's safety and wellbeing. This represents a counterpoint to what more commonly occurs, which is government-controlled data that represents a government narrative about the status and performance of the system, not the wellbeing of the children within it.

Implications for practice

Reducing the disproportionate representation of Aboriginal and Torres Strait Islander children entrenched in Australia's child protection systems demands that professionals and agencies across human services understand the systemic causes of over-representation and its adverse impacts on children and families. The causes involve a wide range of historical and current factors, including the material and social circumstances of families and the communities in which they live, and the psychosocial conditions of life. These factors extend to income, employment, poverty, housing, education, access to community facilities, and demographic factors such as gender and age. In practice settings, it is critical to not only address individual problems but also to understand and address underlying factors. This requires service provision from a number of siloed services and systems, so collaboration and partnering with other workers and agencies, particularly community-controlled organisations, is necessary. Good practice partnership principles identified by SNAICC (2012) include respect for cultural knowledge, history, and lived experience; shared responsibility and accountability for the vision and operation; commitment to redressing inequality and discrimination in the partnership; and an openness to working differently to traditional mainstream ways.

Accountability to children and families means adopting the Child Placement Principle as the fundamental framework to guide practice, program, and policy development. Family-led decision-making processes are a key instrument of participation and therefore self-determination. Commitment to Aboriginal and Torres Strait Islander self-determination is fundamental to working with Aboriginal and Torres Strait Islander children, families, and communities. Such a commitment underpins every interaction, action, inaction, and decision. It is foundational to children being raised by family, connected to community, culture and country, and to an Aboriginal and Torres Strait Islander child's perception of permanence, belonging, and identity development. Commitment to self-determination and community control can be demonstrated across legislation, policy, programs, processes, and practice.

Aboriginal and Torres Strait Islander children, adults, families, and communities have been and continue to be directly and indirectly impacted by trauma. Practitioners are obligated to embrace trauma-informed approaches that understand the impacts of historical trauma on the individual and their community. Atkinson (2013) refers to relationship building and self and community empowerment for healing and recovery, prioritising individual and cultural safety, client self-determination, and integrated supports as elements of a trauma-informed approach. As stated earlier, Aboriginal and Torres Strait Islander children are often removed from parental care for reasons of neglect. Causes have been attributed to factors from parenting deficits to environmental factors such as poverty and lack of opportunity. Statutory agencies tend to be more concerned with a parent-focused approach to child neglect, such as a family's living situation and parenting behaviours, without contextualising these within the role and impact of the historical trauma they and their community have and do experience (Newton 2019). When services are not resourced to address structural disadvantage and only treat individuals and families, chronic or systemic community-level issues continue to contribute to the underlying causes of child neglect in Aboriginal and Torres Strait Islander communities. For these reasons, Newton (2019) argues that child neglect within Aboriginal families and communities should be responded to in the context of historical trauma.

It is important for professionals to understand differences in applying the 'best interests' requirement in decision making about children. Often the discourse around rights in child protection is presented as a false dichotomy: child rights or parental rights; rights to cultural connection posited as separate to a child's right to safety and wellbeing. A singular approach to determining the best interests of a child in decision making for Aboriginal and Torres Strait Islander children is problematic. Critically, the differences for Aboriginal children and for Torres Strait Islander children (e.g. temporary or ongoing care by kin and traditional adoption of Torres Strait Islander children) must be understood (Victorian Law Reform Commission 2015). The five elements of the Child Placement Principle must be taken into account, particularly respect for the cultural authority of family and community members in decision making about, for example, who is kin to a child, cultural support planning, and placements (e.g. Queensland Aboriginal and Torres Strait Islander Child Protection Peak 2017). There are also differences in child-rearing practices of Aboriginal and Torres Strait Islander families and communities (Long & Sephton 2011). Respecting Aboriginal and Torres Strait Islander children's rights also involves regarding culture as a protective factor rather than a risk to a child's safety.

Strengths-based approaches have particular resonance for child protection practice with Aboriginal and Torres Strait Islander children, families, and communities as a child or family's culture or connection to culture are often dismissed or de-valued. When considered as strengths, enabling and problem-solving approaches can be utilised to support families to care for their children. Principles of strengths-based child protection practice include (Oliver 2017):

- The family is a partner in creating safety for the child;
- Every family has strengths that can be harnessed;
- The goal of the work is the future safety of the child;
- Clients will be motivated to achieve their own goals by inviting maximum collaboration;
- Building an effective alliance between clients and workers is key to finding solutions; and
- Coercion and partnership are not mutually exclusive when power and authority is used purposefully.

Systems factors must be considered, such as reporting policies; the conduct of investigations and initial assessments; bias in risk assessment tools; and the availability, mix, and suitability of service provision. Risk assessment and intervention plans should respond to individual parent factors (e.g., drugs and alcohol, domestic violence, mental health) as well as structural issues such as poverty, unemployment, housing, racism, and marginalisation.

Conclusion

Old approaches to delivering child welfare to Aboriginal and Torres Strait Islander children and families have been ineffective and in some cases destructive to individuals, families, and communities. Disproportionately intrusive interventions and the scale of over-representation mean a new approach is required; one that is rights focused and concertedly tackles the continuing and emerging impacts of inter-generational trauma and the complex interplay of individual-, family-, and community-level factors that underpin safety and wellbeing outcomes for Aboriginal and Torres Strait Islander children.

A commitment to self-determination, not just in respect of individual case decisions but also involvement in system design, implementation, delivery, and review is the foundation of a new approach that would enable Aboriginal and Torres Strait Islander children to grow up safe and cared for in family, community, and culture. Integral to self-determination is understanding and applying the five core elements of the Child Placement Principle – prevention, partnership placement, participation, connection – in legislation, policy, programs, processes, and practice across the child protection continuum. Implemented in conjunction with active efforts, the Child Placement Principle provides a framework to reconceptualise child protection practice and give effect to Aboriginal and Torres Strait Islander children, families, and communities realising their rights.

This chapter sets out actions for policy and practice to tackle both the causes and effects of over-representation. Self-determination would be advanced by increased government investment in community-controlled services, and family-led decision making. Universal and targeted services that support children and parents, and enable families and communities to care safely for their children must be more accessible and culturally safe. Family needs stemming from material and social circumstances such as racism, poverty, and unemployment must be addressed at the same time as individual parent factors such as mental health, drugs and alcohol, or domestic and family violence. Good practice collaborations and partnerships between community-controlled and non-Indigenous agencies can mean the range of child and family needs are addressed. Countering the deficit discourse with less negative and more positive, strengths-based approaches to assessment and working with families is required.

Reflective questions

- What are the main principles that describe your approach to working with Aboriginal and Torres Strait Islander children and families?
- What changes could you make within your agency or practice framework to become less deficit focused and more strengths based?
- Thinking about a recent child protection assessment you were involved with, were both individual and social factors identified, and targeted for intervention?
- What does a rights-based approach to child protection for Aboriginal and Torres Strait Islander children mean to you?

References

Atkinson, J., 2013, 'Trauma-informed services and trauma-informed care for Indigenous Australian children', *Closing the Gap Clearinghouse*, vol. 21, pp. 1–27.

AIHW, 2001, *Child protection Australia 1999–2000, Child welfare series no. 27, Cat. no. CWS* 13, Canberra: Australian Institute of Health and Welfare.

AIHW, 2019, *Child protection Australia: 2017–18, Child welfare series no. 70, Cat. no. CWS* 65, Canberra: Australian Institute of Health and Welfare.

AIHW & The Healing Foundation, 2018, *Aboriginal and Torres Strait Islander stolen generations and descendants: Numbers, demographics, characteristics and selected outcomes*, www.aihw.gov.au/getmedia/a6c077c3-e1af-40de-847f-e8a3e3456c44/aihw-ihw-195.pdf.aspx?inline=true, accessed 14 July 2019.

Bywaters, P., Brady, G., Sparks, T., Bos, E., Bunting, L., Daniel, B., Featherstone, B., Morris, K. & Scourfield, J., 2015, 'Exploring inequities in child welfare and child protection services: explaining the 'inverse intervention law', *Children and Youth Services Review*, vol. 57, pp. 98–105.

Chandler, M. & Lalonde, C., 1998, Cultural continuity as a hedge against suicide in Canada's First Nations, http://reviewboard.ca/upload/project_document/Chandler_and_Lalonde_1998_Paper__1265041839.PDF, accessed 12 August 2019.

Commonwealth of Australia, 2019, Closing the Gap Report 2019, Canberra: Commonwealth of Australia.

Cornell, S. & Taylor, J., 2000, *Sovereignty, devolution, and the future of tribal–state relations*, Cambridge, MA: Harvard University.

Denato, R. & Segal, L., 2013, 'Does Australia have the appropriate health reform agenda to close the gap in Indigenous health?', *Australian Health Review*, vol. 37, no. 2, pp. 232–238.

Department of Social Services, 2018, *National framework for protecting Australia's children 2009–2020 fourth action plan*, Canberra: Department of Social Services.

Featherstone, G., 2017, Because I'm Black: What makes for well-functioning Aboriginal families in Brisbane. PhD Thesis, School of Nursing, Midwifery and Social Work, The University of Queensland, https://doi.org/10.14264/uql.2017.441>, accessed 12 August 2019.

Gilbert, N., Parton, N. & Skivenes, M. (eds), 2011, *Child protection systems: International trends and orientations*, New York: Oxford University Press.

Human Rights and Equal Opportunity Commission, 1997, Bringing them home: Report of the national inquiry into the separation of Aboriginal and Torres Strait Islander children from their families, Sydney: Human Rights and Equal Opportunity Commission.

Ivec, M., Braithwaite, V. & Harris, N., 2012, '"Resetting the relationship" in Indigenous child protection: Public hope and private reality', *Law & Policy*, vol. 34, no. 1, pp. 80–103.

Jenkins, B.Q., Tilbury, C., Mazerolle, P. & Hayes, H., 2018, 'Factors associated with child protection recurrence in Australia', *Child Abuse and Neglect*, vol. 81, pp. 181–191.

Long, M. & Sephton, R., 2011, 'Rethinking the "best interests" of the child: Voices from Aboriginal child and family welfare practitioners', *Australian Social Work*, vol. 64, no. 1, pp. 96–112.

McKenzie, B. & Shangreaux, C., 2011, 'From child protection to community caring in first nations child and family services', in B. McKenzie & K. Kufelt, *Child welfare: connecting research, policy, and practice*, 2nd edn, Canada: Wilfred Laurier University Press, pp. 323–338.

Newton, B.J., 2019, 'Understanding child neglect in Aboriginal families and communities in the context of trauma', *Child and Family Social Work*, vol. 24, pp. 218–226.

O'Donnell, M., Taplin, S., Marriott, R., Lima, F. & Stanley, F.J., 2019, 'Infant removals: The need to address the over-representation of Aboriginal infants and community concerns of another "stolen generation"', *Child Abuse and Neglect*, vol. 90, pp. 88–98.

Oliver, C., 2017, *Strengths-based child protection: Firm, fair, and friendly*, Toronto: University of Toronto Press.

Queensland Aboriginal and Torres Strait Islander Child Protection Peak, 2017, *Position statement for Aboriginal kinship care*, Brisbane: Queensland Aboriginal and Torres Strait Islander Child Protection Peak.

SNAICC, 2012, *Opening doors through partnerships: Practical approaches to developing genuine partnerships that address Aboriginal and Torres Strait Islander community needs*, Melbourne: SNAICC.

SNAICC, 2017, *Understanding and applying the Aboriginal and Torres Strait Islander Child Placement Principle: A resource for legislation, policy and program development*, Melbourne: SNAICC.

SNAICC, 2019, *The Family Matters Report 2018: Measuring trends to turn the tide on the over-representation of Aboriginal and Torres Strait Islander children in out-of-home care in Australia*, Melbourne: SNAICC.

United States Department of the Interior, 2016, *Guidelines for Implementing the Indian Child Welfare Act*, Washington DC: The author.

Victorian Law Reform Commission, 2015, Adoption Act: Consultation paper, www.lawreform.vic.gov.au/content/6-aboriginal-and-torres-strait-islander-children-and-best-interests-principle, accessed 11 August 2019.

Zubrick, S.R., Silburn, S.R., Lawrence, D.M, Mitrou, F.G., Dalby, R.B., Blair, E.M, Griffin, J., Milroy, H., De Maio, J.A. & Li, J., 2005, *The Western Australian Aboriginal Child Health Survey: The social and emotional wellbeing of Aboriginal children and young people*, Perth: Curtin University of Technology and the Telethon Institute for Child Health Research.

Chapter 19

Engaging first mothers, fathers and grandparents in the care continuum

Elizabeth Fernandez and Ros Thorpe

Introduction

Out-of-home care provides a service to protect the needs of children whose parental care has been considered inadequate or unsafe. Such services have come to be increasing in demand over the last decade, particularly as a result of an escalation in the rates of reported child abuse and neglect and statutory removals of children to protective care. Although parents are usually subject to the interventions of the State, they are now increasingly being recognised as partners or participants in the child protection system who have their own needs and role to play in informing the best outcomes and interventions for vulnerable children (Farmer & Owen 1995; Ivec 2013). This perspective is consistent with a wider interest in participatory and consumer perspectives in both policy as well as child welfare research. However, despite the recognition of the important role and perspectives of birth or First Parents,[1] research into this area remains under-developed and in need for further investigation (Harries 2008; Ross et al. 2017; Smithson & Gibson 2017).

This chapter examines current research to understand what is known about the characteristics of birth or First Families; the state of relationships between First Families and their caseworkers; their relationship with those caring for their children and their experiences of contact with their children in care. It also examines the personal impact of being involved in the child protection decisions, and the availability of services to address their needs, particularly in relation to when children are reunified with their First Families.

The challenging circumstances of First Families

Child welfare research shows that the biological parents of children in care are disproportionately drawn from disadvantaged socio-economic backgrounds as well as single mother households (Bebbington & Miles 1989; Fernandez 1996; Harries 2008; Lindsey 1995; Fernandez et al. 2019). Many live in poverty or are supported by welfare payments; have low education levels and limited employment opportunities; and are living in government housing, transitional accommodation or are homeless. There is also often a higher than average prevalence of physical and or intellectual disabilities; mental health problems; substance abuse; and sometimes periods of criminal activity and incarceration (Fernandez 1996; Harries 2008; Marcenko, Lyons & Courtney 2011; Palmer, Maiter & Manji 2008; Sykes 2011; Taplin & Mattick 2014; Wells 2011). Other commonly reported circumstances include domestic violence and high rates of physical, emotional or sexual abuse in childhood as well as periods in statutory care (Taplin & Mattick 2014; Wells 2011).

It is noteworthy that most of the households with these characteristics involved single mothers without the support of a partner which is known to be a factor that increases the risk of child removal (Sykes 2011; Wells & Marcenko 2011). The cluster of problems described makes it difficult for mothers to balance caring and household responsibilities and there are usually few financial resources available to obtain the service of baby-sitters as might be the case in middle-class families (Hanmer & Statham 1988). Their situation is further exacerbated upon the removal of their children because this removes their entitlement to many government benefits and often coincides with threats to their housing security if they are offered less rental support and are currently unemployed. All of these factors are known to conspire to make the entry of children into care more likely, but also to reduce the likelihood of reunification once children are in care (Broadhurst & Mason, 2017; Welbourne 2012). On top of all these problems are the bureaucratic demands of government payments, obtaining welfare benefits and negotiating the employment market.

Involvement in child protection decisions

There are a number of particular areas where the child welfare system can have a significant impact on First Parents.

Legal issues and the Court system

In the United States, England and Australia, legislative reform in the area of child protection has seen a shift towards permanency planning, particularly in the case of young children who have been removed. In these reforms, this translates to a shorter allotted time frame for parents to demonstrate to the court that they can effect changes in the parenting environment and provide a safe, stable environment for their children (Broadhurst & Mason 2017; Fernandez 2013). For example, under the Children and Young Person's (Care and Protection) Act 1998 (NSW), while restoration to First Families is the first preference for permanency, First Families now have six months to demonstrate change if their child is under two years of age, and 12 months if their child is over the age of two. These reforms have long-term consequences for First Families arising from failure to demonstrate significant change in parenting capacity in a shorter time frame, leading to their child being placed permanently in a foster family or adopted. As a result, parental status is altered irrevocably and the parents' inability to access rehabilitative services serves to increase the risk of removal of any other children in the home (Broadhurst & Mason 2017; Ross et al. 2017).

Involvement in Court proceedings is frequently an inherently alienating experience for First Families. For example, Ross et al. (2017), using a mixed methods study of parents involved in the child protection system and court proceedings, found that parents were not commonly involved as active participants in decision-making processes. The findings of this and other studies reported that parents have few opportunities to be involved in proceedings, particularly due to the legal jargon and protocols that were unfamiliar, and a lack of knowledge about their rights during the process, including the right to have an advocate or support person or where to find information about their rights (Broadhurst

& Mason 2017; Fernandez 1996; Harries 2008; Ross et al. 2017; Thorpe 2008). Parents reported feeling misunderstood and misrepresented in documents submitted to the court detailing their inability to parent and which included sensitive details about their personal lives that could be discussed during proceedings and that they might be questioned about should they wish to contest removal (Broadhurst & Mason 2017; Ross et al. 2017). For these reasons, social workers can play an important role in supporting parents to navigate the legal system and interpret legal jargon while also providing emotional support to them in dealing with the grief and loss on removal of their child (Forrester et al. 2008; Kemp et al. 2013).

Engagement and inclusion

While literature and policy advocates that workers treat families/parents as partners, parents are rarely involved in decision making even though they have to live with the consequence of decisions. The absence of opportunities for communication through formal or informal mechanisms compounds their alienation from the care process. Studies have found that some workers were inclined to disparage parental capacities and not involve them in decision making or give them opportunities to express their views (Fernandez 1996; Thorpe 1980). This is despite evidence that an atmosphere of trust, openness and partnership in which workers share information, decisions and power with parents is known to contribute more effective child welfare processes and outcomes (Thoburn, Lewis & Shemmings 1995). Although there is some evidence of effective collaborative relationships between child protection agencies and First Families in some jurisdictions, the overwhelming characterisation of the relationship is one of 'us and them', where child protection agencies and workers hold all the power and could control families' lives (Harries 2008). This dynamic is reinforced by Thorpe's (2008) review of the literature discussing the inclusion of First Families in the child protection system, citing one study that made reference to a parent who called child protection workers the 'Gestapo' based on her perception of their use of power (MacKinnon 1998 cited in Thorpe 2008). Parents felt that they were expected to be subordinate and subservient, to simply accept the decisions that were being made for them by caseworkers without eliciting their contribution (Thorpe 2008; Smithson & Gibson 2017). Evidence has shown that the fear of becoming involved with the child protection system prompts families to avoid seeking help from other organisations at the risk of being reported to the statutory child protection department and subsequently having their children removed (Thorpe 2008). Accordingly, Ankersmit (2016) suggests that to address the power imbalance between families and child protection agencies, the model of engagement should be one that works from a strengths-based foundation to build on existing capacity of parents that supports restoration.

The experiences of First Families' inclusion in case conferences and reunification decisions reflects further concern. Smithson and Gibson (2017) conducted qualitative research that explored the perceptions of First Families' experiences of child protection conferences and identified concerns about the expectations and demeanour of caseworkers. Caseworkers were considered to pose obstacles to reunification rather than supporting the process, suggesting they were required to undertake more actions than they felt necessary, the undertakings required were vague, the relevance of such expected actions being poorly explained. Some were of the view that caseworkers often scheduled programs and activities that would interfere with their contact schedule (Ross et al. 2017: Smithson & Gibson 2017).

Relationships with caseworkers

First Parents are usually engaged with child protection caseworkers over an extended period of time from the initial assessment before a child is removed to determine parenting capacity and safety of the home environment, to developing and implementing case plans once a child is removed, and during permanency planning processes related to either reunification or guardianship or adoption. During this process caseworkers face the dual task of supporting the family and protecting the child (Hojer 2011). In circumstances where there is a positive relationship between the caseworker and First Families, parents are usually able to identify the attributes that have fostered this good relationship. Such factors include: treating the family humanely; taking a genuine interest in them; maintaining good communication, working to build rapport; and, applying an empathic style of practice (Smithson & Gibson 2017). Parents also find it helpful when caseworkers acknowledged the limitations of the service and established a collaborative and transparent relationship with them (Palmer, Maiter & Manji 2008; Slettebø 2013).

However, the majority of parents involved in research eliciting their perspectives rarely report supportive responses from their caseworkers. Research by Hojer (2011), for example, conducting focus groups with First Families and social workers to discuss their experiences of the child protection system, found that mothers reported feeling they were continually being punished by their caseworker for failing to take care of their child. Mothers reported having had experienced caseworkers who questioned their parental knowledge and knowledge of their child; had experienced breaches of confidentiality and broken promises particularly regarding contact schedules; had services and information withheld from them and been excluded from decisions; or had workers who failed to follow through with decisions made at case planning meetings (Hojer 2011; Fernandez 1998, Palmer, et al. 2008; Sykes 2011; Smithson & Gibson 2017; Thorpe 2008). In a similar vein, Sykes (2011) found, in a qualitative study of 16 mothers, that caseworkers prefer to work with the 'reforming parent' so parents take on a version of that role to appease the caseworker while still resisting the process of complying with expectations and ticking boxes on case plans (Sykes 2011).

Another qualitative study conducted by Palmer, Maiter and Manji (2008) included interviews with 61 First Parents involved in two Child Protective Services agencies in Ontario to explore the experiences of First Parents in the child protection system and how the experiences could be used to shape practice. It highlighted the low rate of caseworkers providing emotional support to First Families whose child has been removed despite it being a central tenet of social work intervention. Those who received support spoke of workers who were easy to get in touch with, who listened without judgement, and who praised them for seeking help.

Across a number of studies, it appears that the majority of parents reported how outward manifestations of their grief at losing their child – anger, outbursts, and emotionally loaded statements – could be used against them as evidence of being emotionally unstable and unsuitable caregivers. Depression, often resulting from the trauma of engagement with child protection services, was often seen as evidence of parents being lazy or unmotivated (Hojer 2011; Thorpe 2008). Such a tendency towards misinterpretation and lack of attention towards the emotions of First Families is thought to be due to the bureaucratic approach to child protection that prioritises risk assessment and procedural documentation over a relational approach (Palmer et al. 2008).

Other concerns expressed in some studies is that case-worker support is often not consistent or available once children are in care. For example, parents report that, once children have been placed permanently and the case as been closed, contact with caseworkers decreased or ceased despite it being a time when parents wanted more support to process the grief from permanently losing their child (Hojer 2011). As a counter-point to examples of poor practice, a study by Dumbrill (2006) highlighted how more engaged practice can lead to better outcomes for First Parents. They reported that clients reported greater satisfaction and parental engagement when social work interventions aligned with parents' goals for reunification, had clear expectations, prepared them for meetings, advocated for them, respected their culture and supported their active ongoing participation in decisions. Stronger parent–worker relationships are also identified as being beneficial outcomes for their children.

In summary, although some parents may be predisposed to view the worker apprehensively because of initial child protection interventions, it is evident that this predisposition is reinforced by interactions with caseworkers during the care experience. The anger, sadness and powerlessness they experience from coercive court interventions and being separated from their children contributes to the distortion of the relationship and their perceptions and expectations of workers. In the absence of positive encouragement from workers, parents may feel that their parenting capacity may be undermined rather than given the supportive encouragement needed to break the pattern of alienation and marginalisation they experience (Fernandez 1996). This necessitates working with parents in partnership to sustain their continuing involvement in their children's lives when they are in care and facilitating reunification or permanent forms of shared care.

Relationship with carers

When a child is removed from their First Family the foster or kinship family with whom the child is placed either temporarily or permanently becomes an important part of the placement configuration. Typically, an 'exclusive' model of care is employed, meaning that the caseworker mediates the arrangement between the carers and First Families who may never meet each other Three studies exploring First Families' relationships with carers are of interest (Ankersmit 2016; Harries 2008; Ross et al. 2017). Harries's (2008) exploration of the lived experience of First Parents involved in the child protection system through in-depth interviews with 42 First Parents identified the issues that parents had with carers which prevented a constructive relationship from developing. Ankersmit (2016)'s research which utilised the perceptions of caseworkers regarding the relationship between parents and carers highlights the different positions in the relationship – active participant versus passive observer – that influence the potential for collaborative relationships.

The parents interviewed in the study of Ross et al. (2017) acknowledged the importance of carers in their children's lives, but often felt as though they were viewing their child's life from the outside and found the experience very isolating. They spoke about the difficulty of hearing their child call their carer 'mum' or 'dad', and of wanting to share important information about their child's interests or services with carers but not being able to do so, or having it rejected. There were particular challenges for First Parents whose child was placed in kinship care placements in having to navigate a new and unfamiliar familial relationship. If a relationship had been established between carers and First Parents, it was seen to have been initiated by the carers as they held the power in the situation due to having parental responsibility of the child (Ross et al. 2017).

In comparison, a study by Ankersmit (2016) which utilised the perceptions of caseworkers regarding the relationship between carers and First Families focused primarily on how to develop a positive relationship and made little mention of the emotional impact the situation can have on First Parents. It acknowledges the probability of distrust and animosity between parents and carers, further encouraged by stories featured in the media and from friends who have been in a similar situation. However, the main findings of the study were that to establish a positive relationship between carers and First Parents, foster carers must have trust in the reunification process and those involved, must be motivated and willing participants, and that clarity of the responsibilities and roles of each party will help to build trust. Foster carers can be influential in maintaining biological bonds when they are active in the visitation and reunification process (Sanchiro & Jablonka 2000). However, such carers need to be supported in both their task of building relationships with their foster child but also in promoting the child's need for an active relationship with their First Parents and extended family (Fernandez 2009).

Experience of contact

Grounded in a theoretical understanding of attachment, family contact is viewed as essential to nurturing the parent–child connection, building and maintaining attachments (Scott, O'Neill & Ming 2005) and fostering children's identity and their wellbeing (Bullen et al. 2017; Haight, Kagle & Black 2003; Salveron & Arney 2013). As Tregeagle and Mason (2008) point out, an important element of case-work and legal decision making is determining the frequency of contact between children and their First Family and recognising the type of contact is integral to future stability of placements and permanency outcomes.

In practice, parental participation in their child's life is often restricted following removal and usually only involves contact visits, phone calls and emails (Ross et al. 2017), and this is generally consistent with the United Nations Convention on the Rights of the Child which provides that children should have the right to maintain relationships with their parents, unless it is not in their best interests (United Nations General Assembly 1989, cited in Saini, Van Wert & Gofman, 2012). In their review of the literature available regarding supervised visitation between First Parents and their child in both a custody dispute and child welfare context, Saini, Van Wert & Gofman (2012) highlighted the purpose of contact visits is to facilitate relationships between parent and child, and to allow for evaluation of interaction by caseworkers. First Parents play a significant role in their children's lives in care through contact. Children's right to contact is outlined in the United Nations Convention on the Rights of the Child in article 9.3.

Studies have shown that maintaining children's contact with their biological families yields important benefits for children, including fewer placements, stability of care, lower risk of mental heath difficulties, strengthened emotional and behavioural development and increased potential for reunification (Broadhurst & Sen 2011; Fernandez & Atwool 2013; McWey, Acock & Porter 2010). Contact provides an opportunity for parents to exercise some parental responsibility and participation (Atwool 2013). Thus, by supporting parents through contact arrangements, out-of-home care systems can enable families to 'remain an important potential source of support for their children especially when support from State care is withdrawn in later adolescence' (Taplin 2005: 16).

Most studies of family contact have been focused on the impact that it has on the child involved, and very little attention is paid to the experience of the First Families involved in contact visits. This is true of the research studies involved in this review. Most studies drew reference to attachment theory as the principal theoretical foundation for contact visits on the assumption that family connections can assist in decreasing the distress experienced by children when they are separated from their primary caregiver, and that contact visits can help to foster a sense of identity and emotional and behavioural development in children, and help to stabilise a placement (Saini et al. 2012; Taplin & Mattick 2014). At the same time, the studies also presented the contrasting view that contact visits can also be seen to be detrimental to children's well-being if they lead to disruptions in the development of a relationship with their principal carer and are emotionally challenging for the children contributing to disruptions in behaviour following the visits (Saini et al. 2012; Taplin & Mattick 2013).

A number of studies have examined family contact. For example, Taplin and Mattick (2013) presented findings from a larger cross-sectional study on 171 mothers who had been involved in an Opioid Treatment Program in Sydney. Through interviews and data collected from child protection records, it was found that supervised contact was likely to occur less frequently than unsupervised contact, children in kinship care were likely to have contact frequently, and that mothers who reported regular cannabis use were more likely to have supervised visitation which meant less frequent contact. However, as the study was cross-sectional in nature, it was difficult to determine whether the drug use led to supervised contact or whether supervised contact led to increased drug use (Taplin & Mattick 2013). Where parents were questioned about their experiences of contact, it was apparent that they were unsure of their role during contact, and that they tried to squeeze as much direct care into a session as the sessions were insufficient for them to help build a proper parent–child relationship (Ross et al. 2017; Saini, et al. 2012).

Bullen et al. (2017) reported that the family contact literature currently available is generally mostly descriptive. In response to this concern, the authors conducted a systematic review of the limited quantitative studies available examining supervised visitation. Of the 12 eligible studies, when examined using the model in Hudson et al. (2010) to grade the evidence according the rigour of study design and analysis, eight studies received the lowest grade, often for not including comparison groups, clear explanation of their evaluation methods or detailed child outcomes. The study concluded that, while there are some interventions that appear to be beneficial in improving supervised visitation, more research is required with particular focus on parents who are unlikely to have their children restored (Bullen et al. 2017; García-Martin et al. 2019). Another study by Davis et al. (1996) took a more holistic view of reunification and emphasised the importance of children being able to re-establish a sense of belonging and connection to the family on an emotional, psychological and physical level. Such findings challenge the assumption that parental contact is merely important to effect reunification, overlooking its importance in enabling the child to re-establish a sense of belonging and continuing engagement. Other reported positive outcomes of contact include building long-term attachments, better psychosocial wellbeing, fostering a sense of culture and identity and helping children resolve issues of loss and trauma (Broadhurst & Sen 2011).

Personal impact

The removal of children can also impose specific personal costs on parents. Some of the most important of these are as follows.

Grief and loss

As already noted, a significant consequence of the removal of children from the family home is the grief and loss experienced by First Families. It is common for First Families to experience ambiguous loss due to the uncertainty of the period immediately following removal, and then to experience further loss if the child is permanently placed in another family. This ambiguous loss can stall the onset of grieving and prevent coping mechanisms and decision-making skills from working (Boss 2007). Parents also grieve the loss of the daily interactions with children, especially around special events and occasions, and the loss of seeing their child grow and develop (Thorpe 2008). People grieving often look to their support networks for solace; however, parents who have had their children removed often feel very isolated from their support networks due to the stigma and shame associated with the removal of a child. This can be exacerbated when a child is placed in a kinship placement as the relationships have been forced to change (Broadhurst & Mason 2017; Ross et al. 2017). Manifestations of this grief could include anger, and emotional outbursts which, as previously mentioned, can be viewed as evidence of an emotionally unstable parent incapable of suitable parenting (Ross et al. 2017).

Identity

Furthering the notion of loss is the loss of identity that a mother experiences when they are no longer taking care of their child on a regular basis. As there is a lack of available research about First fathers, it is the mother who is labelled as a 'bad parent' (Harries 2008). At the point of removal, a mother has already lost the identity of being considered a 'good mother'. This is a moniker that they will struggle to regain and the label that they are an 'unsuitable' mother will likely follow them in any other child protection cases (Broadhurst & Mason 2017). To reconcile the loss of the label of 'good mother', mothers will distance themselves from the allegations of child maltreatment and reject the child protection agency's reason for intervention. They will also distance themselves from association with what they consider to be 'bad mothers' and highlight the worse aspects of other cases (Sykes 2011). Being labelled as a 'bad mother' commonly sees mothers stigmatised by their families and communities as they seem to have 'failed' what it means to be a responsible adult. Evidence has shown that stigma can increase aggression and self-defeating behaviour which can impact the chances of reunification (Wells 2011).

Trauma

Many First Parents who become involved in the child protection system have experienced trauma in their life before they have contact with child protection agencies. Adolescent trauma has been proven to have an impact on adult relationships and parenting capacity. If unaddressed, the trauma can manifest as troublesome behaviours which may be used as evidence to support removal of their child (Broadhurst, Mason & Webb 2018; Ross et al. 2017). The removal of a child is a traumatic experience in itself and can trigger maladaptive coping mechanisms which can hinder the possibility of reunification (Broadhurst et al. 2018). Some research participants also found court proceedings to be traumatic as they compounded the impacts of other trauma experiences in their history (Ross et al. 2017). Experiences of trauma while involved in the child protection system can serve to alienate First Families from services that are trying to support their reunification with their children.

Access to services

Parents who felt they had been working with a good caseworker identified receiving good referrals to appropriate services to counselling, education and treatment, and concrete help such as food, financial assistance and shelter, as important factors that demonstrated to them that their worker was also working towards reunification of their child (Palmer et al. 2008). Unfortunately, the research reviewed demonstrated that this was an uncommon experience among parents whose children had been removed. Marcenko et al. (2011), for example, conducted a cross-sectional study of the demographic and psychosocial characteristics and service needs of primary caregivers in Washington State who had had an open welfare case within 30 to 120 days prior to the study. Their results showed that parents were more likely to have their service needs met when their child was still in the home than once the child was removed as child protection agencies were working to keep at-risk children in their home (Marcenko et al. 2011). This idea was reinforced in Broadhurst and Mason's (2017) review of the literature available regarding the impact of child removal on First Parents and the development of a comprehensive framework for practice. While children are in care, the absence of adequate services emerged as a common theme and this is known to be detrimental for parental wellbeing and reduces the prospect of reunification (Broadhurst & Mason 2017). Other problems include high worker turnover (Harries 2008; Palmer et al. 2008) or the problem of parents not wanting to ask for support as they fear it being used against them as evidence of poor parenting capability in court proceedings (Thorpe 2008).

As previously discussed, legislative reforms promoting permanency planning have led to a shortened time frame in which First Parents can demonstrate change supporting the reunification of their children, so the cessation of important rehabilitative services occurs earlier (Broadhurst & Mason 2017). This has long-term impacts for First Parents as within the shortened time frames they are unlikely to have resolved all of the issues that led to removal of their child so if they have another baby, it will likely re-involve child protection services in their life, or they may have another child already in their care removed (Broadhurst & Mason 2017).

Grandparents and extended family

As the environment of child protection services includes First Parents, grandparents, foster carers and other professionals it is crucial that social workers deliver support in a way that evaluates all ecological systems and is inclusive of all the child's networks.

As child protection services increasingly seek placements with kin, grandparents are challenged by new full-time caring responsibilities while surviving on limited economic resources and social supports. Social workers need to work closely with grandparents to support their parenting capabilities, and in particular be attuned to a gender lens, and address the needs of grandmothers who are disproportionately burdened by caring responsibilities with sparse support (Bunch et al. 2007).

Gender and child protection

The experience of mothers in the child protection system has been a concern and is the subject of a body of literature (Callahan & Lumb 1995; Swift 1991) which examines the dominant assumptions underpinning child welfare interventions, given the strong presence of women as clients, carers, frontline workers and that child welfare focuses on women's domain of caring for children. Swift (1995) argues for a reconceptualization of child welfare as a feminist issue, challenging the dominant ideologies and assumptions underpinning child welfare interventions and the institution of motherhood and its socially determined conditions. Mothers carry several visible and invisible responsibilities and are not allowed to fail these obligations. Chesler (1987) observes that the ideal mother is expected to choose married motherhood, become pregnant, give birth, bond with, assume full responsibility for her child's physical, emotional, economic and safety needs, and asserts mothers more than fathers are condemned for being psychologically imperfect, for performing parental work inadequately and for failing the parental ideal. The assessment of mothers as being inadequate reflects assumptions that 'normal' mothers cope (Parton 1990). The realities of parenting are rarely acknowledged. Material disadvantage such as poor housing, financial difficulties and the lack of emotional and social support for parenting tasks and threatened and actual violence contribute to physical and emotional stress that compromise their physical and mental health, their parenting potential and the care of their children (Fernandez 1996).

Conceptions of mothers and attitudes to them range from holding them responsible for the outcomes of their children to portraying them as inadequate and incapable of protecting them. The Social Science literature portrays them as primarily responsible for the quality of care of their children. Since Bowlby's (1953) early conceptions viewed parenting in terms of rigid sex role conceptions with mothers having continuous responsibility for child care in the early years, the psychopathology of the child is attributed to mothers. This is reinforced in the legal literature, as King and Trowell note 'It is, to mothers that the system looks as having primary responsibility for any harm that might have been caused, and to rectify that harm' (King & Trowell 1992: 21).

Issues in research

Although there is limited research available on the experiences of First Families involved in the child protection system, there are common issues evident in the studies that have been conducted. Some studies utilised child protection caseworkers and client files as a means of obtaining information about the First Parent experience. This creates a risk of misinterpretation as it is a second-hand view of the client's experience, and it can be clouded by bias if the caseworker had a poor working relationship with the client. In circumstances where First Families were involved in the research study, it was common for them to be recruited through the caseworkers or the programs they had been referred to by caseworkers. It is possible that having caseworkers involved in the recruitment process may have prevented First Parents from speaking freely about their experiences as they feared potential consequences of speaking negatively. However, it was noted that First Families were more likely to be involved in a study if they had a negative experience (Hojer 2011). Despite these potential biases, recruiting participants through caseworkers and parenting programs is currently the most effective means as First Families are a difficult population to access for research for several reasons, such as a general mistrust of the system, fear of further 'punishment' for speaking out, and a desire to move on from their experience (Ankersmit 2016). The sample populations of the studies reviewed which involved members of First Families predominantly consisted of mothers who had had their children removed which may be representative of the tendency of child protection agencies' focus on mothers as primary caregivers and thus in need of the most support (Sykes 2011; Palmer et al. 2008; Sykes 2011). However, studies commonly ignore the experience of First Fathers involved in the child protection system who may have an ongoing impact in the life of their child after removal. This tendency towards samples of predominantly mothers also excludes the experience of the extended family, such as siblings and grandparents. In particular cultures, such as Aboriginal and Torres Strait Islander, and in some Asian cultures, the extended family has a large role in the upbringing of a child, so they are likely to have an important role in the child protection process. As there is an over-representation of Aboriginal and Torres Strait Islander children in Australia in out-of-home care (OOHC) currently – Aboriginal children enter OOHC at ten times the rate of non-Indigenous children, it is important that research also explores the experiences of extended family members (Burns, Burns & Menzies 2004; CFCA 2019; Davis 2018).

While there is a breadth of research available in the area of child protection, and research available examining the impact of the involvement of First Families in the lives of children who have been removed, there is limited research currently available that explores the child protection process through the eyes of the First Parents. The information that is available is often informed by the views of caseworkers and official documents, or the parents that have participated in the research have been recruited through caseworkers and programs, so are unlikely to speak freely for fear of retribution. The overwhelming feeling from First Families is that they are often excluded from the system due to their lack of knowledge and power, and are not given the opportunities to demonstrate or improve their parenting capabilities. The research reviewed also demonstrated that little focus is given to the First Fathers or extended families of children who have been removed which is a significant gap in the research, particularly due to the overwhelming number of Aboriginal and Torres Strait Islander children in OOHC in Australia and the importance the cultures place on the role of the extended family in raising a child (Bamblett & Lewis 2006; McDowall 2016).

Implications for policy, programs, practice and further research

Notwithstanding issues in the research with First Families involved with the child protection system, there is sufficient consistency among the findings of the studies reviewed to be able to identify some salient implications for improvements, not only in direct practice with First Families but also at the levels of program development, and policy formulation.

Implications at a structural, broader policy level are particularly significant in relation to the challenging circumstances in which many First Families live before, during and following child protection intervention. Poverty is a continuing issue for families in which children are seen to be at risk and, while Parenting Payments in Australia are barely adequate for day to day living, the requirements of the *ParentsNext* program make life harder for many single parents (mostly single mothers) of pre-school aged children, and the penalties can lead many families into deepening poverty. When children are taken into care, parents are forced off Parenting Payments onto the NewStart Allowance which they find is grossly inadequate to cover shelter and food, let alone costs associated with complying with requirements laid on them to work towards their children returning home. Social advocacy with regard to securing improvements in the income security and housing systems is thus a clear, highly desirable implication for action emerging from the research. Meanwhile, programs and practice need to be ever mindful of the structural reasons for families living in poverty and, when specifying requirements placed on First Families, consider the realities of living in poverty. Judgements and unrealistic or punitive expectations are harmful rather than helpful. Moreover, the need for material and practical assistance at times (including trauma cleaning and regular ongoing home help – in the past called *Family Aides*) should be regarded as invaluable, given the structural constraints which blight families' socio-economic circumstances and may lead to debilitating depression.

With regard to direct practice, child protection workers' lack of (or limited) experience of living in poverty indicates a need to work hard at critical reflexivity in order to walk in their families' shoes to achieve a greater understanding and acceptance of physically oppressed living conditions and the possible lack of skills a worker may regard as 'common sense', like hygiene or budgeting. Clearly, cross-cultural understanding is also vital in order to appreciate the use, meaning and value of different, but culturally appropriate, strategies for coping with poverty. Far greater culturally aware practice is needed urgently as part of a range of strategies to reduce the massive over-representation of Aboriginal and Torres Strait Islander children in care.

Research findings in relation to gendered issues in child protection add another important dimension to the need for greater awareness of structural forces largely beyond the immediate control of individuals. On top of living in poverty, traditional expectations of women, and superficial analyses of domestic violence and family abuse provide a 'mother blaming' pitfall for front line child protection workers and their supervisors. Hence there also is an urgent need for direct practitioners to be better informed by critical analyses of motherhood and by the latest reviews of research on family abuse (see, for example, Hill 2019) in order to work with women in strengths-based, empowering ways rather than imposing the pejorative label 'failure to protect'. In addition, moving from the personal to the political, there is a need for child protection workers to add their voices to social action campaigns for policy changes with regard to domestic violence and child protection, and for changes to the Family Court Act, given that 'mother blaming' is a salient feature in many current Family Court judgements when mothers are often typecast as liars and/or mad (Hill 2019). The need is pressing for professionals in child protection, be they social workers, police, psychologists, lawyers or Family Report writers, to have in-depth knowledge of the complexity of domestic abuse and be alert to their own exposure to being 'groomed' by perpetrators, who may present as rational and calm in contrast to their ex partners who are battle worn and desperate for the welfare of their children.

Plainly, at the direct practice level, there is a need to fully understand the personal impacts which First Parents experience when child protection agencies get involved in their lives. Fear and anxiety become added to the stress of living with poverty and/or with domestic abuse, and when children are removed into care loss, grief and long-term chronic sorrow are to be expected. While for many decades research with First Families has identified loss and grief as highly significant (initially referred to as *filial deprivation* (Jenkins & Norman 1972), the recognition of trauma as important in the previous life experience of First Parents has only recently become explicit. For many, this may result from one or more of childhood abuse, childhood or adult sexual assault, and childhood or adult domestic abuse. For Aboriginal and Torres Strait Islander First Parents, trauma may also result from the intergenerational trauma of the Stolen Generations, plus past and ongoing racism in society generally and sometimes, also, in child protection processes themselves. The need for direct practice to be trauma-informed is pressing in order to enable First Parents to become active survivors, enabled to resume care for their children (Atkinson 2002; Herman 1997).

Practitioners need understand the inevitability of First Parents becoming deeply depressed and/or angry and not label these as indications of unsuitability to care for their children. Reaching out to the distressed person behind the depression or anger is an essential, advanced skill in building a respectful relationship which, research studies consistently have found, is a key to working constructively with First Parents.

Respect for the dignity and worth (AASW 2010 clause 3.1) of First Parents is a foundation for every aspect of child protection casework, be it facilitating First Parents' active participation in legal proceedings and case planning, having good contact with their children in care, working together with carers and, in a timely manner, accessing services which provide assistance and support. The research studies reviewed in this chapter provide clear guidance on what works more effectively and, importantly, provide insight into what doesn't work well and should be avoided in practice.

Since research findings indicate that less than best practice appears to be widespread, there is a need to identify the conditions which might facilitate improvements in direct practice with First Parents. Conditions in working environments – government and non-government – can often stifle good practice through managerialist requirements of workers and supervision which is largely organisational and administrative rather than professional. One implication from research findings is to focus attention within organisations on building a working environment which is conducive to and supportive of research-informed good practice. Encouraging a knowledge of relevant research findings and their application in practice through, for example, discussion lunches is a practice we have seen in one government office; enabling professional (rather than bureaucratic) supervision within or external to the organisation is another practice which some non-government agencies use. A further implication for child protection organisations might be to enable good practitioners to remain working at the front line but with remuneration which recognises their advanced skills, particularly in working with First Families. While new workers may have energy and commitment, their limited experience is often a stumbling block to good practice. Rather than expected to adapt to what may be an entrenched office culture, new child protection workers need to be enabled by the organisation to examine their own possibly unhelpful attitudes and values, and be supported in working respectfully and in culturally appropriate ways with First Families, including First Grandparents who may become kinship carers.

Respectful relationship-based social work practices (Ruch, Turney & Ward 2018), as indicated by the findings from the research studies reviewed, not only are greatly appreciated by First Families, they also lead to better outcomes for children and families and, even when children and young people remain in care, First Families are enabled to have a more constructive approach to maintaining contact with family, community, culture and country. They also may be less prone to crippling levels of chronic sorrow and better able to rebuild their lives.

This latter hypothesis is an area for future research, since to date, it has been difficult to find enough First Parents with such positive experiences to undertake meaningful research beyond isolated qualitative case studies.

Other areas warranting further research have been identified throughout this research review, including an emerging impression that research with First Parents to date has been culturally bland. Given the huge over-representation of Aboriginal and Torres Strait Islander children removed into out-of-home care there is a need for studies which focus specifically on Indigenous Australian extended First Families' experiences of the full range of child protection processes. While Aboriginal and Torres Strait Islander child protection workers are able to articulate the needs and interests of their people, the whole discourse underpinning new research needs to be re-framed within an appropriate non-western cultural perspective.

Another neglected area of research is that of First Fathers (Campbell et al. 2015; Gordon et al. 2012; Scourfield, Cheung & MacDonald 2014). This should include not only biological fathers who may have had little or no involvement in caring for their child/ren, but also step-fathers who may be important psychological parents of the children with whom they have highly significant attachments which, too often, may be disregarded in child protection processes. Instead, once in care, children may be introduced to their little or unknown biological father who may have perpetrated violence against their mother and even themselves. While, arguably, it is important for all children in care or adoption to know their biological origins, it also is important for their ongoing well-being to maintain important relationships with significant other father figures The complexities surrounding fathers and stepfathers of children entering care need to be explored in detailed research in order to identify implications for practice which are in a child's best interests, emotionally as well as biologically.

A fourth area for further research identified in this review is the experience and impact of contact for First Parents themselves. Thus far, most research has focused on whether and how contact affects children, with beneficial effects identified regardless of whether reunification is accomplished. The perspective of First Parents and their wider family has yet to be explored in depth, particularly with regard to their experience when children are in long term or permanent care. As always, such research needs to be culturally appropriate in full recognition of the significance of wider family and community for Aboriginal and Torres Strait Islander children, and also adapted appropriately for children in care in Australia from diverse other cultural backgrounds with different values and traditions.

Conclusion

In this chapter the state of research knowledge concerning First Parents of children at risk of entry into state care, or already in care, has been reviewed, with implications for direct practice, programs, policy and further research explored. With the trend for child protection agencies around Australia to focus on permanency planning for vulnerable children, the time frame for First Parents to change sufficiently for their children to return to their care has shortened and, accordingly, practice needs to become more intense in order to enable as many children as possible to return home safely to their First Families in a timely manner. While always there is a need for further research, already enough is known to be able to transform child protection processes to work more constructively and effectively with First Families. What is needed is vision and courage on the part of organisations and individual practitioners to implement changes to a truly family-focused approach to child-centred practice.

Note

1 In this chapter the term First Parents is used to refer to what more commonly in academic and professional literature are called Biological parents or Birth parents. Both of these latter terms can have the effect of minimising the reality that First Parents, grandparents and significant others have ties that bind with their children way beyond biological heredity or merely the act of giving birth/life. Invariably, First Parents are the child's psychological parents and important primary attachments connect them and their children. Even when such attachments are new (as at birth) or complicated, First attachments confer a sense of belonging to family, community, culture, and country. Just as First Nations People are the custodians of the land and all that is sacred so, we argue, First Parents are custodians of a Child's identity, the sacredness of which must be supported. In our view, the term First Parents conveys the importance of this truth far more strongly than the terms used hitherto.

References

Australian Association of Social Workers (AASW)2010, *Code of ethics*, Canberra: Australian Association of Social Workers.

Ankersmit, L., 2016, 'The reunification partnership: engaging birth parents and foster carers as collaborators in restoration casework', *Australian Social Work*, vol. 69, no. 3, pp. 273–282.

Atkinson, J., 2002, *Trauma trails: Recreating song lines*. Melbourne: Spinifix Press.

Atwool, N., 2013, 'Birth family contact for children in care: How much? How often? Who with?', *Child Care in Practice*, vol. 19, no. 2, pp. 181–198.

Bamblett, M. & Lewis, P., 2006, 'Embedding culture for a positive future for Koorie kids', *Developing Practice: The Child, Youth and Family Work Journal*, vol. 17, pp. 58–75.

Barber, J. G. & Delfabbro, P. H., 2004, *Children in foster care*, London: Routledge.

Bebbington, A. & Miles, J., 1989, 'The background of children who enter local authority care', *British Journal of Social Work*, vol. 19, no. 5, pp. 349–368.

Boss, P., 2007, 'Ambiguous loss theory: Challenges for scholars and practitioners', *Family Relations*, vol. 56, no. 2, pp. 105–110.

Bowlby, J., 1953, *Child care and the growth of love*. Harmondsworth: Penguin Books.

Broadhurst, K., Mason, C. & Webb, S., 2018, 'Birth mothers returning to court: Can a developmental trauma lens inform practice with women at risk of repeat removal of infants and children?', in M. Shaw & S. Bailey (eds), *Justice for children and families: A developmental perspective*, Cambridge: Cambridge University Press, pp. 59–67.

Broadhurst, K. & Mason, C., 2017, 'Birth parents and the collateral consequences of court-ordered child removal: towards a comprehensive framework', *International Journal of Law, Policy and The Family*, vol. 31, pp. 41–59.

Broadhurst, K. & Sen, R., 2011, 'Contact between children in out-of-home placements and their family and friends' networks: A research review', *Child and Family Social Work*, vol. 16, no. 1, pp. 298–309.

Bullen, T., Taplin, S., McArthur, M., Humphreys, C. & Kertesz, M., 2017, 'Interventions to improve supervised contact visits between children in out of home care and their parents: a systematic review', *Child and Family Social Work*, vol. 22, pp. 822–833.

Burns, A., Burns, K. & Menzies, K., 2004, 'Strong state intervention: The stolen generation', in J. Bowes (ed.), *Children, families and communities: Contexts and consequences*, London: Sage, pp. 190–209.

Callahan, M. & Lumb, C.R., 1995, 'My cheque and my children: The long road to empowerment in child welfare', *Child Welfare*, vol. LXX1V, no. 3, pp. 795–817.

Campbell, C., Howard. D., Rayford, B. & Gordon, D., 2015, 'Fathers matter: involving and engaging fathers in the child welfare system process', *Children and Youth Services Review*, vol. 53, pp. 84–91.

Chesler, P., 1987, *Mothers on trial: The battle for children and custody*, New York: McGraw Hill.

Child Family Community Australia (CFCA), 2019, *Child protection and Aboriginal and Torres Strait Islander children*, Canberra: Australian Institute of Family Studies, Canberra.

Davis, I., Landsverk, J., Newton, R. & Ganger, W., 1996, 'Parental visiting and foster care reunification', *Children and Youth Services Review*, vol. 18, no. 4–5, pp. 363–382.

Dumbrill, G.C., 2006, 'Parental experience of child protection intervention: A qualitative study', *Child Abuse & Neglect*, vol. 30, no. 1, pp. 27–37.

Farmer, E. & Owen, M., 1995, *Child protection practice: Private risks and public remedies –decision making, intervention and outcome in child protection*, London: HMSO.

Fernandez, E.A., 1996, *Significant harm: Unravelling child protection decisions and substitute care careers of children*, Aldershot, UK: Ashgate.

Fernandez E., 1998, 'Realities of women's caring: Rethinking child welfare interventions', in *Women participating in global change: An international collection*, Hong Kong: International Association of Schools of Social Work (IASSW) Women's Symposium.

Fernandez, E.A., 2009, 'Children's wellbeing in care: Evidence from a longitudinal study of outcomes', *Children & Youth Services Review*, vol. 31, no. 10, pp. 1092–1100.

Fernandez, E., 2013, *Accomplishing permanency: Reunification pathways and outcomes for foster children*, Dordrecht: Springer.

Fernandez, E.A. & Atwool, N., 2013, 'Child protection and out of home care: Policy, practice and research connections Australia and New Zealand', *Intervencion Psicosocial*, vol. 22, no. 3, pp. 164–175.

Fernandez, E., Delfabbro, P., Ramia, I.O. & Kovacs, S., 2019, 'Children returning from care: The challenging circumstances of parents in poverty', Special Issue, *Children & Youth Services Review*, vol. 97, pp. 100–111.

Forrester, D., McCambridge, J., Waissbein, C. & Rollnick, S., 2008, 'How do child and family social workers talk to parents about child welfare concerns?', *Child Abuse Review*, vol. 17, no. 1, pp. 23–35.

García-Martín, M., Fuentes, M., Bernedo, I., & Salas, M., 2019, 'The views of birth families regarding access visits in foster care', *Journal of Social Work*, vol. 19, no. 2, pp. 173–191.

Gordon, D., Oliveros, A., Hawes, S. Iwamoto, D. & Rayford, B., 2012, 'Engaging fathers in child protection services: A review of factors and strategies across ecological systems', *Children and Youth Services Review*, vol. 34, no. 8, pp. 1399–1417.

Haight, W., Kagle, J. & Black, J., 2003, 'Understanding and supporting parent–child relationships during foster care visits: Attachment theory and research', *Social Work*, vol. 48, no. 2, pp. 195–207.

Hanmer, J. & Statham, D., 1988, *Women and social work: towards a woman centred practice*, London: The Macmillan Press.

Harries, M., 2008, *The experiences of parents and families of children and young people in care*, Perth: Family Inclusion Network Western Australia.

Herman, J., 1997, *Trauma and recovery*. New York: Basic Books.

Hill, J., 2019, *See what you made me do: Power, control, and domestic abuse*. Melbourne: Black.

Ivec, M., 2013, *A necessary engagement: An international review of parent and family engagement in child protection*, Hobart: Anglicare.

Jenkins, S. & Norman, E., 1972, *Filial deprivation and foster care*. New York: Columbia University Press.

Kemp, S., Marcenko, M., Lyons, S. & Kruzich, J., 2013, 'Strengths-based practice and parental engagement in child welfare services: An empirical examination', *Children and Youth Services Review*, vol. 47, pp. 27–35.

King, M. & Trowell, J., 1992, *Children's welfare and the law: The limits of legal intervention*. London: Sage.

Lindsey, C., 1995, 'Systemic and developmental aspects of contact' in H. Argent (ed.) *See you soon*, London: British Agencies for Adoption and Fostering.

Marcenko, M., Lyons, S. & Courtney, M., 2011, 'Mothers' experiences, resources and needs: The context for reunification', *Children & Youth Services Review*, vol. 33, pp. 431–438.

McDowall, J., 2016, 'Connection to culture by indigenous children and young people in out-of-home care', *Communities, Children & Families Australia*, vol. 10, no. 1, pp. 5–26.

McWey, L., Acock, A. & Porter, B., 2010, 'The impact of continued contact with biological parents upon the mental health of children in foster care', *Children & Youth Services Review*, vol. 32, no. 10, pp. 1338–1345.

Palmer, S., Maiter, S. & Manji, S., 2008, 'Effective intervention in child protective services: Learning from parents', *Children & Youth Services Review*, vol. 28, pp. 812–824.

Parton, C., 1990, 'Women, gender, oppression and child abuse', in The Violence against Children Study Group (ed.), *Taking child abuse seriously: Contemporary issues in child protection theory and practice*. London: Unwin Hyman, pp. 41–62.

Ross, N., Cocks, J., Johnston, L. & Stoker, L., 2017, *'No voice, no opinion, nothing': Parent experiences when children are removed and placed in care*, Newcastle: University of Newcastle.

Ruch, G., Turner, D. & Ward, A., 2018, *Relationship-based social work: Getting to the Heart of practice*, 2nd edn. London: Jessica Kingsley.

Saini, M., Van Wert, M. & Gofman, J., 2012, 'Parent–child supervised visitation within child welfare and custody dispute contexts: An exploratory comparison of two distinct models of practice', *Children and Youth Services Review*, vol. 34, pp. 163–168.

Salveron, M. & Arney, F., 2013, 'Chapter 12: Parents with Children in Care', in F. Arney & D. Scott (eds). *Working with vulnerable families: A partnership approach*, New York: Cambridge University Press.

Sanchirico, A. & Jablonka, K., 2000, 'Keeping foster children connected to their biological parents: The impact of foster parent training and support', *Child and Adolescent Social Work Journal*, vol. 17, no. 3, pp. 185–202.

Scott, D., O'Neill, C. & Minge, A., 2005, 'Literature review: Contact between children in out-of-home care and their birth families', Melbourne: School of Social Work, University of Melbourne.

Scourfield, J., Cheung, S. & MacDonald, G., 2014, 'Working with fathers to improve children's well-being: Results of a survey exploring service provision and intervention approach in the UK', *Children and Youth Services Review*, vol. 43, pp. 40–50.

Slettebø, T., 2013, 'Partnership with Parents of Children in Care: A Study of Collective User Participation in Child Protection Services', *British Journal of Social Work*, vol. 43, no. 3, pp. 579–595.

Smithson, R. & Gibson, M., 2017, 'Less than human: a qualitative study into the experience of parents involved in the child protection system', *Child and Family Social Work*, vol. 22, pp. 565–574.

Swift, K., 1991, 'Contradictions in child welfare neglect and responsibility', in C. Baines, P. Evans & S. Neysmith (eds), *Women's caring: Feminist perspectives on social welfare*, Toronto: McLellend & Stewart, pp. 234–271.

Swift, K., 1995, 'Missing persons: Women in child welfare', *Child Welfare*, vol. LXXIV, no. 9, pp. 486–502.

Sykes, J., 2011, 'Negotiating stigma: Understanding mothers' responses to accusations of child neglect', *Children and Youth Services Review*, vol. 33, pp. 448–456.

Taplin, S., 2005, 'Is all contact between children in care and their birth parents "good" contact?', Ashfield, NSW: NSW Department of Community Service.

Taplin, S. & Mattick, R., 2014, 'Supervised contact visits: Results from a study of women in drug treatment with children in care', *Children and Youth Services Reviews*, vol. 39, pp. 65–72.

Thoburn, J., Lewis, A. & Shemmings, D., 1995, *Paternalism or partnership: Family involvement in the child protection process*, London: Studies in Child Development, HMSO.

Thorpe, R., 1980, 'The experiences of children and parents living apart: Implications and guidelines for practice', in J. Triseliotis (ed.), *New developments in foster care and adoption*, London: Routledge & Kegan Paul.

Thorpe, R., 2008, 'Family inclusion in child protection practice: Building bridges in working with (not against) families', *Communities, Families and Children Australia*, vol. 3, pp. 4–18.

Tregeagle, S. & Mason, J., 2008, 'Service user experience of participation in child welfare case management', *Child & Family Social Work*, vol. 13, no. 4, pp. 391–401.

United Nations General Assembly (UN), 1989, Convention on the Rights of the Child, Geneva: United Nations, Treaty Series, vol. 1577, no. 3.

Welbourne, P., 2012, *Social work with children and families: Developing advanced practice*, New York: Routledge.

Wells, K., 2011, 'A narrative analysis of one mother's story of child custody loss and regain', *Children and Youth Services Review*, vol. 33, pp. 439–447.

Wells, K. & Marcenko, M., 2011, 'Introduction to the Special Issue: Mothers of children in foster care', *Children and Youth Services Review*, vol. 33, pp. 419–423.

Chapter 20

Responding to carers' needs

Jill Duerr Berrick

In most countries, child welfare policy is clear: Children should be cared for safely in their home of origin. Some circumstances, however, compromise children's safety or well-being such that they must be separated from their birth parents or other caregivers. In these instances, children are typically placed in out-of-home care while their parents or caregivers make changes to the circumstances that precipitated the separation. These substitute care arrangements may be with a relative or close family friend (referred to as relative care or kinship care), with a non-relative (a stranger to the child), or children may be placed in a congregate care setting with 24-hour staff. In most Western, industrialized countries, kinship caregivers and non-relative foster caregivers are preferred placement settings for children and will therefore be the focus of this chapter. They will be referred to, globally, as 'foster care', or 'foster caregivers', though they may be referred to as 'carers' or 'resource families', depending on the country context in which they reside.

In Australia, approximately 55,000 children were living in out-of-home care in 2017–18, or about 1 in every 100 children (AIHW 2018). Of these, about half were living with relatives and almost 40% were living with foster parents (less than 10% were in residential/group care). Similar to the U.S. and England, Australian infants and other young children predominate in out-of-home care. This, in contrast to many Western European nations where older children are more likely to be in the out-of-home care system (Berrick, Gilbert & Skivenes 2021). And similar to other Western industrialized nations, indigenous children in Australia were heavily over-represented in care at a rate 17 times greater than non-indigenous children (AIHW 2018).

Foster care is designed as a temporary caregiving arrangement until children can be reunified with their birth parent or, if impossible, they are transitioned to a permanent alternative living situation. In some countries, foster care is designed as a short-term arrangement (e.g., England, U.S.A.); whereas in other countries (e.g., Australia, Norway), foster caring may be a long-term setting for children who are unlikely to go home. In Australia, for example, over two-thirds of children in out-of-home care have been there for over two years (AIHW 2018). In a typical foster care arrangement, custody is transferred from the birth parent to the state with the foster parent acting on the state's behalf to secure the child's safety and promote his/her well-being.

Children are placed in foster care either voluntarily or involuntarily. Some countries rely more heavily on voluntary care (e.g., Finland) than involuntary care (e.g., Australia). Involuntary cases proceed upon the recommendation of a child welfare professional and the concurrence of a judge or other judicial decision maker. During the time children reside in foster care, their birth parent is usually required to participate in services designed to secure the child's safe return. These services might include drug treatment, parent training, counseling, or other customized activities. In many countries, regular agency or court reviews assess whether circumstances in the birth home have changed sufficiently to ensure children's safe return.

As the foundation for children's substitute care, foster care should be recognized as the backbone of the child welfare system. Without it, children would either remain with parents who were unable or unwilling to provide safe care, or they would be placed in congregate care settings, largely viewed by child development experts as inappropriate settings for the large majority of children served by the child welfare system. Because of its centrality to the child welfare system and to children's health and well-being, this chapter examines the nature of the care required of foster carers, who provides this care to children, and their needs for social work supports.

Roles and responsibilities of foster parents

Foster carers play two essential roles in the lives of children; they also play contested roles in relation to child welfare professionals. With regard to children, foster parents have both a 'bureaucratic' and a 'familial' role (Berrick 2015). With regard to child welfare professionals, foster parents may be considered a colleague, a contractor, or even a client.

In the *bureaucratic*, or 'public role' (Rymph 2017) vis-à-vis children, foster parents serve as agents of the state, attending to the needs of the child and responding to the needs of the system on behalf of the government. Ideally, they serve as a 'professional team member' (Rymph 2017: 185), working in collaboration with child welfare professionals. In their bureaucratic role, foster carers might be required, for example, to transport a child to therapy or visitation sessions with the parent. They are also required to fulfill all of the requirements of the case plan, to file appropriate documents with child welfare professionals, or to attend meetings at the child welfare agency. If the child's court-mandated case plan includes reunification, the foster carer is required to support the birth parents in their efforts to reunify with their child.

In the *familial* or 'private' role, foster parents serve as substitute parents to the child, engaging in behaviors that would be typical among highly effective parents. Features of 'successful' foster carers suggest that they are warm and child-centered; they are stable, loving, nurturing, fair, respectful, and their relationship is enduring (Sinclair & Wilson 2003). Caregivers support children's development, their cultural heritage, and the birth and extended families (Buehler et al. 2006; Shlonsky & Berrick 2001). Since the majority of studies on carers focus on foster mothers, an emerging literature on foster fathers also suggests that they may play a particularly intentional role in offering foster children a positive role model, and in showcasing a range of parenting tasks in which men can be involved (Riggs, Delfabbro & Augoustinos 2010). In addition to these parenting qualities, it is widely understood that the requirements of foster parents extend beyond typical parenting (Megahead & Soliday 2013). The circumstances of children's separation from their parents, the court and child welfare agency's involvement with their family, and the unique behavioral and emotional challenges posed by children who have usually experienced trauma create an exceptional care environment, referred to by some authors as 'parenting plus' (Berrick & Skivenes 2012).

Children in foster care may exhibit a range of physical, emotional, and educational challenges that require greater than average advocacy on the part of foster parents. According to one U.S. study including a nationally representative sample of children having contact with the child welfare system, almost one-third (27%) of children entering foster care have a chronic or recurrent health condition (Administration on Children and Families 2007). Two-thirds of children have a significant cognitive, social, or behavioral need in the clinical range (Administration on Children and Families 2007). One study indicated the prevalence of five mental health conditions among children ages 12–17.5. Findings suggested that 43% of youth reported at least one mental health concern including substance abuse/use (23%), ADHD (19%), suicidality (14%), anxiety (14%), or depression, (9%) (Horwitz et al. 2012). Children and youth in out-of-home care typically evidence higher rates of mental health problems than peers of a similar age not in care (Leslie et al. 2000; Sawyer et al. 2007). And depending on the study, between 35% and 85% of all children in out-of-home care suffer from a mental health condition (Farmer et al. 2001; Vasileva & Petermann 2016). These circumstances not only require a thoughtful parenting response in the home, but they also require significant advocacy efforts to ensure children's needs are met by a range of service providers in the community (Fergeus et al. 2018).

Given children's special needs, the demands placed on foster carers are significant, but perhaps none so great as the emotional requirements of care. Foster carers are asked to make an unconditional commitment to the children in their care, loving them as though they were a child from their original family. At the same time, foster parents are expected to release the child to the birth parent if reunification is required by the courts. Approximately half of children placed in foster care in the U.S. are reunified with their birth parent (Child Welfare Information Gateway 2011). Although data regarding reunification in Australia are not as clear, approximately one-third of children remain in care for fewer than two years, suggesting that most of these children likely return home (AIHW 2018). Given these data, it's clear that foster parents, in general, experience a high degree of loss and resulting grief in the reunification process (Buehler, Cox & Cuddeback 2003; Rhodes, Orme & Buehler 2001). As such, the familial role they play is essential to children's development and well-being, but it exacts a toll on caregivers when they are required to say 'good-bye'.

Foster parents' role vis-à-vis child welfare agencies is less clear. While the academic literature suggests that foster parents can and should be considered important partners, collaborators and colleagues with child welfare professionals, relied on for their knowledge, expertise, and relationship to the child (Buehler et al. 2006), the evidence suggests that many foster parents do not experience that role when they are in contact with child welfare professionals (Hudson & Levasseur 2002). Instead, many foster parents experience their role as a hired contractor, serving children largely in isolation with little support or recognition for their efforts (Shlonsky & Berrick 2001). Public messaging about the foster parent role is also ambiguous. Foster parents who are treated as contractors in the intimate process and experience of care nonetheless largely serve as volunteers, receiving a modest subsidy for some of the expenses incurred, but they typically do not enjoy the advantages of employment that might include a salary and associated benefits. Because the typical foster parent cares for challenging children, many foster parents need advice, help, and support from child welfare professionals. In that regard, they may sometimes be viewed as additional clients of the child welfare system whose needs also require the time and attention of busy social workers.

Characteristics of foster parents

Who are these adults who step in to care for children? It is difficult to make cross-national comparisons of foster parent characteristics as limited information is available from most countries. We know, however, that the majority of Australian carers are middle income, with no post-school education, and they are between ages 35 and 54 (McHugh et al. 2004). Kinship caregivers are typically about ten years older, on average, than foster parents (Butcher 2005). The majority of Canadian carers are Caucasian and married, with one parent working outside of the home (Rodger 2006). And in Norway, the typical foster home consists of a two-parent heterosexual couple, both of whom work outside the home. About two-in-five have a high school diploma and another two-in-five have completed college. About half of foster parents in Norway would be characterized as middle class (Berrick & Skivenes 2012). Non-relative and kinship foster carers in the U.S. are, on average, socio-economically vulnerable compared to average U.S. parents. Studies suggest that they are older, have a lower level of education, and have lower incomes (Barth et al. 2008; Berrick & Boyd 2016; O'Hare 2008).

Research on caregivers' motivations suggest that carers are generally altruistic (Colton, Roberts & Williams 2008; Kirton, Beecham & Ogilvie 2007). Foster parents serve because of their love of children, because they want to make a difference (Tyebjee 2003), and in some cases because their own children have grown and left their home and they want to continue the parenting role (Gillis-Arnold et al. 1998). No doubt a substantial proportion of caregivers offer children a caring environment that matches foster parents' aspirations for positive care. In fact, a review of studies highlighting the characteristics of 'successful caregivers' (those whose care promoted permanency or placement stability) for older youth indicated the following qualities associated with success: having a sense of humor, belief in a higher power, the capacity to tolerate rejection, and having flexible expectations (Day et al. 2018).

Of concern, however, some evidence suggests that a minority of U.S. caregivers do not offer children the sensitive caregiving environment they require. According to one study, about one-fifth of caregivers in the U.S. have 'problems in their home environment, family functioning, and parenting' (Orme & Buehler 2001:12). Other studies indicate that a similar proportion of caregivers can be characterized as 'highly aggravated' or living with poor mental health (Kortenkamp & Ehrle 2002). On average, the home environment of foster care is considered 'much less stimulating' than the average U.S. household (Barth et al. 2008). Although a minority of caregivers, these data are concerning and suggest that greater efforts may be required to recruit adults who are likely to provide effective care, and to support caregivers in this essential work.

Support for effective foster parents

Foster caregiving is typically a lonely activity as caregivers conduct their work in private homes across many communities. In Australia, children who live in remote or very remote areas of the country are twice as likely to be in out-of-home care (AIHW 2018). These foster parents likely experience considerable isolation. But a significant body of evidence suggests that foster parents need support in order to routinely care for children thoughtfully and responsively. Unlike typical professionals whose employment is limited to certain hours or days of the week, foster carers 'work' every day and night, throughout the year, usually with few or any breaks.

In addition to the isolation and constant nature of the experience, the work itself is very challenging. The children, many with special needs, have high demands for care; relationships with birth parents may be difficult; children may be taken from their care with little notice; and some children, upset or confused by their circumstances, may lodge child maltreatment allegations against the caregiver. Caregiving also takes its toll on the foster carer's family. Studies show that caregiving can increase family and marital conflict (Brown & Calder 2000; Poland & Groze 1993; Seaburg & Harrigan 1999). Caring for others' children while caring for one's own also poses challenges. Research indicates that caregivers worry about the effects foster children may have on their own children: Will their children feel a need to compete for their attention? Will their own children be prematurely exposed to mature life circumstances? Will their children learn inappropriate behaviors (Broady et al. 2010; Pugh 1996; Younes & Harp 2007)? Studies of birth children indicate that they feel the effects of foster children on their family life, noting a reduced sense of closeness among family members and increased family tension (Thompson & McPherson 2011). When carers already have birth children at home, children's foster care placements are more likely to be disrupted and this can lead to placement instability (Rock et al. 2013). Substantial evidence suggests that instability – moving from one home to another during a spell in out-of-home care – is especially hard on children, leading to a range of deleterious short- and long-term effects (Rubin et al. 2007). Among foster carers, serial caregiving – caring for multiple children over a long period of time – is especially hard on children and families as new routines and activities must be employed to respond to the unique needs of each individual child (Seaburg & Harrigan 1997; 1999).

In spite of these difficulties, other evidence suggests beneficial effects on carers' birth children. Carers describe their children as more empathic, accepting, generous, and mature following a foster child's placement (Broady et al. 2010; Hojer 2004; Younes & Harp 2007). Carers who remain in the field, after reflecting on the challenges and their successes, routinely point to their love for the children in their care as the fundamental reason they stay (Buehler, Cox & Cuddeback 2003: Coakley et al. 2007).

The sometimes turbulent emotional landscape of family life requires thoughtful support and consideration, from child welfare professionals, family, friends, and other treatment team providers. Foster parents can benefit from support groups with others, and intentional responsiveness from child welfare professionals.

Implications for child welfare professionals

Because foster carers play such a vital role in children's care and protection, child welfare professionals, agency managers, and researchers should consider four areas where targeted, intensive efforts could reap rewards. Efforts to improve *recruitment, screening, support*, and *retention* would have lasting effects for children.

New *recruitment* strategies are necessary if we hope to change the dismal supply/demand equation in foster care. Ample evidence suggests that the supply of available foster parents does not meet the demand for care (Kelly et al. 2018), and that this phenomenon is global (Ciarrochi et al. 2012). In addition to the shortage of foster parents in most jurisdictions, only a minority of caregivers in any given community provide care to the majority of children. These 'vital few', estimated at about one-fifth of the foster parent pool, care for about three-quarters of the foster children needing care. These caregivers are especially important to the child welfare system as the children in these homes experience fewer placement changes, and the care they receive is considered more effective than the care provided by the large majority of foster parents. In addition, the vital few are especially likely to accept children with special needs, so they are particularly responsive to the population served by child welfare agencies (Cherry & Orme 2013; Orme & Cherry 2015).

Recruitment for effective caregivers must target adults who are likely to offer highly responsive care. A growing body of evidence informs our understanding of the characteristics of those most likely to show interest in caring (Ciarrochi et al. 2012), and the characteristics of those most likely to provide effective care (Berrick, Shauffer & Rodriguez 2011). This research helps in targeting an appropriate recruitment message. But in spite of these important advancements, we know little about the messaging that would be most likely to appeal to prospective caregiver applicants.

Because the applicant pool is usually limited, child welfare agencies typically use rather few criteria for *screening* applicants. In the U.S., each state sets licencing criteria that focus largely on the safety of the caregiver's home. A child welfare professional usually conducts a home study to assess the parenting of the caregiver using a 'minimum adequacy' standard. Although some have argued that standards of care should be raised to ensure that only the most effective caregivers are selected as foster parents (Crea, Griffin & Barth 2011), there is an equal reluctance to do so out of concern that higher standards will further shrink the pool of available caregivers (Colton, Roberts & Williams 2008). Screening tools have been developed by researchers that include positive aspects of care such as commitment, confidence, affection, and acceptance. They also include negative qualities or behaviors that might suggest areas of concern (Orme et al. 2007). In spite of the promise these tools offer the field, they are not in widespread use, and standardized cut-off points for eligibility have not yet been established.

Among the adults who step forward to serve, many will need *support* to provide the effective care that children need. In a cross-national study of effective foster parents in the U.S. and in Norway (Berrick & Skivenes 2012), the authors determined that the nature of foster parents' care for children can be characterized as having *affective* and *behavioral* components (similar to Polgar's assessment of caregivers' *abilities* and *capacities* (2001)). The *behavioral* qualities of care (i.e., *capacities*) – including advocacy skills, transition planning, and positive reinforcement strategies – may be responsive to training. Alternatively, child welfare staff may find that the *affective* qualities of care (i.e., *abilities*) – including empathy for children, or parenting with respect and humility – may be characteristics adults bring to care naturally. Adults may be able to learn these traits, but perhaps not so readily.

Research involving foster carers routinely indicates a preference for responsive support. In most jurisdictions, however, caregivers receive little support to prepare them for their role and responsibilities. In many countries, foster parents are required to participate in basic training. In a study conducted in Queensland, Australia, however, the majority of kinship caregivers and an important minority of foster parents (15%) had received no training prior to a child's placement in their care (Butcher 2005). Recent research suggests benefits may accrue to caregivers who participate in training including perceptions of improved parenting skills (Akin et al. 2017), increased satisfaction with the foster parenting role (Randle, Miller & Dolnicar 2017), reductions in children's behavior problems (Solomon, Niec & Schoonover 2017), and stronger relationships with children's birth parents (Cooley & Petren 2011). Research on two of the most widely used training models in the world, PRIDE and MAPP, however, show few effects (Dorsey et al. 2008). Instead, new research is emerging indicating that caregivers and children may first benefit from training, but thereafter experience positive effects from close consultation and ongoing coaching from social work staff (Linares et al. 2006; McNeil et al. 2005; Timmer, Urquiza & Zebell 2006). These programs, showing effects when delivered to foster carers or to birth parents, reduce children's behavior problems and improve positive parenting behaviors. The programs are usually delivered *in vivo* so that parents can practice newly developing skills and receive feedback and support to strengthen and reinforce these skills (Chamberlain & Mihalic 1998; Dozier, Dozier & Manni 2002; Dozier et al. 2002; 2006). Implementation of the KEEP program (a modified version of Multidimensional Treatment Foster Care (MTFC)), involving a 16-week training program, regular telephone calls and homework, has shown important effects in randomized trials, increasing positive parenting, placement stability, and improving the odds of reunification (Chamberlain et al. 2008; Price et al. 2008).

In addition to the support caregivers need in responding to their foster child's special needs and behavioral difficulties, they may also need assistance managing the emotions associated with the role. Carers may need to consider how the introduction of a foster child will change their role as a parent, and how they will introduce and support a foster child into their existing family. Relationships with family members and with friends may change. Therefore, having formal and informal support can help to reduce foster parent stress, and co-parenting stress in couples (Richardson et al. 2018). Developing new support networks among other foster parents can also be helpful. In fact, some evidence suggests that support networks are critical for some groups. The work of Brown et al. (2013) indicates that Aboriginal foster parents may be especially responsive to a supportive network.

But beyond training, coaching, and articulated models of support, ample evidence shows that foster carers need to enjoy a relationship with the child welfare professional that is built on respect, accurate information, and responsiveness. In short, they need the child welfare professional they work with to visit and to listen; to offer advice about the children in their care and about community resources; to follow through on their commitments; and to serve as an effective problem solver (Fisher et al. 2000). Moreover, they want the care they provide to children to be well informed. For these reasons, they want timely and accurate information about the child and his or her family circumstances and history (Geiger, Hayes & Lietz 2013; MacGregor et al. 2006), and they want to enjoy a relationship of clear and open communication (Denlinger & Dorius 2018).

Caregiving is emotionally gratifying, but the work is difficult. As a result, many of the best foster carers leave the field. Turnover rates of between 30% and 50% are not uncommon (Christian 2002; Whenan, Oxlad & Lushington 2009), and the median duration foster carers remain in the field is only 8–14 months (Gibbs & Wildfire 2007). *Retention* is fueled, in part, by the bureaucratic features of foster care that do not correspond with the familial experiences of raising children (Rindfleisch, Bean & Denby 1998; Shlonsky & Berrick 2001). In addition, many public and private foster care agencies struggle to treat caregivers in ways that carers would prefer: with respect as valued team members or with appreciation for caregivers' heroic efforts (Burgess, McDonald & Smith 2003; Fisher et al. 2000). And seemingly simple acts of professional courtesy, for example, promptly returning phone calls, appear to be a perennial problem (Rhodes, Orme & Buehler 2001; Triseliotis, Borland & Hill 1998). Of course, reimbursement rates that are so low that carers must subsidize children's care can contribute to a caregiver's difficulties continuing in the field (Ahn et al. 2018; Rhodes, Orme & Buehler 2001).

Nations across the globe now rely heavily upon kinship or relative carers to provide children with care and support. But most child welfare systems will always rely on foster care with non-relatives for some children. Given the central role foster care plays in the child welfare system, improved efforts to recruit, screen, support, and retain the best among these will serve child welfare agencies and the children and families in their care.

Case study

Kay and Steven Denton called to inquire about foster parenting after they saw a sign about foster care on a local bus stop. First, they filled out lots of forms and then they participated in a lengthy interview with a social worker to determine their appropriateness to serve as foster parents. The social worker wanted to know a lot about the physical safety of their home; she only asked a few questions about how they saw themselves as parents. Kay and Steven knew they would be good caregivers, though, as they had both performed a lot of babysitting when they were young. Once approved, they installed locks on their medicine closet and attended to other safety hazards in their home; they also participated in the 30-hour foster parent training course. Kay and Steven thought they were ready to take on the challenge of foster care.

Tabitha and her little brother, Roger, were four and two respectively when they came to live with the Dentons. Everything about Kay and Steven's home was foreign to the siblings. The foods, smells, and sounds of the home were different, the routines were different, their clothes, toys, and books were different. Nonetheless, the children settled into their new routine fairly quickly and the Dentons felt pretty confident in their caregiving.

Steven was away at work most days, leaving Kay to tend to the children alone. She called her social worker a couple of times a week during the first few weeks. She had all sorts of unanticipated questions about the children, about what she was allowed (and not allowed) to do, and how she should handle certain situations. She knew her social worker was busy, so she was unsurprised that most of her voice mail messages were left unanswered.

As the weeks turned to months, Kay fell in love with the children. They were sweet and funny, and each of them had their own, unique personality. Her feelings of affection seemed to carry her through the difficult moments: a crying fit, an angry outburst, a defiant 'no!' But in spite of her generally positive feelings, Kay felt as though she could benefit from more structured and intentional strategies to manage the children's behavior. What was that she had learned about positive reinforcement in her foster parent training? When was it appropriate to use a time-out? Should she expect different behaviors from little Roger than from his big sister? She called her social worker a couple of times to find out more about support groups or extra training. She got a call back, once, with a promise to send some brochures, but they never arrived.

Kay shuttled the children to weekly visits with their mother, Diana. Kay was shy and didn't know if she could or should interact with her. Kay wanted to talk with Diana and reassure her about her children's well-being; she wanted to ask Diana about her children's needs and desires; and she wanted to offer Diana support as she imagined the difficulties of her circumstances. But they hadn't been formally introduced and she didn't know what role was appropriate, so she usually waited in the car while the children enjoyed time with their mother.

The social worker visited Kay and Steven's home about once a month. She regularly inquired about the children, their health and well-being. But she always ran out of time, and infrequently asked about Kay, Steven, or about their views of the family and the family's needs. Kay thought that foster parenting was going to be a partnership. She thought that she had been invited onto a team to help Diana and her family. Instead, she felt like a poorly paid employee, minus the pay or the benefits. She noticed that her social worker rarely expressed her appreciation to either Kay or Steven.

One evening, at the end of a lovely visit with their mother, Tabitha and Roger did not want to go home with Kay. They cried and begged to be left with their mother. Diana couldn't have been more helpful. She told the children how much she loved them and that she would see them soon; she helped transfer them to the car seats in Kay's car; and she assured them that Kay would take good care of them in her absence. Crying turned into screaming as the children called out for the mother, but Diana assured Kay that they would settle down. Diana hugged the children one more time and walked away.

The children didn't settle down. Their screaming was relentless. Steven was working late, so Kay knew there was no one to help her at home. She pulled the car over for a moment to call her social worker. No answer. The on-call social worker assured her the children would settle down as soon as they got home. As they pulled into the driveway, Kay wondered what her neighbors might think. Tabitha screamed as she was pulled out of her car seat; Roger wailed as Kay carried him into the house. Nothing worked. Storytime, songs, an evening snack, nothing. Kay felt helpless, isolated, and utterly incompetent. She vowed to herself that she would call the agency in the morning and quit.

Kay remembered a neighbor down the street who once told her he was a children's therapist. At the end of her rope, she called, desperately hoping he might offer a suggestion or at least a friendly, adult voice. He came over, quietly offered Kay some suggestions about how to respond to the children's emotions and behaviors. Kay tried them out, and within a short time, the children were quiet, they were snuggled in bed, and they were fast asleep.

1. Kay and Steven learned about foster care from a public sign. What other strategies might be employed to *recruit* highly effective foster parents?
2. The social worker who screened Kay and Steven applied a 'minimal adequacy' standard. What additional standards, if any, should be applied in the *screening process*?
3. What are some of the emotional challenges of care Kay is experiencing?
4. What could the social worker do to offer Kay a *collaborative* role in supporting Diana, Tabitha, and Roger?
5. What are some of the positive, *affective characteristics* Kay brought to her caregiving?
6. What are some additional *behavioral characteristics* Kay could have benefitted from learning?

7 What type of *support* could have helped Kay respond effectively to Tabitha and Roger during their especially difficult evening?
8 What strategies might the social worker employ to *retain* Kay and Steven as foster parents?

References

Administration on Children and Families, 2007, Who are the children in foster care? National Survey of Child and Adolescent Well-being: Research Brief No. 1, www.acf.hhs.gov/sites/default/files/opre/children_fostercare.pdf, accessed 12 August 2019.

Ahn, H., DePanfilis, D., Frick, K. & Barth, R.P., 2018, 'Estimating minimum adequate foster care costs for children in the United States', *Children and Youth Services Review*, vol. 84, pp. 55–67.

Akin, B., Yan, Y., McDonald, T. & Moon, J., 2017, 'Changes in parenting practices during Parent management training Oregon model with parents of children in foster care', *Children and Youth Services Review*, vol. 76, pp. 181–191.

AIHW, 2018, *Child protection Australia, 2017–18*, Canberra: Australian Institute of Health and Welfare.

Barth, R.P., Green, R., Webb, M., Wall, A., Gibbons, C. & Craig, C., 2008, 'Characteristics of out-of-home caregiving environments provided under child welfare services', *Child Welfare*, vol. 87, no. 3.

Berrick, J.D., 2015, 'Research and practice with families in foster care', in S. Browning & K. Pasley (eds), *Contemporary families: Translating research into practice*, London: Routledge.

Berrick, J.D. & Boyd, R., 2016, 'The financial well-being of children in family-based foster care: Exploring variation in income supports for kin and non-kin caregivers', *Children & Youth Services Review*, vol. 69, pp. 166–173.

Berrick, J.D., Gilbert, N. & Skivenes, M., 2021, in press, *International handbook of child protection systems*, New York: Oxford University Press.

Berrick, J.D. & Skivenes, M., 2012, 'Dimensions of high quality foster care: Parenting plus', *Children & Youth Services Review*, vol. 34, no. 9, pp. 1956–1965.

Berrick, J.D., Shauffer, C. & Rodriguez, J., 2011, 'Recruiting for excellence in foster care: Marrying child welfare research with brand marketing strategies', *Journal of Public Child Welfare*, vol. 5, no. 2, pp. 271–281.

Broady, T.R., Stoyles, G.J., McMullan, K., Caputi, P. & Crittenden, N., 2010, 'The experiment of foster care', *Journal of Child & Family Studies*, vol. 19, pp. 559–571.

Brown, J. & Calder, P., 2000, 'Concept mapping the needs of foster parents', *Child Welfare League of America*, vol. 79, pp. 729–746.

Brown, J.D., Ivonova, V., Mehta, N., Skrodzki, D. & Gerrits, J., 2013, 'Social needs of aboriginal foster parents', *Children & Youth Services Review*, vol. 35, pp. 1886–1893.

Buehler, C., Cox, M. & Cuddeback, G., 2003, 'Foster parents' perceptions of factors that promote or inhibit successful fostering', *Qualitative Social Work*, vol. 2, pp. 61–83.

Buehler, C., Rhodes, K., Orme, J. & Cuddeback, G., 2006, 'The potential for successful family foster care: Conceptualizing competency domains for foster parents', *Child Welfare*, vol. 85, pp. 523–558.

Burgess, C., McDonald, P.S. & Smith, K., 2003, 'A support team for foster carers: The views and perceptions of service users', *British Journal of Social Work*, vol. 33, pp. 825–832.

Butcher, A., 2005, 'Upping the ante: The training and status of foster carers in Queensland', *Children Australia*, vol. 30, no. 3, pp. 25–30.

Chamberlain, P. & Mihalic, S., 1998, *Blueprints for violence prevention*, Boulder, CO: Center for the Study and Prevention of Violence.

Chamberlain, P., Price, J., Leve, L.D., Laurent, H., Landsverk, J. & Reid, J., 2008, 'Prevention of behavior problems for children in foster care: Outcomes and mediation effects', *Prevention Science*, vol. 9, pp. 17–27.

Cherry, D. & Orme, J., 2013, 'The vital few foster mothers', *Children & Youth Services Review*, vol. 35, pp. 1625–1633.

Child Welfare Information Gateway, 2011, *Family reunification: What the evidence shows*, Washington, DC: Children's Bureau.

Christian, S., 2002, 'Supporting and retaining foster parents. Washington, D.C.: National Conference of State Legislators', *State Legislative Report*, vol. 27, no. 11, pp. 1–11.

Ciarrochi, J., Randle, M., Miller, L. & Dolnicar, S., 2012, 'Hope for the future: Identifying the individual difference characteristics of people who are interested in and intend to foster-care', *British Journal of Social Work*, vol. 42, pp. 7–25.

Coakley, T.M., Cuddebak, G., Buehler, C. & Cox, M.E., 2007, 'Kinship foster parents' perceptions of factors that promote or inhibit successful fostering', *Children & Youth Services Review*, vol. 29, pp. 92–109.

Colton, M., Roberts, S. & Williams, M., 2008, 'The recruitment and retention of family foster carers: An international and cross-cultural analysis', *British Journal of Social Work*, vol. 38, pp. 865–884.

Cooley, M.E. & Petren, R.E., 2011, 'Foster parent perceptions of competency: Implications for foster parent training', *Children & Youth Services Review*, vol. 33, no. 10, pp. 1968–1974.

Crea, T.M., Griffin, A. & Barth, R.P., 2011, 'The intersection of home study assessments and child specific recruitment: The performance of home studies in practice', *Children & Youth Services Review*, vol. 33, pp. 28–33.

Day, A., Willis, T., Vanderwill, L., Resko, S., Patterson, D., Henneman, K. & Cohick, S., 2018, 'Key factors and characteristics of successful resource parents who care for older youth: A systematic review of research', *Children & Youth Services Review*, vol. 84, pp. 152–158.

Denlinger, M. & Dorius, C., 2018, 'Communication patterns between foster parents and case managers', *Children and Youth Services Review*, vol. 89, pp. 329–339.

Dorsey, S., Farmer, E. M. Z., Barth, R. P., Greene, K. M., Reid, J. & Landsverk, J., 2008, 'Current status and evidence base of training for foster and treatment foster parents', *Children & Youth Services Review*, vol. 30, no. 12, pp. 1403–1416.

Dozier, M., Dozier, D. & Manni, M., 2002, 'Attachment and biobehavioral catch-up: The ABCs of helping infants in foster care cope with early adversity', *Zero to Three*, vol. 22, pp. 7–13.

Dozier, M., Higley, E., Albus, K. & Nutter, A., 2002, 'Intervening with foster infants' caregivers: Targeting three critical needs', *Infant Mental Health Journal*, vol. 25, pp. 541–554.

Dozier, M., Peloso, E., Lindhiem, O., Gordon, M. K., Manni, M., Sepulveda, S. & Ackerman, J., 2006, 'Developing evidence-based interventions for foster children: An example of a randomized clinical trial with infants and toddlers', *Journal of Social Issues*, vol. 62, pp. 767–785.

Farmer, E.M., Burns, B.J., Chapman, M.V., Phillips, S.D., Angold, A. & Costello, E.J., 2001, 'Use of mental health services by youth in contact with social services', *Social Service Review*, vol. 75, no. 4, pp. 605–624.

Fergeus, J. Humphreys, C., Harvey, C. & Herrman, H., 2018, 'Supporting foster and kinship carers to promote the mental health of children', *Child & Family Social Work*, vol. 24, no. 1, pp. 1–7.

Fisher, T., Gibbs, I., Sinclair, I. & Wilson, K., 2000, 'Sharing the care: Qualities sought of social workers by foster carers', *Child & Family Social Work*, vol. 5, pp. 225–233.

Geiger, J.M., Hayes, M.J. & Lietz, C.A., 2013, 'Should I stay or should I go? A mixed methods study examining the factors influencing foster parents' decisions to continue or discontinue providing foster care', *Children & Youth Services Review*, vol. 35, no. 9, pp. 1356–1365.

Gibbs, D. & Wildfire, J., 2007, 'Length of service for foster parents: Using administrative data to understand retention', *Children & Youth Services Review*, vol. 29, pp. 588–599.

Gillis-Arnold, R., Crase, S.J., Stockdale, D.F. & Shelley, M.C., 1998, 'Parenting attitudes, foster parenting attitudes, and motivations of adoptive and nonadoptive foster parent trainees', *Children & Youth Service Review*, vol. 20, no. 8, pp. 715–732.

Hojer, I., 2004, 'What happens in the foster family? A study of fostering relationships in Sweden', *Adoption & Fostering*, vol. 28, no. 1, pp. 38–48.

Horwitz, S.M., Hurlburt, M.S., Heneghan, A., Zhang, J., Rolls-Reutz, J., Fisher, E., Landsverk, J. & Stein, R.E., 2012, 'Mental health problems in young children investigated by US child welfare agencies', *Journal of the American Academy of Child & Adolescent Psychiatry*, vol. 51, no. 6, pp. 572–581.

Hudson, P. & Levasseur, K., 2002, 'Supporting foster parents: Caring voices', *Child Welfare*, vol. 81, no. 6, pp. 853–877.

Kelly, J., Heimpel, D., Loudenback, J., Renick, C., Phagan-Hansel, K., Green, E., Pham, S. & Zarate, M., 2018, *The foster care housing crisis*, Los Angeles, CA: The Chronicle of Social Change.

Kirton, D., Beecham, J. & Ogilvie, K., 2007, 'Gaining satisfaction? An exploration of foster carers attitudes to payment', *British Journal of Social Work*, vol. 37, no. 7, pp. 1205–1224.

Kortenkamp, K. & Ehrle, J., 2002, *The well-being of children involved with the child welfare system: A national overview*, New Federalism Series B., no. B-43, Washington, DC: Urban Institute.

Leslie, L.K., Landsverk, J., Ezzet-Lofstrom, R., Tschann, J.M., Slymen, D.J. & Garland, A.F., 2000, 'Children in foster care: Factors influencing outpatient mental health service use', *Child Abuse & Neglect*, vol. 24, no. 4, pp. 465–476.

Linares, L.O., Montalto, D., Li, M. & Oza, V., 2006, 'A promising parenting intervention in foster care', *Journal of Consulting & Clinical Psychology*, vol. 74, pp. 32–41.

MacGregor, T.E., Rodger, S., Cummings, A.L. & Leschied, A.W., 2006, 'The needs of foster parents: A qualitative study of motivation, support, and retention', *Qualitative Social Work*, vol. 5, no. 3, pp. 351–368.

McHugh, M., McNab, J., Smyth, C., Chalmers, J., Siminski, P. & Saunders, P., 2004, *The availability of foster carers: Main report*, Sydney: Social Policy Research Centre, University of New South Wales.

McNeil, C., Herschell, A.D., Gurwitch, R.H. & Clemens-Mowrer, L.C., 2005, 'Training foster parents in parent-child interaction therapy', *Education and Treatment of Children*, vol. 28, pp. 182–196.

Megahead, H. & Soliday, E., 2013, 'Developing a conceptual framework of foster family placement', *Journal of Family Psychotherapy*, vol. 24, pp. 48–63.

O'Hare, W., 2008, *Data on children in foster care from the Census Bureau*, Baltimore, MD: Annie E. Casey Foundation.

Orme, J. & Buehler, C., 2001, 'Foster family characteristics and behavioral and emotional problems of foster children: A narrative review', *Family Relations*, vol. 50, no. 1, p. 12

Orme, J. & Cherry, D.J., 2015, 'The vital few foster parents: Replication and extension', *Children & Youth Services Review*, vol. 56, pp. 33–41.

Orme, J., Cuddeback, G., Buehler, C., Cox, M. & LeProhn, N., 2007, 'Measuring foster parent potential: Casey Foster parent inventory-Applicant version', *Research on Social Work Practice*, vol. 17, pp. 77–92.

Poland, D.C. & Groze, V., 1993, 'Effects of foster care placement on birth children in the home', *Child & Adolescent Social Work Journal*, vol. 10, pp. 153–164.

Polgar, A., 2001, *Conducting parenting capacity assessments*, Hamilton, Ontario: Samdriam.

Price, J., Chamberlain, P., Landsverk, J., Reid, J., Leve, L. & Laurant, H., 2008, 'Effects of a foster parent training intervention on placement changes of children in foster care', *Child Maltreatment*, vol. 13, pp. 64–75.

Pugh, G., 1996, 'Seen but not heard? Addressing the needs of children who foster', *Adoption & Fostering*, vol. 20, pp. 35–41.

Randle, M., Miller, L. & Dolnicar, S., 2017, 'What can agencies do to increase foster carer satisfaction?', *Child & Family Social Work*, vol. 32, no. 2, pp. 212–221.

Rhodes, K., Orme, J. & Buehler, C., 2001, 'A comparison of family foster parents who quit, consider quitting, and plan to continue fostering', *Social Service Review*, vol. 75, pp. 85–114.

Richardson, E., Futris, T.G., Mallette, J.K. & Campbell, A., 2018, 'Foster mothers' parenting stress and coparenting quality: An examination of the moderating role of support', *Children & Youth Services Review*, vol. 89, pp. 77–82.

Riggs, D., Delfabbro, P.H. & Augoustinos, M., 2010, 'Foster fathers and carework: Engaging alternate models of parenting', *Fathering*, vol. 8, no. 1, pp. 24–36.

Rindfleisch, N., Bean, G. & Denby, R., 1998, 'Why foster parents continue and cease to foster', *Journal of Sociology & Social Welfare*, vol. 25, no. 1, pp. 5−24

Rock, S., Michelson, D., Thomson, S. & Day, C., 2013, 'Understanding Foster Placement Instability for Looked After Children: A Systematic Review and Narrative Synthesis of Quantitative and Qualitative Evidence', *British Journal of Social Work*, vol. 45, no. 1, pp. 177–203.

Rodger, S., 2006, 'Who is caring for our most vulnerable children? The motivation to foster in child welfare', *Child Abuse and Neglect*, vol. 30, no. 10, pp. 1129–1142.

Rubin, D.M., O'Reilly, A.L., Luan, X. & Localio, A.R., 2007, 'The impact of placement stability on behavioral well-being for children in foster care', *Pediatrics*, vol. 119, no. 2, pp. 336–344.

Rymph, C.E., 2017, *Raising government children: A history of foster care and the American welfare state*, Chapel Hill, NC: University of North Carolina Press.

Sawyer, M.G., Carbone, J.A., Searle, A.K. & Robinson, P., 2007, 'The mental health and wellbeing of children and adolescents in home-based foster care', *Medical Journal of Australia*, vol. 186, no. 4, pp. 181–184.

Seaberg, J.R. & Harrigan, M.P., 1997, 'Family functioning in foster care', *Families in Society*, vol. 78, pp. 463–470.

Seaberg, J.R. & Harrigan, M.P., 1999, 'Foster families' functioning, experiences and views: variations by race', *Children & Youth Services Review*, vol. 21, pp. 31–55.

Shlonsky, A. & Berrick, J.D., 2001, 'Assessing and promoting quality in kin and nonkin foster care', *Social Service Review*, vol. 75, pp. 60–83.

Sinclair, I. & Wilson, K., 2003, 'Matches and mismatches: The contribution of careers and children to the success of foster placements', *British Journal of Social Work*, vol. 33, pp. 871–884.

Solomon, D.T., Niec, L.N. & Schoonover, C.E., 2017, 'The impact of foster parent training on parenting skills and child disruptive behavior: A meta-analysis', *Child Maltreatment*, vol. 22, no. 1, pp. 3–13.

Thompson, H. & McPherson, S., 2011, 'The experience of living with a foster sibling as described by the birth children of foster carers: a thematic analysis of the literature', *Adoption & Fostering*, vol. 35, no. 2, pp. 49–60.

Timmer, S.G., Urquiza, A.J. & Zebell, N., 2006, 'Challenging foster caregiver-maltreated child relationships: The effectiveness of parent-child interaction therapy', *Children & Youth Services Review*, vol. 28, pp. 1–19.

Triseliotis, J., Borland, M. & Hill, M., 1998, 'Foster carers who cease to foster', *Adoption and Fostering*, vol. 22, no. 2, pp. 54–61.

Tyebjee, T., 2003, 'Attitude, interest, and motivation for adoption and foster care', *Child Welfare*, vol. 82, no. 6, pp. 685–706.

Vasileva, M. & Petermann, F., 2016, 'Attachment, development, and mental health in abused and neglected preschool children in foster care: A meta-analysis', *Trauma, Violence, & Abuse*, vol. 19, no. 4, pp. 1–16.

Whenan, R., Oxlad, M. & Lushington, K., 2009, 'Factors associated with foster carer well-being, satisfaction and intention to continue providing out-of-home care', *Children & Youth Services Review*, vol. 31, pp. 752–760.

Younes, M.N. & Harp, M., 2007, 'Addressing the impact of foster care on birth children and their families', *Child Welfare*, vol. 86, no. 4, pp. 21–40.

Index

Page numbers in *italics* refer to figures. Page numbers in **bold** refer to tables.

AAI *see* Adult Attachment Interview
Aboriginal and Torres Strait Islander (ATSI) children: child placement principle 57, 292; factors causing over-representation of 295; Family Matters campaign and 293–294; formal kinship care 180; intergenerational trauma 293–294; measures to address disparities in access to services by 57–58; in OOHC 84; over-representation in child welfare system 6, 8, 12–13, 57–58, 289–290; placement in out-of-home care 290; rights framework for 291–293; self-determination commitment 8, 291, 295, 297
Aboriginal Care Circles 281
Aboriginal Child Placement Principle 13, 114–115, 116, 181
Aboriginal children 296; in OOHC 310; reunification patterns 229; transfer into white care 44
Aboriginal parenting, Bowlby's theory of attachment 32
'absent parenting' 211
'absent presence' *see* child neglect
abuse *see* child abuse
abusive behaviour towards child: attachment-based trauma and 74; defence mechanism to cope with 74; triggered by baby cry 73
accommodation process 28
ACEs *see* Adverse Childhood Experiences
ACEs adults 40
ACLSA *see* Ansell-Casey Life Skills Assessment
ACT *see* Australian Capital Territory
Action for Children 68
'Active efforts,' concept of 293
activity scheduling and play therapies 139–140
actuarial approaches 103, 104
Additional Child Care Subsidy for Grandparents 178
adoption 11; associated questions 243–244; attachment impact on 244–245; challenges to 241; developmental recovery in 249–250; development of 241–242; evolution of 249; growth of 242; lawful 246; legal status of 242; lifelong impact on child 242–243; origins in UK 241; risk factors of 244
Adoption of Children Act 1926 242
Adult Attachment Interview 33
Adverse Childhood Experiences 40, 41, 246
advocacy coalitions 280–281
affectional bonds, disruption of 32
affectional relationships 34
after-care support 253
age of children: age of 5–6 29; age of 10–12 29; age of 15–17 29; and reunification patterns, link between 228–229
Ages and Stages Questionnaire 106
Ainsworth, Mary 31
alternative education 212
ambiguous loss, grief reactions associated with 33
anger management 138
Ansell-Casey Life Skills Assessment 106
ASQ *see* Ages and Stages Questionnaire
assimilation process 28
attachment: Aboriginal parenting 32; behaviours, complexity of 31; *vs.* bonding 33–34; Bowlby's conceptualisations of 32; and brain development, link between 39–40; classification across cultures 31; cognitive theory of 30–31; definition of 30, 140; development phases 31; ethological theory of 30; learning theory of 31; manifestations of 31; nurturing and supporting 32; for optimum development 30; psychodynamic theory of 30; relationship and mentalization 74; stages of 31; *see also* child welfare

attachment-based trauma 75
attachment disorder 135
attachment-style interviews 33
attachment system 31
attachment therapy 140–141
Australia 53–54; Care and Protection orders 7; Children's Courts in 123–124; feminist activism 81; NSW advertising campaign 79; social democratic welfare model 55–56; TRC pilot program 194–197, 201–203
Australia, kinship care in 175; children in 176–177; formal 179–185; informal 178–179; lack of government support 179; perspectives of children and parents 185–186; services to families 176
Australian Association of Young People in Care 273
Australian Capital Territory: legislative basis for cumulative harm 125–126; mandatory reporting requirements 124
Australian Family Law Act 1975 59
Australian Government: children's participation in court 59–60; measures to address disparities 57; neoliberal and market-oriented policies 56; programme to support parents 56; responses to CSA 91–92; Third Action Plan (2015–2018) 56
Australian Personal Safety Study (PSS 2016) 82
Australian 'social investment state' 56

'baby farming' 242
balancing perspectives 45–46
'battered child syndrome' 4
Behavioural and Emotional Scale 106
behavioural problems, in CP populations: 'attachment disorder' 135; behavioural therapy for 135–136; cognitive-behavioural therapy for 137; internalising problems 135; multidimensional treatment foster care for 136–137; prevalence of 134
behaviour modification 135–136
Berrick, Jill Duerr 318
Berry Street 252, 256
BERS *see* Behavioural and Emotional Scale
best interest principle/standard *see* child's best interests, standard of
Best Interests Case Practice Model 277
Better Outcomes, Brighter Futures approach 155
biological parents *see* First Families
birth parents *see* First Families
bonding 32; *vs.* attachment 33–34; definition 33; early and extended contact on 34; empirical and sociological bases of 34; factors influencing assessment of 34; theorising 33–34
book-gifting programmes 216
brain alterations and child abuse, relationship between 41
brain development: and attachment, link between 39–40; trauma impact on 39–41
brain regions and stress managing functions 39
brainwashing 72

CAF *see* Common Assessment Framework
California Family Risk Assessment 105
CAPI *see* Child Abuse Potential Inventory
Care and Protection Orders 7
caregivers 67
care leavers: assistance to 255; backgrounds and experiences 252–253; classification of 253; from disadvantaged families 253; experiencing inadequacies in state care 253–254; experiencing poor outcomes 256; family relationships 263–264; funding available to 255–256; lack of family support to 254; 'moving-on group' 253; public inquiries 256; reasons for vulnerability of 253–254; social exclusion barriers to 252; 'strugglers' 253; 'survivors' 253; transition from care plan 255; Victorian policy and 255–256; *see also* leaving care
CARE model 204n2
'caretaker' movement 273
case management 114
Casey Family Services Demonstration project 234
CASPARS *see* Clinical Assessment Package for Assessing Clients' Risks and Strengths
CBT *see* cognitive behavioural therapy
CCYP *see* Commission for Children and Young People
CDI *see* Child-Directed Interaction
Central Statistics Office 154
Centrelink 178
CFRA *see* California Family Risk Assessment
child abuse 35–36; and brain alterations, relationship between 40–41; definitions of 4, 5, 6; difficulty in deciding matters of 127–129; at institutional and structural levels 5; reporting pattern 6; reports 7; *see also* child sexual abuse
Child Abuse Potential Inventory 110
child and childhood self, connection between 73
child behaviour management strategies 139
child behaviour therapy 135–136
child-centred and child-inclusive research 35
child development: attachment and bonding 29–33; attachment impact on 244–245; contextual relationships influencing 36; of intelligence 28; key features of 245; proponents of stages of 27–28; risk and

protective factors affecting 38; stage theory 28; *see also* developmental theories
Child-Directed Interaction 141
childhood: conceptualized as vulnerable 272; sociology of 35
childhood abuse 153
childhood adversity: definition of 40; examples of 40; responses to 41
childhood trauma: effect on brain development 39–41; neurological harm associated with 39; stimuli in context of 40
child maltreatment 14, 107; ATSI children 290; 'battered child syndrome' 4; definitions of 3, 4, 5; exposure to physical, sexual and emotional abuse 4; framed in legislation 125–126; impact on child developmental health 245–246; longer-term negative outcomes of 153; and low-income families, association between 5; parental inadequacies in 9; protective factors in relation to 152; reporting pattern 6; reporting requirements 5; risk factors for 153; social conditions associated with 112; state and media interest in 6; stressful stimuli 40; structural bases of 5; and structural disadvantage, link between 5; trauma from 4–5; *see also* child abuse
child needs: changes in 27; and family needs, sociological frameworks of 36; lack of awareness of 71
child neglect: case examples of 69–76; case review issues 69; cumulative harm associated with 128–129; definitions of 67; generalised assessments 70; of identity 70; impact on brain development 40; lack of awareness of needs 71; legislation connected to 68; parameters of 67; prevalence in UK 68; psychological and physical consequences of 5; 'relational poverty' 67; reporting pattern 6; re-referral rate of 69
Child Placement Principle 13, 57, 114–115, 116, 181, 292, 293
child pornography 5
child protection 10, 14, 271; agenda mobilisation 4; approach 38; concerns 126; co-production in 283; framework of Australia 125; historical context and trends in 6–10; ideological goals of 11; interventions in 96; jurisdiction 126; lists of actions 71; neglect as ground for 128–129; notifications 125; participation principle in 277–278; reports/notifications for 96; stages of 277; State and Territory governments role in 96; work in divided society 42–43
Child Protection Act 1999 126
child protection assessment 34, 96; analytical 115; approaches to 99; child-centred approach to 116–117; conceptualisation of 100–101; culturally appropriate 113–115; definition of 97; ecological approach to 112; engaging parents 117; in environment of uncertainty 112–113; factors with respect to child and family 100–101; family assessment 107–111; focus of 97; in linear model 98; nature of 97–98; need for best practice in 100; qualitative and quantitative methods 99; questions to be considered in 101; responding to diversity 113–115; risk assessment 101–105; safety assessment 100; sequential steps 98; structured decision-making tools for 105; using knowledge in 115–116; wellbeing asessment 105–107
child protection intervention: ATSI children 289–290; effectiveness and impact of 8; as legal enterprise 125; and removals 13; statutory legal powers 125
child protection legislation 124; Australian 124; child abuse matters and 127–129; child maltreatment framed in 125–126; legal criterion of significant harm 128; and legal systems, tension between 126
child protection national policy 9
child protection practices: advocacy coalitions 280–281; children and practitioners positioning in 275–277; focus on risk of harm to children 272; relational participation in 278–279; rising demand for 125; and socio-economic disadvantage, relationship between 126; threats of risk to children 272
child protection systems 3, 5, 125, 127, 277, 290; challenges in design and delivery of 7; changes in 10; deficits and inadequacies 7–8; dilemmas confronting 3; discourses around operation of 7; First Families involved with 301–313; forensically dominated responses to 7; paradigm shift in operation of 9–10; preoccupation with focus of 7; public interest in 9; review of 7, 126–127; systemic failures in 56
children: conceptualisations of 35; looked after by local authority, special needs of *169*
Children, Youth and Families Act 2005 126, 256
Children and Young People Act 2008 126
Children and Young Persons Act 1933 68
Children and Young Persons (Care and Protection) Act 1998 277, 301
children in out-of-home care (OOHC), educational progress of: in Australia 209, 211; education liaison personnel 215; in England 209–213; foster carer/family-focused interventions 217–218; mentoring programme 216; policy and practice implications 218–219; poorer outcomes 210; provision for supporting 211–212; reading

interventions 216–217; systemic interventions for 212–215; trauma training 213; tutoring programmes 215–216; in US 209–211; young people's experience 210; *see also* out-of-home care
children's capacities and age, link between 28
Children's Court for Care and Protection Orders 7
Children's Courts: challenges to 129–131; innovations in jurisprudence approaches 126; judicial officers 129–130; jurisdiction in Australia 123–124; need for shared enterprise 131; operation of 129–130; problem-solving approach 126–127; problem-solving courts 130; workload of 130
children's participation 271; analytical models for 274–275; in care and protection system 273; in child protection and care systems 272; deliberative democracy and 281–283; in protective care continuum 12; relational 278–279; rights in court proceedings 59–60; typology relating to techniques of 275
children's rights: arguments for 43; and child liberation 43–44; codification in Convention 274; and leaving care 61; and parental duties 42; to participate in assessment 116–117; to participate in decision making 59–60; to participation in care systems 272–275; to protection 271–272; recognition of 12, 55; significance of awarding 53; to voice, liberal conceptualization of 273
children's rights movement 4, 35; patriarchal view of society 52; self-determination claims 52; and UNCRC 53, 55
children's wishes and feelings 59
child safe organisations 84
child safety problems 57
child's best interests 58–59, 129
child's best interests, standard of: alternative approaches to implementation of 45; indeterminacy of 44–45, 58; open-endedness of 44; significance in decision making 44
child sexual abuse: definitions of 80–82; disclosure of 80, 85–86; feminist activism 81; gendered nature of 80; grooming and 86–87; harmful sexual behaviour and 89–90; issues surrounding 81; journey to recovery from 88; NSW advertising campaign 79; prevalence of 82, 92; recognition of 81; resistance to 79, 80; responses to, in Australian context 91–92; vulnerable populations at risk of 82–85 *see also* child abuse; child sexual abuse
child sexual assault 80
child sexual exploitation 5
child's network, membership determinants of 152
child's perception of security and personal adequacy 28
child's viewpoint 43
child trafficking and institutional abuse 5
child welfare 14; central element of 3; inequality 154, 289; resilience and strengths-based approaches in 37–38; strengths-based practice 38–39; trauma and neurobiological perspectives 39–41; variation for children population 27; *see also* attachment
child welfare continuum: definition of 3; priority in 3–4; variations in 4
child welfare legislation 131; *see also* child protection legislation
child welfare policy 14, 42, 44, 155, 223, 292, 318; conditions influencing 3; focus of 11
child welfare practice 4, 5, 6, 9, 35, 37, 46, 96, 151; ecological principles relevant in thinking about 37; focused at tertiary level 9; important points of 29; for mentalization 75, 76; *see also* resilience-based approaches; reunification; strengths-based practice; value frameworks, child welfare
child welfare professionals, implications for 322–325
child welfare system 7, 27; entry into 125; with indigenous families 13; orientation of 291
child wellbeing assessment 105–107
child with complex needs 36
'Circle of Security' 32
client gender considerations 114
Clinical Assessment Package for Assessing Clients' Risks and Strengths 110
cognitive behavioural therapy 76, 137, 200
cognitive development: children under 12 29; environmental stimuli for 28; epigenetic stages of 28–29; key stages of 28; *see also* child development
cognitive reframing 139
collaboration 99
colonisation legacy, indigenous and non-indigenous wellbeing 13
Commission for Children and Young People 197, 202
Common Assessment Framework 111, 117
'community caring' model 291
complex behaviour 37, 39, 141, 199, 257; *see also* behavioural problems, in CP populations
concrete operations 28
conditioning *see* grooming of sexually abused children
conflict resolution 138
consensus-based approach to risk assessment 102–105
conservative model of social policy systems 55

corporativist model *see* conservative model of social policy systems
court proceedings 129; children's participation rights in 59–60; experience of First Families 301, 308; legal vs welfare approaches 124–125; *see also* Children's Courts
CP *see* child protection
CREATE Foundation 12, 273
CSO *see* Central Statistics Office
cultural awareness 114
culturally appropriate assessment 113–114, 311, 313
culture-appropriate case management 115–116
cumulative harm 101, 125; associated with neglect 128–129; legislative basis to address 128

DBT *see* Dialectical Behavioural Therapy
defence of birth family and parent rights 43
deinstitutionalisation 128, 192
Delfabbro, Paul 3, 27, 134, 223
Devaney, Carmel 151
developmental approach for child welfare 27
developmental disorders 29
developmental processes of personality and thinking 14
developmental tasks 27–28
developmental theories: caution when applying 116; childhood 35; contextual approaches 36; epigenetic stages of development 28–29; Eurocentric bias 116; knowledge of 115; *see also* child development
development of children *see* child development
Dialectical Behavioural Therapy 200
disclosures of CSA 85–86
Double Orphan's Allowance 179
Driscoll, Jennifer 52

early developmental harm, dealing with 139
early intervention approaches, for child maltreatment 9–10, 14; content and focus of 151–152; family structures and 152; focus on family practices 152; in Ireland 155–160; outcomes of 153; protective factors and 152; shift of investment towards 153; social and economic conditions 154–155; support for parents 152; timing importance in 153
early relationships 34
EBP *see* evidence-based practice
ecological approach to assessment 112
ecological principles 37
ecomaps 109
educational interventions, in OOHC: education and schooling issues 11; education liaison personnel 215; foster carer/family-focused interventions 217–218; mentoring 216; policy and practice implications 218–219; reading interventions 216–217; systemic 212–215; tutoring programmes 215–216
Education Champions 217–218
education liaison personnel 215
emotional abuse: case examples of 69–76; definitions of 68; forms of 71–72; legislation connected to 68; and neglect, transmission rates of 72–73; prevalence in UK 68; reporting pattern 6; towards eldest child 75
emotional and behavioural development 40
emotionally abused child 28
Empowering Parents, Empowering Communities 58
English Children (Leaving Care) Act 2000 256
EPEC *see* Empowering Parents, Empowering Communities
epigenetic stages of development 28–29
Erikson's developmental theory 28–29
Escape from Childhood (Holt) 52
European Union (EU) Survey on Income and Living Conditions (SILC) 154
evidence-based practice 201
exchange model 99
'exclusive fostering' 43
explicit online material, harm from 91
extended care 254
eye movement desensitization and reprocessing (EMDR) therapy 76

FACN *see* Framework for the Assessment of Children in Need and their Families
FAF *see* Family Assessment Form
Families First 235
family and child welfare challenges 3
family assessment: challenges 107; cross-cultural perspective 116; disadvantaged families 107–108; frameworks 108–111; purpose of 107, 108; strengths and protective factors 108
Family Assessment Form 110
family-based, early intervention 9, 11
family-based foster care 10
Family Centred Out of Home Care Program 234
Family Court of Australia 91
Family Drug Treatment Courts 126
family functioning, environmental factors influencing 35–36
family group conferences 58, 281
Family Matters campaign 293–294
family practices, notion of 152
family preservation programme 108, 127, 234–235
family relationship, minimal intervention and intrusion into 42

family reunification *see* reunification
Family Reunification Service 234
Family Strengths and Needs Assessment 105
family structure and reunification patterns 230
Family Support orientation 7
family support services 108, 125
Farmer, Elaine 175
Fattore, Tobia 271
Federal Circuit Court of Australia 123
Fernandez, Elizabeth 3, 27, 96, 223, 300
First Families: access to services 308; engagement and inclusion 302–303; family contact 305–307; grief and loss experienced by 307, 312; involvement in court proceedings 301–302; issues in research of 309–310, 312–313; legal issues affecting 301; loss of identity 307; need for material and practical assistance 311; poverty of 311; relationships with carers 304–305; relationships with caseworkers 303–304; respect for dignity and worth of 312; restoration to 301; socio-economic circumstances of 300–301, 311; traumatic experience 307–308
formalised risk assessments systems 100
formal kinship care 175–176, 179; care arrangements 182–183; child and carer, relationship between 181; children's contact with parents 183–184; children's restoration to parents from 184; financial support for carers 183; Indigenous children 180; permanency planning legislation 185; pressure to keep children out of 185; regulation and support 181–182; stability and quality of care 184
formal operations 28
foster carers: affective and behavioural qualities of 323; applicant screening criteria 323; family-focused interventions 217–218; parenting assessment 323; recruitment strategies 322–323; roles and responsibilities of 319–321; training programs for 323–324
foster family care 4, 10, 42, 211; child's experience in 45; custody in 318; reunification from 230–231; services and birth parent 319; significance of 319; state-provided 163; voluntary and involuntary 318
foster family care service: children and families requiring 163–165, **164**, **165**; foster care roles and tasks 165–166; foster carers 166–167; informal 163; long-term 167; 'mixed economy' of provision 166–167; scoping the research on 168–171; services required to support 167; wellbeing outcomes 167–168
foster parents: case study 325–327; characteristics of 321; support for 321–322
Framework for Reunification (tool) 233–234
Framework for the Assessment of Children in Need and their Families 111
FRS *see* Family Reunification Service
FSNA *see* Family Strengths and Needs Assessment
'future risk of emotional harm,' notion of 68

gender and child protection 309
genogram 109
'ghosts in the nursery,' experiencing 73
Grandparent Advisor program 178
grandparent care 177–179
'Grandparent Inquiry' 179
grief reactions 33
grooming of sexually abused children 86–87
Guardian's Allowance 178

Harding, Fox 42–43
harmful sexual behaviour 80; of children towards other children 89–90; exposure to explicit online material 91
holistic ecological assessments 105
Holt, John 273
HOME *see* Home Observation for Measurement of Environment
home-based care 211
home-based tutoring programme 216
HOMEBUILDERS program 235
'home-grown model' 194
Home Observation for Measurement of Environment 110
HSB *see* harmful sexual behaviour
human development, normative course of 27
Human Rights (Parliamentary Scrutiny) Act 2011 53
'hypo arousal' state 74

identity, Erikson's theorising on 29
'inclusive fostering' 43
Incredible Years programs 142
indigenous children: formal kinship care 180; in out-of-home care 10; overrepresentation in child welfare system 12–13, 125, 290; role of relatives in care of 116; wellbeing of 13
indiscriminate attachment 31
individual differences and resilience 37
infants, attachment in: developmental phases of 31; development theories of 30–31; manifestations of 31
informal foster care 163
informal kinship care 176, 178–179
insecure attachment 31
institutional forms of care 4
intelligence, development of 28
interactionism 37

inter-generational abuse 12
intergenerational trauma 293
international child welfare literature 5
inter-professional collaboration 127
interventive approaches 41
'invisible trauma' *see* child neglect
Ireland, prevention and early intervention in practice in 155–160; family-based care placements 155; foster care arrangements 155; Meitheal activity 156–160; Prevention, Partnership and Family Support (PPFS) 156; Tusla and 155–156

KEEP program 324
kinship care 211, 318; benefits of 177; challenges for carers in 177–178; definition of 175; *vs.* foster care 177; kinship foster care 10–11, 166; reunification from 230–231; terminology 175
kinship care, in Australia and UK 175; children in 176–177; formal 175–176, 179–185; informal 178–179; lack of government support 179; perspectives of children and parents 185–186; services to families 176
Kiraly, Meredith 175
KITS programme 217
knowledge, child protection assessments 115–116
Kor, Kenny 192

laissez-faire value position 42
lawful adoption 246
leaving care: definition of 252; extended till at least 21 years of age 254; legislative provisions 255–256; Stand By Me program 256–260; *see also* care leavers
legal approaches, for child protection cases 124–125
legislation and agency policies 99
Letterbox Club (Griffiths), The 216
Lewis, Natalie 289
liberal model of social policy systems 55
local authority care 211
Locke, John 272–273
London Fostering Achievement 217
looked-after children 211
Loving, Alice 67
loving caregivers 40
lower socio-economic areas: difficult living circumstances in 36

magistrates 126
maltreatment *see* child maltreatment
mandatory reporting requirements 124
marginalisation 8
Mason, Jan 271
maternal bonding: concept 30; development of 33–34
maternal deprivation thesis 30
maternal infant attachment, theory of 29–30
McNamara, Patricia 192
'Meitheal' model 156–160
Mendes, Philip 252
mental health treatment approaches 200–201; implications for policy 202–203; implications for practice 201–202; milieu-based and 194
mentalization and parenting 74–76
mentoring 216
milieu-based models: aims of 197; implications for policy 202–203; implications for practice 201–202; key findings of 197–198, **198**; strengths and limitations 199–200; young people's experience 198
mind-control techniques 72
minority status and reunification patterns, link between 229
mother–infant bond *see* maternal bonding
MST *see* multisystemic therapy
MTFC *see* multidimensional treatment foster care
multidimensional treatment foster care 136–137
multisystemic therapy 37, 143, 235

natal and neonatal experience, humanising 34
National Association of Young People in Care 273
National Child Protection Framework Action Plan for 2015–18 255
National Framework for Protecting Australia's Children 9, 56, 58–59, 125
National Institute for Clinical Excellence (NICE 2017) 68
National Office for Child Safety 92
National Society for the Prevention of Cruelty to Children (NSPCC 2014) 68
National Survey of Child and Adolescent Wellbeing 105
NCFAS *see* North Carolina Family Assessment Scale
NCFAS for Reunification 109–110
NCFAS-R *see* NCFAS for Reunification
neglect *see* child neglect
neglected child: cognitive development 28; smaller brain of 41
neglectful emotional experiences 73
neglectful parenting 69
neoliberal policy 55
neurobiological perspective, child welfare decision making 41
neuroscience 246–249
'new sociology of childhood' 273
New South Wales 81; legislative basis for cumulative harm 125–126

2006 New South Wales Aboriginal Child Sexual Assault Taskforce Report 81
New Street Services in NSW 90
non-Aboriginal societies, over-representation of 13
non-Indigenous children 6, 10, 57, 180, 229, 255, 290, 310
non-mainstream schools 212
North Carolina Family Assessment Scale 109–110, 231–233, *232*
Northern Ireland: foster children in 217; milieu-based models evaluated in 197–200, **198**; reading interventions 216
NSCAW *see* National Survey of Child and Adolescent Wellbeing
NSW Association of Child Caring Agencies 273
NSW Care and Protection Practice Standards 277
nuclear family and child protection 152

Office of the Victorian Ombudsman 126
online technologies, sexual development associated with 90–92
OOHC *see* out-of-home care
optimum parenting, materially favourable environment for 43
Osborn, Alexandra 134
out-of-home care 4, 155, 163, 255, 300, 318; ATSI in 84; carers 84; CSA prevention in 84; CSA risk for children in 83–84; difficulties in leaving 12; formal and informal care 10–11; goals of 11; growing numbers of children in 224; intensive approaches to 11; outcomes 11; pattern of disproportionality 10; placement consideration 7; quality and instability of 42; *see also* children in out-of-home care (OOHC), educational progress of

paired reading 216
parental employment and reunification patterns 230
parental engagement 117
parental separation: article 9 of UNCRC and 54; factors associated with negative effects of 30; types and lengths of 30
parental skill training: Incredible Years programs 142; multisystemic therapy 143; Parent–Child Interaction therapy 141; parent management training 142; positive parenting program 143–144
Parent–Child Interaction therapy 141
parent child relationship 42
Parent-Directed Interaction 141
parent–infant bond 34
Parent–infant psychotherapy 76
parenting 32, 36, 117
Parenting Payments 311
Parenting Stress Index 110
parent management training 142
Parent Partner Program 235
parents: and carers, responses to children by 87–88; primary responsibility of 54, 55; rights and defence of birth family 43
ParentsNext initiative 56, 311
paternalism 44, 55
PCIT *see* Parent–Child Interaction therapy
PDI *see* Parent-Directed Interaction
PEP *see* Personal Education Plan
permanency planning legislation 185
Personal Adviser (PA) model 257
Personal Education Plan 211–213
personality traits: of excessive frustration 28; of overly indulged gratification 28
physical battery, phenomenon of 4
Piaget's stage theory 27–28
Play therapy 139–140
PMT *see* parent management training
Poor Law Amendment Act of 1868 68
pornography and harmful sexual behaviour, link between 90
positive parenting program 143–144
poverty: and child abuse, link between 5, 36; reunification affected by 229–230; SILC figures on 154
PPFS *see* Prevention, Partnership and Family Support
PPP *see* positive parenting program
preoperational development 28
preventative and supportive services 8
Prevention, Partnership and Family Support 156
preventive and supportive work with families and children 43
preventive interventions, for child maltreatment: content and focus of 151–152; family structures and 152; focus on family practices 152; in Ireland 155–160; outcomes of 153; protective factors and 152; shift of investment towards 153; social and economic conditions 154–155; support for parents 152; timing importance in 153
private spaces, CSA in 84
privatisation 55, 56
procedural model 99
Protecting Children: The Child Protection Outcomes Project 126
Protecting Victoria's Vulnerable Children Inquiry 128
protectionism 272
protective care continuum, guiding principles in decision making in 58–60
PSI *see* Parenting Stress Index
psychoeducation 139

psychological disturbance 5
psychometric instruments 103–104
psychosocial development of children 27
PTSD-type symptoms 73
public care 9
public health 9–10, 14
Pupil Premium Plus grant 212
Purtell, Jade 252

qualitative and quantitative assessment methods 99
Queensland: legislative basis for cumulative harm 125–126; reunification patterns in 229
questioning model 99

radicalization processes 71
reading interventions 216–217
reframing 45
relational experiences with caregivers: brain development shaped by 39–40; trusting relationship 117; undermined 88
relational participation 278–279
relational recovery, model for 88
relationships: affectional 34; and resilience 37; trustful 29; unconventional networks of 152
relative care 230–231, 318
Report of the Special Commission of Inquiry into Child Protective Services in NSW 127
residency and reunification patterns 230
residential care, in OOHC context 4, 211; challenges 192; paradox of 192; shift to smaller group homes 192; *vs.* therapeutic residential care 192–193
resilience 37
resilience-based approaches 37–38
'restoration' *see* reunification
restorative justice 89
reunification 11, 32, 211, 236; assessments 115; case-planning and practice issues 231–234; challenge of re-entry to care following 235–236; decision making 109–110; definition of 223, 224; demographic risk factors of 228–229; destination after exit from care 225; duration of 226; *vs.* exit from care 225; familial factors 228–230; framework for 234; legal status 226; outcome 226; passive *vs.* active process 227; screening tool for 231–233; services designed to focus on 234–235; statistical and research issues 227; statistical patterns of 224–225; system factors 228; timing 226
'rights-based' approach to children issues 53
rights framework 291–292
risk assessment: actuarial approaches 103, 104; balanced approach 113; in child abuse 101–102; consensus-based approaches 102–104; constraints 112–113; decision-making tools 290; definition 100; environment of 112–113; ethical considerations 104–105; evidence-based frameworks 104; identification of situational hazards 102; likelihood of harm estimation 100, 101; models 128; practitioners' decision making 113; psychometric instruments for 103–104
risk management 38
role-modelling 138
Royal Commission into Institutional Responses to Child Sexual Abuse 79, 192; definition of child sexual abuse 81–82; limitations of 91
'rule of optimism' 42

SA *see* Safety Assessment
Safety Assessment 105
SAICA *see* Social Adjustment Inventory for Children and Adolescents
SBM program *see* Stand By Me program
school climate 212
SDM *see* structured decision-making tools
Sebba, Judy 209
secure attachment 31–32
'selective social smiling' 31
self-assertiveness training 138
self-discipline and obligations 138
sensorimotor development 28
separation and loss, notions of 33
separation anxiety 31
separation at birth 34
sex education 91
sexual abuse 12, 71; *see also* child sexual abuse
sexual behaviours 81–82
sexual development, with online technologies 90–91
sexual exploitation gangs 71–72
sexually abused children: grooming of 86–87; harming person facilitating recovery of 88–89; journey to recovery for 88; response from parents or carers 87–88
'sexually harmful behaviour' 80
sexual safety of children 80
SGOs *see* Special Guardianship Orders
Sheehan, Rosemary 123
Shemmings, David 67
sibling sexual abuse 83
Signs of Safety 111
SILC *see* Survey on Income and Living Conditions
Simmonds, John 241
single parents, situational prevention for 84–85
situational prevention 84–85
skin to skin contact to infants 33–34
Social Adjustment Inventory for Children and Adolescents 106

social and economic conditions 154–155
social-behavioural problems 139
social care and education, liaison between 215
social competency and resilience issues 137; activity scheduling and play therapies 139–140; attachment therapy for 140–141; early developmental harm 139; social skills training for 137–138; trauma-informed counselling 139
social democratic welfare model 55
social learning 138
socially acceptable behaviour 28
social policy systems, models of 55
social skills training 137–138
Social Support Networks map 109
social welfare policies 55
social work practitioners 69, 134
social work with children and families 7
socio-economic disadvantage and contact with child protection services, relationship between 126
socio-economic stress and maltreatment, link between 6
South Australia: children in OOHC in 229; Children's Courts 123, 129; kinship carers 183; reunification patterns in 229
Special Guardianship Orders 181
'specific attachment' 31
'spotters' 71–72
'stage,' concept of 27
standard model of family life and operation 152
Stand By Me program 252, 265; aims and objectives of 256–257; case study 260; evaluation 257–259; family relationships 263–264; holistic support 259–260; leaving care and post-care anxiety reduction 259; leaving care planning and implementation 259; SBM worker roles 257; strengthened housing assistance 262–263; worker–client relationship 259
state duties, to support child care 54–58; prioritizing resource allocation 55; social policy models and 55–56; support to parents 55
state institutions, investment in 55
state intervention 291; birth family defence and parent rights 43–44; child family relationship and 42; for child protection 42–43; children's right to protection through 271–272
state paternalism and child protection position 42–43
Statutory child protection agencies 124
Staying Put extended foster care program 254
stranger anxiety 31
'Strange Situation' framework 31
strengths-based practice 38–39
stressful early experiences and brain development 39
stress managing functions, brain regions associated with 39
stress responsive systems 40
structured decision-making tools 105
Survey on Income and Living Conditions 154

Tasmania: Children's Courts in 123; reunification patterns in 211, 224, 229
teenager, child welfare needs of 27
TF-CBT *see* Trauma-Focused Cognitive Behavioural Therapy
therapeutic residential care: case study of 203–204; definitions of 193, 194; *vs.* general residential care 192–193; home-grown approach 194–197, **196**; implications for policy 202–203; implications for practice 201–202; mental health treatment approaches 200–201; milieu-based models approach 197–200, **198**; principles for designing and implementing 193; research evidence 193–194
therapeutic residential care pilot program 194; *vs.* general residential care group **196**; implications for policy 202–203; implications for practice 201–202; mental health and wellbeing outcomes 195; strengths and limitations 195–197; young people's perspectives 195
Third Action Plan (2015–2018) 56
Thoburn, June 163
Thorpe, Ros 300
TILA *see* Transition to Independent Living Allowance
Tilbury, Clare 289
'token economy' procedure 136
Tolliday, Dale 79
'trait trap' 37
transactionism 37
Transition to Independent Living Allowance 255
trauma *see* childhood trauma
Trauma-Focused Cognitive Behavioural Therapy 200
trauma-informed care 41
trauma-informed counselling 139
traumatic childhood abuse 72–73
traumatic memories 73
TRC pilot program *see* therapeutic residential care pilot program
triangulation of knowledge 45–46
trustful relationships 29
Tusla 155–156
TutorBright 216
tutoring programmes 215–216

UK, kinship care in 175; children in 176, 177; formal 179–185; informal 178–179; perspectives of children and parents 185–186; services to families 176
UK family assessment frameworks 111
UK Looking After Children Initiative 107
UN Committee on the Rights of the Child 2013 58–59
UN Convention on the Rights of the Child 44
United Nations Convention on the Rights of the Child 15, 53, 272; article 2 of 59; article 3–1 of 58; article 4 of 55; article 9 of 54; article 12 of 59, 116; article 12–1 of 59; article 18 of 54; article 18–2 of 55; article 26 of 55; article 27 of 55; children's rights and 52–53; child's best interests in 58; core principles of 35; on disparities in access to services 57; General Principles of 53; implications 62; incorporated into domestic law 53–54; prioritization of 'early intervention approaches 53; recommendations to strengthen family support 53; reporting mechanism 54; state's duties to support children care 54–58
USA mental health treatment approaches 200–201

value frameworks, child welfare 41; children's rights and child liberation 43–44; defence of birth family and parent rights 43; laissez faire 42; state paternalism and child protection 42–43
Verso 194
Victoria: child protection system 127; children on care and protection orders in 125; legislative basis for cumulative harm 125–126; mandatory reporting requirements 124; reunification patterns in 229
Victorian Law Reform Commission 126, 131
Victorian policy 255–256
Virtual Schools 211–213
vulnerable children 82; policies to protect 272; resilience 37; sibling sexual abuse 83; and young people 83
vulnerable families of children: risk factors experienced by 8; trend of ignoring 7, 8

'welfare to work' model 56
wellbeing of child 11
wellbeing of indigenous children 13
Western Australia: Children's Courts in 123, 129; mandatory reporting requirements 124
'Who Cares' conference, 273
'whole of community' approach 125
'women's movement' 4

'Young People in Care Speakout' 273

For Product Safety Concerns and Information please contact our EU
representative GPSR@taylorandfrancis.com
Taylor & Francis Verlag GmbH, Kaufingerstraße 24, 80331 München, Germany

www.ingramcontent.com/pod-product-compliance
Ingram Content Group UK Ltd.
Pitfield, Milton Keynes, MK11 3LW, UK
UKHW052224190926
475702UK00007B/1196
* 9 7 8 0 3 6 7 6 3 9 1 7 4 *